Facilitating Emotional Change:
The Moment-by-Moment Process

Facilitating Emotional Change:
The Moment-by-Moment Process

Leslie S. Greenberg
Laura N. Rice
Robert Elliott

The Guilford Press
New York   London

Library of Congress Cataloging-in-Publication Data

Greenberg, Leslie S.
    Facilitating emotional change : the moment-by-moment process / Leslie S. Greenberg, Laura N. Rice, and Robert Elliott.
        p. cm.
    Includes bibliographical references and index.
    ISBN 0-89862-994-2.—1-57230-201-1 (pbk.)
    1. Experiential psychotherapy. 2. Cognitive-experiential psychotherapy. I. Rice, Laura North, 1920– . II. Elliott, Robert, 1950– . III. Title.
RC489.E96G74   1993
616.89′14—dc20   93-7562
                                                                 CIP

And so each venture
Is a new beginning, a raid on the inarticulate
And what there is to conquer
By strength and submission, has already been discovered
Once or twice, or several times, by men [sic] whom one cannot hope
To emulate—but there is no competition—
There is only the fight to recover what has been lost
And found and lost again and again:
For us, there is only the trying. The rest is not our business.

T. S. ELIOT, "East Coker," *Four Quartets*

PREFACE

This work is the product of our years of experience as clinicians and as researchers and is our attempt to explicate some of our implicit understanding of how change takes place in therapy. It appears to us that ours is first and foremost an approach to change that emphasizes the emotional process and its facilitation. It is the emphasis on the moment-by-moment experiential process and the facilitation of a next step that distinguishes what we do from many other therapeutic approaches. As opposed to emphasizing particular contents of the psyche or to using techniques to teach or modify, we emphasize facilitating the client's moment-by-moment affective/cognitive process in order to facilitate shifts in meaning. When we practice as therapists, what is uppermost in our minds are the details of our client's moment-by-moment experience and expression. We are absorbed in the process and with how to facilitate a next step rather than with an attempt to understand recurring maladaptive patterns or to try to achieve predetermined behavioral change goals. In our view, the therapist is expert in knowing how to facilitate particular kinds of exploration of experience rather than knowing what the client is experiencing.

Ours is an approach that integrates an "organismic" view of human functioning, which emphasizes certain innate biologically based aspects of functioning, with a "process-structural" view, which emphasizes how functional mental structures are involved in generating preformance (Pascual-Leone, 1976c, 1984, 1987). In attempting to explain change, we emphasize the biological role of both the evolutionarily based aspects of emotion and the organismic tendency toward growth; we emphasize as well the role of internal cognitive/affective structures (schemes) and processes (attending to, symbolizing, and reflecting on experience) involved in the moment-by-moment generation of experience and behavior.

Our view of emotions is crucial in understanding our approach. We believe that an important goal of therapy is to help people articulate their feelings and needs, for it is through this that people gain access to what is emotionally significant to them. An important aspect of therapy is becoming aware of the implicit emotion schemes that guide experience and action. We do not see emotion as synonomous with heightened arousal or intense expression. We do not see emotion as disruptive of cognition or behavior; nor do we view emotions merely as internal feelings. Rather, we believe emotions constitute an organized, meaningful, and generally adaptive action system. The biological function of emotion is to ensure survival and reproduction of the organism by providing feedback about reactions to situations to aid adaptation and problem solving. Culturally, however, emotion has been cast in a negative light and has received bad press—emotion is viewed as disorganizing, people are described as being "too emotional" and are viewed as needing "to control their emotions." People are often ashamed if they show too much emotion, and believe that they are being immature if they are emotional.

Although at times emotions are connected to dysfunction because of maladaptive emotional learning, the effects of emotion in general are positive and adaptive. They generally guide people to meet important needs and motivate effective action. Rather than generally being disruptive, emotions are rich informational outputs of a complex processing system that evaluates both what is significant to us and whether or not we can attain what is significant. It is through becoming aware of and articulating our emotions and needs that we gain knowledge of the significance things have for us. Thus, by being aware of our emotions, we truly get to know ourselves, that is, our appraisals of what is significant to us.

We wish to comment here on our use of the concept of scheme and emotion schemes throughout the book. This is not meant to reify this structural construct to the status of an existing entity in the head. We have used this concept as a tool to capture our view that an internal organizing process exists. Our perspective does not stand or fall on the use of this concept. If and when schemes are replaced by another concept such as distributive processing, or neural nets, or some other complex patterning process, this will not perturb our theory which relies only on the notion of some modular internal organization of experience.

Of interest to us in presenting a book that emerges from the Experiential Therapy tradition is the current convergence in the field of different approaches to psychotherapy. This convergence is most clearly reflected in the development of the Society for the Exploration of Psychotherapy Integration and the increasing number of publications on integration. Methods of integrating different approaches as well as identifying commonalities across approaches have also promoted respect for, and learning from, differences in approaches. Both identifying commonalities and recognizing differences are important aspects of this development.

In this spirit, we note the convergence represented in this book between aspects of the experiential perspectives and aspects of both cognitive and object relations perspectives. This convergence occurs particularly at the level of theory, in which internal representations or schemes and the role of the emotions are of strong and growing interest in all areas. Our theory bears definite similarities to those cognitive approaches that emphasize the importance of core beliefs and the construction of meaning as central in guiding people's behavior, and definite similarities to object relations theory in seeing people as constructing internal representations of affectively based early interactions. Similarities to self psychology are also highly apparent, both in the importance placed on the self, and self-esteem regulation, and in the role of empathy in strengthening the self. We believe for this reason that this book will speak to both cognitive and psychodynamically oriented therapists.

However, rather than presenting this effort as a book whose primary aim is integration, our goal in writing it is to articulate an approach within an Experiential Therapy framework. We believe that a volume of this type is important both to revive interest in what this tradition has to offer and to present the distinguishing features of the approach we have developed. In this book we offer a perspective on how to differentially facilitate different affective/cognitive processes that lead to the resolution of different types of emotional-processing difficulties. We believe that the specification of these processes and of the features of our approach will in the long run be helpful in promoting integration, since it clearly defines how our approach differs from other approaches and therefore specifies more clearly what an Experiential perspective may have to offer to an integrative endeavor.

We wish to comment on our use of transcripts. Some of the contents of a number of the transcripts have been somewhat altered to remove identifying features, to maintain confidentiality, and to improve clarity. We have attempted however in so doing to retain the essential client process that occurred in each episode and to tamper with therapist interventions as little as possible in order to convey as faithfully as possible the interactions that actually occurred.

Finally, we would like to thank all of our colleagues and students who have directly and indirectly contributed to our thinking and to this book. More specifically, we benefited greatly from the feedback of Art Bohart, Irene Elkin, Germain Lietar, Tracy Mayne, and Bill Stiles. We also benefited greatly from conversations with Juan Pascual-Leone, who has significantly influenced our theoretical views on human functioning. In addition, many colleagues and students contributed to the development of the ideas in this book both directly and indirectly. We gratefully acknowledge the input of our colleagues Sue Johnson, David Rennie, and Shake Toukmanian, and our many students, most currently Claudia Clark, Florence Foerster, Rhonda Goldman, Ruth Rohn, Hadas Wiseman, Sandra Paivio, Renee Rhodes, and Jean Watson. Finally, we wish to extend our sincere gratitude to Zehra Bandhu, our always helpful secretary, who tirelessly typed and retyped our endless refinements. To all these people and to our clients who have helped us to learn what we know about therapy so that we may impart that knowledge to others, we offer our thanks.

CONTENTS

PART I

INTRODUCTION

CHAPTER 1

INTRODUCTION TO
THE APPROACH

I N THIS BOOK we present the theory and methods of an emotionally focused, process-facilitative approach to therapy, an approach oriented toward the construction of new emotional meaning. In this approach the therapist is viewed as facilitating the client's moment-by-moment processing of experiential information by guiding the client's attention so as to enable the client to construct new personal meanings.

It is our intent in this work both (1) to embed an experiential approach to therapy in modern theoretical perspectives on constructive information processing and the adaptive role of emotion in human functioning and (2) to provide a manual of specific methods of therapeutic intervention that in the context of an empathic relationship utilize redeployment of attention and other cognitive/affective processes to facilitate change in emotional schemes.

Of crucial importance in this process oriented experiential approach to the facilitation of emotional change is the recognition that all the client's processing operations occur in the present and that the therapist's attention needs to be focused in a fully absorbed manner on the client's present experience and expression. The therapist attempts to hear, see, and understand clients as they are at that moment and to stimulate experiential processing rather than attempting to formulate hypotheses about clients' internal dynamics or to change or modify clients' cognitions or behaviors. In addition to attending to and facilitating specific attention and memory processes occurring in the moment, the therapist continuously attempts to provide an optimal environment for the type of flexible cognitive/affective processing required in therapy. We will argue that the provision of an empathically attuned, respecting relationship, in which the therapist genuinely affirms the client's experience and genuinely prizes rather than appraises the client, promotes a person's trust in his or her own capacities. This enables the person to feel safe enough to allocate maximal processing capacities to the task of exploring and generating new emotional meanings.

In addition to the creation of a particular relational environment, we suggest the use of a number of therapeutic tasks that we have found productive in helping clients resolve specific affective problems. We have observed that particular types of affective problems appear to occur frequently across clients in therapy. These are problems that possess a task-like quality in that clients are continually engaged in active attempts to resolve them. In our view, if therapists are able to recognize when clients are in a current state of struggling to resolve one of these affective problems they will know when and how to intervene most appropriately. Thus, intervention involves recognition and facilitation of the resolution of the affective task in which the client is currently engaged.

In this book we outline six different types of facilitative intervention strategies for six different types of affective problems. This specification of different types of interventions for different types of problems in no way implies that therapy is a deterministic process of applying the correct formula to achieve the correct solution. Rather we see these interventions as highly complex methods of interpersonal facilitation. The interventions we outline are: Systematic Evocative Unfolding, for resolving problematic reactions; Two-Chair Dialogue, for resolving splits; and Two-Chair Enactment, for undoing self interruptions; Focusing, for symbolizing an unclear felt sense; Empty-Chair Dialogue, for resolving unfinished business; and Empathic Prizing at times of intense vulnerability. It is important from the start to understand that we view therapy as the facilitation of the client's creation of new emotional meanings and that we believe that the art of therapy can best be made more understandable by defining and investigating the different kinds of meaning-creation tasks that promote change.

All the above problems, then, are viewed as affective information-processing problems, whose solutions are best facilitated in different ways. Throughout this book, terms such as "affective information processing" or "experiential processing" will be used to mean an active dialectically constructive process of creating emotional meaning, rather than a passive, computer-like processing of information through linear stages to produce predetermined outputs. "Information processing" as we use the term implies a process of generating and attending to emotionally toned information to *create* emotional meaning.

We will argue that the purpose of working with clients' moment-by-moment manner of cognitive/affective processing is to enable clients to achieve change in the way in which they construct their sense of self as well as change in underlying self-relevant cognitive/affective structures. We refer to these underlying structures as *emotion schemes.** We suggest that these complex internal models automatically guide our sense of emotional meaning. Further, we suggest that therapeutic change occurs by means of the reorganization of existing emotion schemes and the creation of new ones.

We define emotion schemes as internal synthesizing structures that preconsciously process a variety of cognitive, affective, and sensory sources of information to provide our sense of personal meaning. This will help us to present a view of people as wholistic, organismic beings, in whom affect, cognition, motivation, and action are continually integrated in everything they do. We contend that emotions are crucial in capturing the wholeness of human functioning in that they are complex, integrative, organismically based reactions to our perceptions of ourselves and the world. They integrate the social and the biological as well as the cognitive, the motivational, and the physiological, into a single complex response that synthesizes a number of levels of processing.

Emotion schemes are thus complex synthesizing structures that integrate cognition (in the form of appraisals, expectations, and beliefs) and motivation (in the form of needs, concerns, intentions, and goals) with affect (in the form of physiological arousal and sensory, bodily feeling) and action (in the form of expressive-motor responses and action tendencies). Together, these form complex internal models of self-in-the-world experience. Although these are complex multicomponent mental models of the world, we call them *emotion schemes* because it is those models that are formed around emotional responses to the world that are most influential in guiding automatic processing of personal meaning. It is these emotion-based schematic structures that automatically integrate propositional, sensory, and proprioceptive information to produce an embodied "sense" or "feeling" of oneself in the world, as opposed to purely cognitive structures that produce only thoughts or ideas. Thus one's feelings of being "on top of the world," "down in the dumps," or of being "unsure of oneself" are all produced by these complex schematic emotional syntheses. Emotion schemes then form supraordinate emotional meaning/action structures that determine our wholistic experience of being-in-the-world. It is these emotion structures that also automatically organize and stabilize our initially transient emotional reactions to provide our enduring sense of self-in-world. And it is these structures that determine what is personally meaningful to us and lead to our immediate

---

*We use scheme here rather than schema to denote an action-producing structure rather than a purely representational structure. We use the term emotion to emphasize that they are schemes that are formed around an emotion nucleus. This will be discussed fully in Chapter 3.

emotional experience of being-in-the-world. It is from our emotional reactions that we can tell what is important to us, how we are appraising our world and how we are coping with it (cf. Oatley, 1992; Lazarus, 1991b; Teasdale, in press).

Therapy, then, is the process of activating and facilitating the reorganization of these emotionally based schemes. Two key features of our therapeutic method for changing emotion schemes are: (1) the therapist's empathic attunement to the client's moment-by-moment emotional experience and (2) the facilitation of particular types of experiential processing, at particular times, to promote the activation and reorganization of the emotion schemes. In our view, in order for emotional change to occur the meaning structures that generate emotional experience need to be activated in therapy so that they are currently governing experience. It is only then that they become accessible to new input and change. Experiencing what is being talked about in the session in an emotionally toned fashion is an indication that the relevant meaning structure has been activated and is amenable to the processing of new information.

Using this approach, the therapist does not attempt to provide the new meaning for the client but, instead, attempts to facilitate those cognitive/affective processes in the client that will enable him or her to reorganize experience and construct new emotional meanings. Thus, the therapist is a facilitator and stimulator of new experience and its exploration and reorganization. The product or content of the reorganization and the new construction come from the client.

As we have said, a core therapeutic process in this approach to changing emotion schemes is the systematic facilitation of the client's attention. This allows the client to bring new elements of experience into awareness and to process them. Because what people attend to serves as the basis of their awareness, facilitating the allocation of attention in particular ways at particular times alters current awareness. Thus, rather than talking about a problem or trying to solve it, rationally, *attending* to a sinking feeling in one's stomach, to the stimulus that generated that feeling, or to the sense of "feeling like a failure" associated with it, in and of itself, reorganizes current experience by changing attentional focus. Change in attentional allocation is highly related to change in both experience and action because it promotes new awareness. The new awareness of feeling disappointed at a loss or angry at being mistreated can lead to semantic/perceptual reorganization and to the possibility of new options and choices. Action generally occurs in response to new perception or understanding of the situation and to new perceived options. Change in awareness therefore is the key to altered action, and differential redeployment of attention is the key to change of awareness.

Emotional awareness is our current organization of what currently matters to us in relation to the ever changing environment. Thus, awareness is dependent both on what is selectively attended to and how this is organized into private meaning. Change any of the elements attended to in current awareness, or change their interpretation, and this will produce a new perspective and new emotional meaning.

The activation of internal emotion structures, the reprocessing of information and its reencoding, thus ultimately leads to change in emotion structures or the generation of new schemes. The therapist's most active role in facilitating the reorganization of emotion schemes is *neither* one of interpreting the meaning of the client's experience nor of attempting to modify the scheme or to challenge it. It is to focus the client's attention on some elements of his or her experience, not in current focal awareness, to symbolize it and to thereby activate scehmes and further process information. This, in turn, promotes *self*-reorganization of experience and the construction of a new view of self-in-the-world.

THE DEVELOPMENT OF THIS APPROACH

The approach to facilitating the emotional processes described in this volume is the product of two major developments in our view of a process-oriented, experiential therapy. One development is related to change in the *actual practice* of therapy at the level of therapeutic intervention; the other is related to change in the *theory of practice* at the level of the explanation of how change occurs.

In our clinical experience, utilizing empathically oriented Experiential Therapy, we became aware of many times when some important client shift in emotional meaning in relation to a personal concern seemed to be taking place, a shift that led to some positive change. At such times, the client had seemed able to engage in particular kinds of noticeable (albeit internal) mental processes. If recognized and facilitated by the therapist, this often led to something new, to a novel view of one's self-in-the-world. An emotional reorganization involving a new perspective on oneself occurred, or an emotional difficulty was resolved, or some shift in awareness and perception took place that seemed important to both client and therapist.

The importance of facilitating client curiosity, exploration of novelty, and new awareness seemed to be some of the central goals of intervention. This observation had two major implications for practice. On the one hand, we viewed empathic reflections of feelings as important interventive tools to convey understanding of meaning. On the other hand, they were also viewed as tools for facilitating different and novel momentary processing. Certain types of reflections seemed to lead to more productive processing at certain times (Rice, 1974). In addition, empathic reflections seemed more accurately characterized as empathic *selections* (Greenberg & Goldman, 1988) in that the response selectively focused on, or emphasized, particular aspects of the client's meaning in a particular manner. Empathic selections seemed designed to enhance both exploration and manner of processing. Rice (1974) had initially suggested that an information-processing model was the best theoretical base for understanding the operations of client-centered therapy and the mechanisms of change involved. This perspective led us to view the therapist as a type of information-processing facilitator who helped the client explore and create novel experience in therapy. In addition to focusing on the therapist's facilitation of moment-by-moment information processing, we also came to see that therapists could facilitate the solution of certain more molar client processing tasks by differential intervention. We labeled these tasks as potential change events and began to study them intensively.

Rice (1974) identified the first change event within the context of a client-centered approach to treatment. This involved the solution of a problematic reaction by means of a specific form of evocative responding. A problematic reaction is an in-therapy state in which a client feels puzzled or troubled by a reaction he or she had to some situation. Rice suggested that it was people's "enduring constructions or schemes that are brought to bear on each new experience" that are troublesome in these situations. In addition, she suggested that the targets of therapy are "the set of schemes that are relevant to the recurrent situations in which the client reacts in unsatisfactory ways" (Rice, 1974, p. 293). Therapeutic intervention was viewed as attempting to evoke an experience from such problem situations in a manner that was relatively undistorted by the scheme, and as facilitating a reprocessing of the experience.

Greenberg (1975), working in a schematic processing framework, went on to identify a second change event drawn from the practice of Gestalt therapy. This involved the resolution of splits in the personality by means of a Two-Chair Dialogue. A split describes an in-therapy statement of a conscious conflict between two aspects of the self. The resolution process was viewed as involving the accessing and bringing into contact of two opposing schemes, or parts of the self, in order to promote an integration of the opposing schemes. The identification of problematic reaction points and splits as markers of affective problems requiring specific types of intervention was the first step in developing a more differentiated approach to experientially oriented intervention. This led to the development of the concept of recurrent change events in therapy and to the identification and intensive study of the processes involved in the different change events (Rice & Greenberg, 1984).

These in-therapy events were defined as possessing an identifiable structure. Events begin with the client's expression, in the session, of a particular type of problem experience, which is viewed as a "marker" of both an underlying emotional processing problem and of the client's readiness for a particular kind of therapeutic exploration. The markers, together with the use of specific sets of interventions suited to facilitating the resolution of the particular processing difficulty, led to a specific type of emotional exploration. This exploration evolved through a series of important client-processing steps that in turn led to resolution of the affective problem. It became increasingly clear to us that, within the "wholeness" of a successful therapy, there were a number of identifiable change events of the sort we have described, events that could be more or less successfully facilitated by different interventions (Rice & Greenberg, 1984; Greenberg, 1986). Research on these change events yielded models elucidating the different types of productive client involvement. The kinds of therapist participation needed to facilitate client involvements at each stage of the event were also defined.

A second development took place at the level of theory of functioning. We had always been impressed both with the human capacity for dynamically organizing emotional experience and constructing meaning and with the importance of these processes in the client's ever-changing perceptions of reality. How people viewed themselves and their worlds seemed to depend very clearly on their ongoing cognitive/affective constructions. Rather than possessing constructs people are constantly constructing meaning. It seemed to us that it was the client's current emotionally toned constructive processes, and the underlying schematic organizations of these, that were the ultimate targets of therapeutic intervention.

From the start, we viewed the markers of emotional-processing problems as representations of the tacit schematic processing that the client was currently engaged in and that needed to be changed. In our view, it was changes in the client's cognitive/affective processing (yielding change in emotional meanings) that ultimately led to therapeutic change. In addition, the manner and type of in-session performance were manifest signs of the type of internal mental operations in which the client was engaged and which needed to be changed. Since change in clients' emotionally based constructions of self and reality was our ultimate concern, we were most interested in the developments in cognitive science and emotion theory (Greenberg & Safran, 1987) that could shed light on the internal operations involved in the therapeutic change process.

We realized that the experiential theories of psychotherapy from which our work derived (Rogers, 1951, 1957, 1959; Perls, Hefferline, & Goodman, 1951; Perls, 1969) were developed in an era when there was not an adequate understanding in psychology of the type of cognitive and affective processes involved in human functioning. At that time, psychoanalysis and behaviorism were the two dominant theoretical modes. On the one hand, human functioning was assumed to be strongly governed by unconscious instinctual drives. On the other hand, behavior was deemed to be controlled by learned stimulus–response links. The role of internal models and automatic processing in the construction of emotional meaning and the nature and role of emotion in human functioning were underdeveloped areas in theoretical psychology. There were no adequate models for the therapeutic phenomena that Rogers and Perls wrote about in their approaches. They were both keenly aware of the importance of the human capacity for self-reflective consciousness and of the roles of awareness, emotional experience, meaning, and choice in determining human behavior. However, there was little cognitive/affective processing theory, at the time, that could do justice to the complexity of real, human functioning in the world. Thus, in their formal theoretical statements of Client-Centered and Gestalt therapy, Rogers and Perls were attempting to construct theories of function, dysfunction, and therapeutic change that would do justice to their beliefs about human agency and the human capacity for change. All this was done without the benefit of modern developments in psychology.

GUIDE TO READING THE BOOK

In this volume we present the theoretical framework of this approach drawn from cognitive science and emotion theory and a manual of the different methods and skills for facilitating different types of processing that lead to change. Part I of the book, of which this chapter forms a part, serves as an introduction to the overall approach. A brief introduction to some of the key elements of the approach and its development has been presented in this chapter. The overall approach to treatment is discussed in the next chapter.

Part II of the book presents the theory underlying the process oriented experiential approach that we will refer to as a process-experiential approach. The chapters in this part discuss the application of cognitive science and emotion theory to the understanding of psychological processes in psychotherapy and present issues related to a theory of emotional functioning and to emotional dysfunction. This part of the book is highly theoretical and will primarily be of interest to psychologists interested in the role of emotion and cognition in personality functioning and those interested in theories of dysfunction.

Part III presents the detailed manual for the implementation of this approach. Those more inclined to reading about practice and not wanting to start with theory could proceed from Part I to Part III, which orients the reader to the treatment approach and provides the manual of skills and tasks. Part IV concludes with a discussion of issues in the application of the approach.

CHAPTER 2

A PROCESS-FACILITATIVE APPROACH TO PSYCHOTHERAPY

IN THIS CHAPTER we describe the central features of the process-experiential approach to psychotherapy. Our basic assumption in this treatment approach is that the barriers to current healthy functioning result from clients' problems in symbolizing their own experience and from the dysfunctional, emotion-laden schemes through which their experience is processed. Therefore, in our view, the process goal of therapy is to enable clients to access these dysfunctional schemes under therapeutic conditions that will facilitate relevant schematic change. The targets of therapy are the meaning-construction processes and the sets of emotion schemes that are relevant to the troubling issues and situations brought to therapy by each client. The goal of this approach is to instigate methods by which clients in therapy can access emotionally relevant schemes, can more adequately symbolize their experience, and can reprocess important experiences relevant to dysfunctional schemes. Emotional processing of this nature leads to the reorganization of the old schematic structures and the creation of new schemes.

Different modes of client processing in therapy are important at two different levels of the client–therapist interaction. The first level concerns the moment-by-moment effects of each therapist response on the following client response. Therapist responses that convey accurate and empathic understanding of the client's message provide a feeling of being understood and truly received. These affirming and understanding responses enable the client to move into difficult issues and to explore them more and more deeply. A second, less obvious but important, feature of the therapist's moment-by-moment reflective responses concerns that aspect of the client's statements on which the therapist leaves the focus. If the focus is on the aspect that seems to feel most alive and poignant for the client at that moment, this maintains the client's focus on this area, leaving the client free to correct it or carry it further. (These issues will be discussed more fully in Chapter 7.)

The second level at which the client–therapist interaction needs to be viewed is the more molar level, at which the therapist is attempting to enable the client to resolve the larger affective problems that present themselves as in-session therapeutic tasks. As we studied the therapeutic process, viewing clients as active problem solvers engaged in attempts to achieve resolution of puzzling or disturbing experiences, we began to identify a number of different types of in-session tasks with which clients seemed to struggle. In this framework, different types of client-processing operations seemed to be useful at different times in order to access different schemes in different ways. These different types of operations, which we refer to later as "modes of engagement," seemed to require different kinds of client in-session involvement. It was apparent that these different styles of engagement could be facilitated by different types of therapist interventions. In investigating these events we concluded that therapists can help clients to resolve particular classes of processing problems by selectively facilitating their engagement in the kinds of exploratory tasks that specifically target the relevant processing difficulties.

Each of the different classes of client tasks is identifiable by the occurrence of an in-session "marker" that indicates the nature of the specific processing difficulty with which the client is struggling and also indicates the client's current readiness for tackling the problem. This "readiness" feature indicates that the client is currently experiencing difficulty and is trying to solve the problem, that is, is engaged in a task and is therefore more receptive to intervention designed to facilitate its solution. We have concluded that task-focused interventions at identifiable readiness markers constitute a useful strategy for helping clients to resolve specific therapeutic tasks.

In this view of therapy the therapist is highly sensitive to the moment-by-moment changing nature of the clients' states and processes. The therapist engages in an ongoing manner in a type of "process diagnosis," identifying in-session processing problems that appear currently amenable to intervention. As noted below, it is important to emphasize that process diagnosis is based on assessment of the current state of the client as indicated by momentary manner and style of expression. It is not a diagnosis of stable states or traits but, rather, an empathic attunement to momentary affective states and to the particular client's orientation toward solving the current problem.

A PROCESS-FOCUSED APPROACH

In a process-facilitative experiential approach to therapy designed to facilitate differential processing, the therapeutic action is seen as occurring in the moment-by-moment transactions between the client and the therapist. Clients are viewed as being engaged in an ongoing process of organizing experience, and of creating new emotional meanings in order to better understand and guide themselves in relation to their world. This experiencing/meaning-creation process involves the construction of meaning from a variety of types of information including sensory, affective, perceptual, memorial, and conceptual information. The resulting organized synthesis of all this processing is the person's conscious experience of being-in-the world. This is the therapist's ongoing referent. The therapist's attention is continually focused on the moment-by-moment shifts in client experiencing and manner of processing.

Thus a client statement such as "I felt so hurt, I just wanted to withdraw. I didn't want to look at them. I needed to protect myself," is the result of a complex process of meaning construction involving the symbolization of an automatic appraisal of a self-situation relationship in relation to an organismic concern and the integration of a large amount of situation and response information processed out of awareness. The therapist, by responding with a statement such as "You felt just wounded inside, and kind of wanting to pull away so you could heal," engages in this process with the client with a particular manner and intent. The manner is empathic and caring. The intent in this response is both to help the client feel understood and to help focus the client on the most poignant aspect of her experience, the tendency to withdraw to protect herself. This, or some other appropriate response, is designed to facilitate certain processing activities that will help the client attend to and symbolize the most lively part of his or her experience. This will help to access appraisals, feelings, needs, and other complex tacit information implicit in that experience. This in turn will aid the client in constructing new emotional meaning and in seeing the world in new ways.

In facilitating emotional experience the therapist does not hold that specific content must be dealt with in order to achieve change. Instead, the focus is on listening to the client's current state and recognizing the mode of facilitating the cognitive/affective processes that would be, at that moment, most helpful in the creation of new meaning. There is no fixed theory of psychological content that dictates that certain material must be dealt with for a successful therapy outcome. No specific material, such as irrational beliefs or unconscious motivations, must be dealt with for therapeutic change to occur. The underlying theory is a *process* theory concerned with the client's current mode of cognitive/affective processing of the content that is most salient for him or her. Therapists' decisions on appropriate interventions are based on attending to *how* clients are currently organizing their experience. What we attempt to facilitate is change in the *manner* in which people are processing, change in both *what* they attend to and *how* they symbolize, rather than the modification or understanding of specific contents.

It is important to reiterate that it is always the *current* emotional meaning-construction processes that are the targets of change, not *traits* or broadly assessed etiological processes of a disorder. We are not attempting to modify an information-processing difficulty associated with a disorder, such as negative thinking or overgeneralization in depression, or vigilance in anxiety. Instead, the therapist is attempting to facilitate some aspect of current processing involved in a person's current emotional meaning-construction process to help clients attend to, symbolize, or reflect on some aspect of experience, and we believe that change in these processes will lead to change in the disorder. Thus, if a client is currently experiencing a sense of hopelessness or threat, the therapist helps the client to attend to or search for the underlying appraisals, to express the underlying emotions to completion, and to acknowledge unmet needs. This helps the client to construct new emotional meaning, and it is this that will lead to change in such things as depression or anxiety.

The therapist therefore begins treatment with an open, process-oriented stance by empathically entering the client's internal frame of reference in order to discover how the client experiences and sees his or her world. It does not impose on the client a theoretical frame of reference or particular contents that need to be dealt with. The goal is to bring to awareness clients' schematic emotional processing, which automatically organizes and creates experience, in order both to help them symbolize their experience and to change the scheme when necessary.

Central in our view is that the client is an active collaborator in the change process and that without this collaboration change will not occur. Our approach involves a combination and a balance between client-centered empathic responding and the process directiveness of experiential and Gestalt therapies. In this approach, the therapist is highly *empathically attuned* to the client's moment-by-moment feelings and experience of being. He or she is also *directive in process*, guiding the client toward engaging in particular types of resolution-enhancing, affective information-processing strategies at different times. Our therapist thus facilitates the client's process, both by responding empathically to the client's experience and by providing directions or suggestions as to the actions or mental operations the client might engage in, at the moment, to enhance processing. The goal is to stimulate new awareness, experiencing, and meaning construction, *not* to provide insight or to modify cognitions. The issue of balancing the relational bond with engaging in therapeutic work will be described in more detail in Part III, where we elaborate a distinction between therapeutic principles specifying the nature of the relationship and therapeutic principles identifying how the therapeutic work is fostered more directly.

The types of processes involved in working on therapeutic tasks are facilitated in a variety of ways that are described in Chapters 8 through 13 of this book. For example, at times the therapist may help the client focus attention on body sensations or a bodily felt sense in order to build a "bottom-up" sense of experience. At other times it is important to facilitate the client's engagement in different types of internal mental operations, such as symbolizing from memory a feature of a specific stimulus to which the client was reacting, or recognizing a currently mobilized need or want associated with an emotional expression.

Within this process-facilitative framework the therapist is viewed as an expert in facilitating the types of processes that will lead to new experience and the possible steps involved in certain affective problem-solving processes. However the client is seen as the expert on what he or she is experiencing, and as an active agent in the change process. Throughout therapy, the therapist, even when being process directive, adopts an inquiring, "not knowing" attitude. This position entails a stance of curiosity and suggestion rather than one of a knowing authority. Therapists' actions and attitudes express a desire to know more about clients' experience, and suggestions are made to help explicate the implicit, rather than to convey that therapists are more knowing and are searching for hidden material. This "less knowing" position, adopted by therapists in a process-experiential perspective, stands in contrast to the adoption of a more knowing position in an interpretive approach in which the therapist operates as an expert on the client's experience, on the basis of theoretical truths or professional knowledge. In being process-directive, the therapist engages with clients not to make meaning for them, nor to identify patterns, nor to ferret out the hidden, nor to suggest better ways of seeing themselves or the world. Rather, the therapist guides or stimulates the client to engage in certain information-processing activities believed to enhance access to schematic information that will aid the client in reorganizing experience and in making new meaning in areas that are troublesome to him or her. It is self-generated reorganization in areas of desired change that best helps people to see themselves, or their world, in a new way.

Our view is that in order to enhance this type of change, the therapist should pay focal attention to the client's moment-by-moment unfolding experiential process. This enables the therapist to recognize and promote shifts in particular experiential states. Two aspects of present client engagement, reexperiencing the narrated past and experiencing the present moment, offer important opportunities for engaging clients in modes of processing that will facilitate the reorganization of inner experience and the construction of new meaning. These two major types of present client experience form the focus of the therapist's attention.

Clients' in-session reexperiencing of the past involves promoting the client's reconstruction and reexperiencing of past events in the present. When clients are talking about an important incident from the recent or more distant past, the therapist attempts to evoke the past feeling in the present. The therapist attends to what seems currently most alive and poignant for the client in this recounting, and intervenes in ways that facilitate the vivid reexperiencing of the immediate stimulus situation and the feelings thus aroused. In this experiential context the client is able to recognize and reprocess this experience in the present.

The second possible focus of the therapist's attention is the client's current experience of what is occurring in the session, without reference to reliving a past experience. Here the client and therapist are not exploring some earlier relationship or incident in the client's life but, rather, are focusing on the client's current experience and construction of meaning as it occurs in the moment. The focus here is on the client's present experience of the present. This may at times involve remembering feelings about the past or feelings about anticipated future events, but the focus is on current experience rather than reliving or anticipating.

PROCESS DIAGNOSIS

In this approach, as we have said, the therapist enters the client's internal frame of reference in order to see how the client experiences and views his or her world. From this perspective, when the therapist hears particular types of client experiential states emerging in the moment, he or she responds in ways intended to facilitate the client's accessing of relevant emotion schemes and the generating of new experience that will lead to the reorganization of the schemes. Based on the recognition of different emerging client states, the therapist intervenes in different ways at different times in order to facilitate particular types of constructive information processing. Thus intervention is guided by a type of "process diagnosis" of the client's current state and by ideas of what would be most helpful at any particular moment in facilitating the client's cognitive/ affective processing.

The therapist therefore joins with the client's phenomenal world, entering into the client's frame of reference, sensing what it is like to be the client in this moment, and then intervening in particular ways at different times to point the information processing in a constructive direction. The therapist is thus *process directive* to facilitate different types of processing at different times. The directiveness is, however, suggestive and experimental rather than authoritative.

The therapist first becomes empathically attuned to the client's experiential world by entering the client's internal frame of reference, attending empathically to the client's inner experience, and communicating this understanding by means of empathic reflections. Both verbally and nonverbally, the therapist's responses capture the client's affective quality and intensity, as well as convey understanding of the content and meaning of their communication. This process of empathic attunement serves two important functions. It conveys to the client a sense of being really *heard* by the therapist, of being nonjudgmentally valued as a person, which is therapeutic in itself. It also serves the function of enabling the therapist to make more accurate and facilitative *process diagnoses*, thus enabling the therapist to make the kind of intervention that would help the client take the next experiential processing step. The therapist listens for the emergence of particular client states that indicate both that the client is currently experiencing a particular type of emotional processing problem and that the client is open to intervention.

Process diagnosis thus involves the identification of "markers" of emotional processing problems. When a marker of a particular type emerges, the therapist facilitates particular types of processing activity, designed to help resolve the currently experienced emotional processing problem. The term "diagnosis" is not used here to mean an act of labeling the client or the client's experience and thereby reifying or adopting a more expert, knowing stance. Rather it is meant to describe the therapist's internal process of noticing the client's focus and type of engagement, and thereby recognizing a "marker" to guide his or her own actions.

The client's content is not the only focus of the therapist's attention in process diagnosis. The client's expressive manner and style of processing are also attended to in order to understand client experience. How clients say what they are saying and the nonverbal and paralinguistic aspects of their expression are crucial aspects of the communication of meaning. It is thus client style and manner that often convey what is significant and will benefit from attention. Therapists thus need to be highly attuned to aspects of expressions such as vocal quality, speech rhythm, breathing, sighs, direction of gaze and postural shifts, as it is the expressive form that often conveys the client's current internal state. It is by dwelling on these subsidiary signs that we can get closest to knowing the mind or experience of another person (Polanyi, 1966).

Although the therapist is process-diagnostic and process-directive, it is important to note that he or she is tracking the client's emerging experience, and the diagnoses and interventions are always guided by whatever is emerging from the client, not by any preformed ideas about the client's problems. The therapist's process diagnosis also involves assessing a client's *current readiness* to engage in a particular operation at this time. Interventions are never imposed on the client, and are always made within the context of the client as the ultimate expert on his or her own experience.

It follows from this that all therapist assessments or interventions are made in a spirit of checking with the client whether or not the therapist's understanding or processing suggestion fits with the client's experience. The therapist is always cognizant of the fact that a therapist can never directly know the client's inner world, and thus needs to check frequently with the client about the accuracy of his or her sensed perceptions and process suggestions and to be guided by the responses received from the client.

A second reason for the therapist to adopt an attitude of tentativeness in developing process diagnoses is the understanding that one cannot direct or modify another's experience by instruction alone. Thus one cannot make the client truly experience a feeling by instructing him or her to feel sad or angry, confident or relaxed, or by interpreting that that emotion is what he or she feels. In other words, the person is a self-organizing system who cannot easily be intentionally modified by another person. Rather, the therapist can only attempt to join with the other and *facilitate* certain self-generated experiences by suggesting that the person try certain processing activities at certain times. It is then up to the client to respond and to organize him- or herself in a new way as a function of the facilitation. A therapist cannot "make" a client spontaneously experience or resolve anything. Only the client can organize his or her own processing so as to experience something in a particular manner.

THERAPIST RELATIONSHIP ATTITUDES

In our view, the client-centered attitudes of empathy, nonjudgmentalness or prizing and genuineness (Rogers, 1957) are central change-producing aspects of the process-experiential approach to therapy; they provide, as well, the optimal conditions for promoting the types of emotional processing we are suggesting. As we elaborate in later chapters, providing an empathic environment does not only involve entering the other's phenomenal world and responding to it. It is also characterized by the therapist's attitude of unconditional valuing of the client's experiencing, thus enabling him or her to feel fully accepted and understood. This sense of the therapist's unconditional prizing is crucial in reducing clients' interpersonal anxiety and enabling them to allocate full attention to the exploratory tasks of therapy. Rather than being concerned with how the therapist may be seeing him or her, the client feels *really* heard and received and experiences the therapist as being able and willing to resolve any interpersonal misunderstandings that may arise in a genuine, congruent fashion. Consequently, the client becomes increasingly confident of the therapist's unfailing positive regard.

The client benefits from the therapist's unfailing positive regard in two ways. First, the experience of being accepted and truly valued is a unique learning experience, which helps to counteract internalized conditions of worth and negative self-evaluations and self-doubts. In addition, removing the need for interpersonal vigilance liberates the client's processing capacity, increasing attentional breadth as well as access to memory. This allows the client to engage more fully in inner exploration. Support of this type thus encourages the client to face more painful and anxiety-provoking material. The reduction of interpersonal anxiety allows the client to tolerate more intrapersonal anxiety in self-exploration, creating an optimal environment for engaging in the cognitive/affective tasks of therapy.

Empathic attunement to clients' ongoing affective experience is a crucial aspect of the essential fabric of the therapist's involvement. Empathic attunement to clients' feelings helps clients to confirm and strengthen their own sense of themselves. It is similar to the way children synthesize their own internal emotional responses to situations. With the caretaker's empathic attunement to their experience, they are able to develop a strong sense of their own selves (Stern, 1985). In a similar way, clients build a stronger sense of their own experience by having their experience recognized, responded to, and thereby validated by their therapists. Having one's own feelings understood and accurately reflected back to oneself in both a verbal and nonverbal manner helps one to experience the feeling more fully and with increased confidence that "this is really what I am feeling." Feelings are often inchoate, emerging from a highly subjective, idiosyncratic, inner world for which there is no formal descriptive language. When the experience is symbolized and shared, it is confirmed as being what it is by the other's understanding of it. The process of empathic attunement therefore leads to the building of a sense of confidence in one's own experience. Thus growth occurs best in the context of empathy. It is important to note here, however, that it is not the specific behavior of reflection of feeling that is meant by being empathic. Rather, it is an *attitude*, and it is ultimately the *client's perception* of the therapist as empathic that is important.

In addition to providing an optimal environment for client growth, empathy is also essential for process diagnosis. Empathic resonance to the client's state fosters the recognition of particular markers. The therapist's stance in making process diagnoses is not observational or diagnostic in the usual sense of objectively assessing the client. Rather, it is one of entering the client's frame of reference, attempting to understand the client's view of his or her experience as if the therapist were the client and, from this perspective, responding to emerging experiential puzzles or struggles. Responding appropriately to a specific marker with a specific intervention thus is a highly empathic act and can be experienced by the client as having been truly understood by the therapist's intervention.

In addition to prizing and empathy, therapist genuineness is a crucial aspect of the therapist's involvement. If empathy and prizing are offered by a therapist in a way perceived as inauthentic by the client, these will not encourage client safety and self-exploration. Thus, as Rogers has so clearly stated (Rogers, 1957, 1961), the therapist must also be genuine and congruent. As Rogers has defined it, congruence means that the therapist is aware of his or her own experience during the session and is thus being nondefensively authentic in his or her communications. This state of congruence in the therapist is necessary to enable the client to experience empathy and prizing as occurring in a real relationship with another human being.

In addition, Buber (1958) has defined the characteristics of an I–Thou relationship as one possessing, among other things, presence, immediacy, and nonexploitativeness. This helps to convey what is meant by us in the terms "genuineness" or "congruence." One can be empathic with many aims in mind, not all salutary, as is the case with people who utilize their empathically based understanding of others' feelings and needs to manipulate them. In our terms, congruence means also nonexploitative, nonblaming, and nondefensive communication of one's essential experience.

The therapist therefore offers the client a real relationship in which he or she continually values the deeper core of the client (Lietaer, 1984). In this process the therapist is constantly attuned to the feelings that flow within him or her in the interaction with the client. What the therapist experiences is available to awareness, can be lived in the relationship, and communicated when appropriate in order to contact the deeper core of the client. In longer-term therapies with more distressed people it is the genuine relationship that becomes the core of therapy. The therapy proceeds by working through the difficulties, the disappointments, and the joys of two people stubbornly struggling to remain authentic and in contact with each other.

The presence of a real, empathic, and prizing therapist in itself provides some of the therapeutic healing, but it also provides the soil in which other specific changes can take place. As we have said, in addition to genuinely and sensitively following the client's moment-by-moment experiencing and providing acceptant prizing, the therapist facilitates experiential processing by offering process directives. These process suggestions or directives are guided by what has just emerged for the client. They are always offered in a nonimposing, collaborative manner, checking against the client's experience, in the context of the client as the expert on his or her own experience and as an active participant in the change process. This emphasis on nonimposing, nonmanipulative offering of suggestions is important in maintaining the collaborative, facilitative relationship environment regarded as so crucial in helping the client engage as much as possible in nondefensive processing. Within this relational framework, it is important to facilitate certain kinds of client processing, a topic discussed in a later section of this chapter.

MANAGING PROCESS DIRECTIVENESS AND THE RELATIONAL ATTITUDES: THE NEED FOR CARE AND BALANCE

The approach described above relies on the provision of an optimally empathic relational environment and on the therapist being optimally responsive to the client's experience. Within this context, however, we suggest that the therapist can also profitably guide the client's processing in certain directions. The balance between responsiveness and directiveness is a central issue for this treatment model, and is at the same time both its strongest and its most difficult aspect.

Issues of control and directiveness are highly important in this approach to therapy and relate directly both to the degree of anxiety experienced by the client and to the degree of collaborative exploration achieved. The optimal situation is a synergistic interaction in which client and therapist are working together, with each feeling neither led nor simply followed by the other. Instead, the goal is an easy sense of mutual collaboration and coexploration. There is one caveat to this, however. At times of disjunction or disagreement, clients are viewed as the experts on their own experience, and it is this experience that is viewed as the ultimate reference point. Therapist interventions are always offered in a *nonimposing, nonauthoritative* manner, as suggestions or offers rather than as instructions or statements of truth.

The combination of directive and responsive styles of intervening adopted in this approach (see Benjamin, 1979) allows us to combine the benefits of both styles and to ameliorate the disadvantages of each. In adopting a more complex and flexible dual style of this sort, balance and judgment are the guiding characteristics. One needs to be constantly assessing the best combination for this client at this time, judging whether more active stimulation or more responsive attunement would be most helpful, all the while keeping the overall balance of autonomy in favor of client-directed exploration. The therapist is recognized as an expert in the types of processing steps that might be facilitative, but it is made clear that ultimately the therapist is a facilitator of the client's discovery and exploration process, not a leader of the expedition or a provider of truth.

A crucial issue in the use of a combination of directiveness and responsiveness is the degree to which the therapist facilitates an experiential discovery process in which clients construct their own idiosyncratic meaning from their own experience. Being too directive can create premature closure of the client's meaning-creation process and suggest that the therapist knows the client's experience better than the client does. This alters the balance of influence too strongly in the direction of the therapist and robs the client of the opportunity to capture his or her own unique experience. As we have said, a process-experiential approach to therapy is based on the assumption that self-generated meaning ultimately leads to the most stable and enduring change. In contrast with the problem of being too directive is the problem of being too passive. By not being sufficiently responsive the therapist does not provide sufficient facilitation of the exploration process. It is the therapist's process suggestions and selective focus that often provide the needed added stimulation that promotes further self-exploration.

The therapist, as we have said, is an expert on process, facilitating specific processes at specific times to help exploration unfold. The therapist, while maintaining the relational attitudes, may direct clients' attention to aspects of their experience such as their breathing, to their inner reaction to a stimulus, or to some current muscular activity or bodily felt sense. The therapist is thus engaged in process facilitation rather than interpretation of the meaning of a client's experience or directing the client to deal with a particular content. Although fuzzy at its boundaries, the process–content distinction is important, with the emphasis in this approach always being placed on process directiveness rather than content directiveness.

In being directive, therapists offer expertise on how to facilitate different types of processes and how these help resolve tasks. They are neither experts on the client's experience nor on the correct resolution of this problem for this particular client. Rather, resolution is a unique self construction. Ultimately, there are many ways to resolve a particular problem. The therapist knows something about what elements are helpful in creating a resolution but does not know the precise form resolution will ultimately take. Thus the therapist, in being directive, leads by facilitating the bringing of material into awareness, but he or she follows the client's direction in creating closure on the stimulated information. The directive attitude is always experimental in nature ("try this and see if it fits"), aiming to promote discovery and self-created meaning rather than encouraging compliance or the adoption of therapist-created meaning.

The more responsive self-discovery oriented style helps clients to learn to trust their own experience. On the other hand, in the more directive style of intervention, the therapist is seen as an expert on certain principles of human functioning. Even so, the therapist is still viewed as helping the client to become aware of aspects of his or her *own* experience. The potential gain from directing people to become aware of specific features of their own process at an optimal moment must always be weighed against the potential loss of the uniqueness resulting from allowing clients to self-select what stands out from them, thereby more independently constructing their own meaning. Construction of one's own meanings helps develop potentially more accurate and differentiated understandings of self as well as fostering greater autonomy and trust in one's own experience. The major guard against the therapist's process directiveness closing down the client's own differentiation of new meaning is the therapeutic attitude of empathic attunement, in which the therapist constantly checks his or her suggestions against the client's current experience to see if they fit.

The crucial judgment in this process is when to lead (direct) or when to follow (respond), and a key, helpful distinction can be made to help guide this judgment. This is the distinction between when clients are in contact with their own experience, that is, engaging in productive emotional processing, and when they are not. When clients are congruently experiencing themselves, it is crucial to follow them and facilitate their own processes of discovery and construction of new meaning. To lead or direct at this time could distort, deflect, or put premature closure on their experience and construction of meaning.

When, however, clients are on the surface of their experience, blocked, or engaged in some interruptive, dysfunctional process, it is helpful for the therapist to lead by stimulating experiencing or suggesting ways clients can become aware of the self-interruptive processing. Thus, therapist process directives are often used to facilitate the generation of new experiential material or to focus clients on the nature of the internal processes that are impeding their exploration or interrupting their experience. New experience is, for example, stimulated by facilitating clients' vivid reentry into problematic situations by helping them imagine the scene or by facilitating the expression or intensification of their expression. Blocks or interruptive processes can, for example, be brought into awareness by clients attending to their physical sensations and muscular tension and by clients' attempts to enact and verbalize their blocking process in an active manner such as enacting the pushing down of one's feelings or the squeezing back of tears.

THERAPEUTIC WORK

In addition to the provision of a safe, growth-producing environment by means of the relationship attitudes, the therapist also facilitates therapeutic work by the client. Central to our approach is the view that different client modes of engagement in therapy are useful at different times and seem to be necessary for the resolution of particular types of problems. It appears that these different modes of engagement enable clients to access, work with, and change underlying emotion schematic structures in particular ways.

Modes of Client Engagement

These different types of engagement can be clustered into four different global modes of processing for accessing emotion schemes. The four dimensions that are crucial to the tasks of process-facilitative therapy are Attending/Awareness, Experiential Search, Active Expression, and Interpersonal Learning.

Attending/Awareness

The focus in this first mode of client engagement is on directly attending to particular elements of sensation, rather than symbolizing complex relational feelings and meanings. Becoming aware of internal sensations (somesthetic and kinesthetic) and external stimuli (visual and auditory) are essential parts of making clear contact with reality. Attending involves making contact with incoming information and provides the person with basic sensory information about self and external reality from which further meaning can be constructed. Attending is at the basis of "bottom-up" processing. It focuses on attending to present sensory reality, often yielding information that is somewhat different from people's anticipations or imaginings about reality.

Learning to attend to basic sensory data from within and without is a style of processing experience that can provide clients access to information that is influencing their current sense of self. Thus, a client may become aware of tightening his or her face, clenching a fist, or tensing in the stomach, or of the more complex sensations of feeling alive, of a surging sense of power, or of feeling passive, tired, or fragile. Attending may also involve clients' becoming aware of external stimuli, including those from the therapist, such as raised eyebrows, a smile on the face, or the tone of the voice.

The therapist may facilitate this process of self-awareness in the present by calling attention to some visible aspect of the client's expression, for example, saying, "Are you aware that you are clenching your fists?" Then, the client may focus his or her awareness on the tight and forceful feel, including a sense of wanting to "lash out" or a "self-controlled" feeling associated with the clenching. Another example might be having a client attend to shifts in gaze while talking (e.g., looking down or away from the therapist). Attending to these may help clients to become more aware of what leads to their reactions. For some clients, and at certain times in therapy, learning to attend to these kinds of inner and outer experience can be extremely important, for they are the raw data from which experience is built and one of the core means of experiencing contact with self and world.

Experiential Search

The second mode of client engagement involves a deliberate turning inward of attentional energy in an attempt to access one's own complex, idiosyncratic inner experience and to begin to symbolize it in words. This process goes beyond the mode of Attending/Awareness described in the previous section. If appropriately facilitated by the therapist, this can be a process of discovery in which clients symbolize a level of tacit inner experience that is influential in guiding their own functioning but is seldom available to self-reflective awareness.

The process of conscious symbolization of complex inner experience may take a number of different forms. For instance, it may involve getting in touch with one's own complex present inner state and being able to describe it in words. Or it may involve retrieving a perceptual experience that has had an impact but had not been fully processed in awareness at the time. Or the Experiential Search process may involve a deliberate attempt to get in touch with a vaguely felt meaning that is sensed as important but that is not currently in awareness or easily accessible. In each of these examples, the client is able to become newly aware of complex feelings and meanings by a process of attending inwardly and symbolizing inner experience. The process of Experiential Search enables the client to access and explore emotion schemes that had not previously been available to self-reflective awareness.

Active Expression

When clients actively and spontaneously express their own experiential reactions, they are provided a unique opportunity to discover and own what it is that they *do* feel. Expression also involves allowing the action tendency to run to completion and brings feelings into *contact* with their appropriate objects. Clients are thus encouraged to try out expressions in therapy in order to recognize what they are actually experiencing and to complete the expression by connecting it to the appropriate object.

Experience is pregnant with meaning that is implicit until it is expressed. By the act of expressing, people take an explicit position in relation to something, thereby creating meaning. Once expressed, the expressed meaning in turn becomes a new stimulus for the person. It becomes available to awareness for reflection and evocation of further internal reactions. Once a statement such as "I needed you" is expressed, it can be considered for its truth value, can be reflected on, and can strongly evoke further experiencing. Therefore by "doing" something, people have an opportunity to experience whether or not the expressed action/meaning fits and to claim what fits as their own. Further, the meaning and the sensory expressive motor aspects generated by expression act as cues that activate new schemes thereby evoking new experience. In addition, Active Expression helps people experience themselves as agents and authors of their experience. Finally, by contacting the environment and bringing the expression into contact with its appropriate target, the expression is brought to completion.

Active Expression can be uniquely effective in establishing contact between aspects of internal experience. For example, when clients express a need such as "I need to rest" or "I need support" to an imagined other or another aspect of self, they begin to recognize and claim the experience as their own. This kind of dialectical confrontation between previously polarized aspects of experience can be especially effective in the differentiation and synthesis of these aspects of experience into a new whole.

Interpersonal Contact

The final mode of client engagement occurs in the context of the relationship itself. The therapist's empathic attunement, consistent unconditional prizing, and genuine presence during the client's process of self-exploration are important elements throughout therapy. These therapist attitudes, plus the emphasis on discovery and growth orientation, consistently convey to clients that the therapist has a basic trust in the clients' own inner experiences as a source of information for guiding their lives. Clients learn from this to *trust their own experience* and to accept their own feelings. In addition, they learn that they are *able to be themselves in relation to another* and that this can be a rewarding experience. They are confirmed in their existence as worthwhile people.

At particular times, specific experiences with the therapist can be crucial in leading to change. In these experiences it is through the here-and-now interpersonal interaction between client and therapist that the client works through his or her relational experience with the therapist and learns something new (Lietaer, 1984). Different relational experiences can provide crucial new learnings for the client by providing important new experiences that disconfirm old, restrictive learnings and beliefs about the difficulties or dangers of being with another. For example, clients can learn that their anger can be heard and will not destroy others or evoke attack from them, that their successes will not be experienced as a threat, and that their weakness will not be scorned. They in addition learn that risking being themselves can be rewarding and healing.

Individual Differences in Typical Processing Style

Different people come to therapy with different typical styles, capacities, and preferred modes of engagement. Clients who are not easily able to turn inward and search inner experience with the help of empathic reflections may benefit more from being guided toward Active Expression of their feelings. A client who has difficulty with Active Expression and is uneasy with such therapist directives may thrive in a more reflectively guided Experiential Search. Thus, within the context of a process-diagnostic approach, the therapist is also aware that different modes of processing may suit, and be more effective, for different kinds of people. Consequently, therapists need to be able to adjust their intervention styles to facilitate the kinds of processing demands that are most suited to that client's style and resources.

In the earlier phases of therapy, the client is facilitated in engaging in different types of in-therapy processing tasks. In this process, the therapist gets a feel for the styles that seem to produce the greatest yield of productive exploration. Also, some people may work best by operating initially at the level of conceptual processing and only later begin to symbolize their preconceptual inner experience, whereas others may thrive on symbolizing or actively expressing inner experience. Still others may find that the interpersonal safety and understanding of the therapist are what prove most helpful in facilitating their learning to become more congruent within themselves. By recognizing that different people can benefit from different modes of engagement, a process-experiential approach to therapy attempts to be more responsive to a wider variety of clients rather than to fit them all into a Procrustean bed of one single type of processing.

Experienced Impacts

Given an empathic, collaborative relationship between client and therapist, most of the work of therapy occurs within the modes of client engagement described above. The work carried out through these processes results in various positive *impacts*, or effects. Clients, on reviewing tapes of their sessions, report three major impacts of process-experiential therapy. These are *changes in perception*, creation of *problem solutions*, and feeling *supported and understood*, (Elliott, James, Reimschuessel, Cislo, & Sack, 1985). These experienced impacts sometimes emerge clearly in the session, while at other times clients only become aware of them later, as they mull over the session or encounter situations that relate to the issues explored in the session. The impacts are discussed below.

Perceptual Change

Clients often report changes in how they view themselves and others. Elliott et al. (1985) identified three types of perceptual changes from client recalls of the significant moments in sessions. First, they found that the client may be more directly or strongly *aware* of a feeling or particular aspect of self or an other. Something may now be "owned" as part of the self (e.g., my feeling of anger) or may be more clearly seen in another (e.g., that my father was actually very frightened inside). Clients may experience this sort of impact as coming into contact or "touch" with a feeling or experience that they partially knew was there before but that is now "known better" or is more clearly recognized.

Clients also report *new understandings* of something about self or another; they may come to understand a connection between their response and a situation, perhaps understanding a reason or cause of their experience or reaction (e.g., "I did this because I felt angry" or "I realize I cover up my hurt with bitterness and anger"). From the client's point of view, this type of impact is often experienced as an insight, or a seeing into self, as if the pieces of a puzzle had suddenly "clicked" into place.

Clients also report developing more *positive evaluations* or acceptance of self or others. Thus, a client may come to feel more self-accepting, less guilty or blameworthy for something that has happened, or may forgive another for a hurt or deprivation. Often, the experience is one of seeing that "I'm not so bad, after all" or feeling compassionate toward oneself. Beyond this, the client may come to see self or other as having positive attributes, as good, well-intended, "doing my best," or as having rights or abilities not previously recognized.

Problem Solutions

In addition to, and as a consequence of, perceptual changes clients also experience changes that relate more directly to solving their problems outside of therapy and to actions they may take outside therapy. For one thing, they may become clearer about what their problems, goals, or tasks are, that is, what they need to "work on." In addition, they may come to decisions, figure out what to do about problems, or commit themselves to taking some action outside therapy. Problem impacts thus contain a *motivational* or energizing component, an organizing of the self toward some goal or action, or a commitment to pursue a goal or take some action. This is a crucial aspect of the process by which clients spontaneously translate what has happened in the session into the rest of their lives.

Problem impacts may occur right at the end of a session as the client prepares to go "back out into the world"; however, they often occur after the session, often as the client reflects further on the issues raised by the session. In addition, problem impacts may emerge from scheme change, as when greater awareness of the seriousness of a problem leads to a resolution to work on it further. When the client experiences problem impacts in the session, he or she orients away from the past and present and toward the future (cf. Bohart et al., 1991). The client may tentatively propose and evaluate different possible courses of action, or he or she may imagine what it would be like to act in a different way (cf. Mahrer, 1989). Sometimes, there is an interest or excitement in "carrying forward" an in-therapy change or shift into the rest of the client's life. In the process-experiential approach the therapist listens for and facilitates these impacts when they emerge from the client, but does not try to "induce" them.

Interpersonal Impacts

In addition to the impacts just described, clients also experience impacts that are interpersonal. They may experience the therapist as being understanding or supportive, or they may come to feel closer to the therapist or more invested in the work of therapy. These interpersonal impacts may occur in combination with the other impact, but they seem to flow most directly from the interpersonal contacting mode of engagement. Often, the client gives no obvious signs in treatment that an interpersonal impact has occurred. At other times, however, the client may comment on feeling understood, supported, and so on, or may give nonverbal signs of relief such as, a large sigh after being understood.

CONCLUSION

Process-experiential therapy is therefore guided by the major assumption that therapy proceeds best by client discovery and construction of meaning. A further assumption is that therapists can best facilitate clients in this process by two means: on the one hand, by being genuinely prizing and empathically attuned, and, on the other hand, by facilitating specific client-processing activities at specific times. The latter involves attempting to mesh with, recognize and understand the type of internal mental operations in which clients are currently engaging in order to facilitate productive moment-by-moment movement toward task resolution.

THEORY: EMOTION AND COGNITION IN CHANGE

PERSPECTIVES ON HUMAN FUNCTIONING

EXPERIENTIAL PERSPECTIVES

Experientially oriented therapies share a belief in the uniquely human capacity for self-reflective awareness, and a theory of human functioning that focuses on the uniqueness of each person's inner experience and meaning construction. Thus they advocate a variety of methods that enable each person to "access in awareness" his or her own inner experience and to express and symbolize previously implicit meanings or blocked feelings.

In this perspective, human beings are viewed as oriented toward growth and full development of their own potentialities. Major elements in dysfunction are the inaccessibility of organismic experience to awareness and the blocking of growth capacities. Therefore, fostering awareness of experience and facilitating attention to the growth tendency are central to experiential therapy. This is done by helping clients to identify and overcome blocks to awareness, and by recognizing and fostering clients' awareness of their inner push toward growth and expansion.

Rogers and Perls were the two major originators of experientially oriented approaches to therapy. Rogers emphasized the relational environment most conducive to therapeutic exploration and change. Perls provided a variety of procedures that were designed to make more vivid the feelings, thoughts, and behaviors that are involved in maintaining rigidity and preventing growth.

Below we briefly review the positions of Rogers and Perls concerning human functioning and change. We will then introduce relevant contributions from cognitive science and modern emotion theory. In the next chapter we will present our development and elaboration of these views of functioning in terms of contemporary schematic and emotional processing perspectives.

CLASSICAL THEORY

Client-Centered Therapy

Rogers' view of healthy, or "ideal," functioning was based on his belief in an inborn, actualizing tendency that leads people to strive not only to meet deficiency needs such as hunger and thirst but to be motivated to develop and expand their own unique personal capacities toward growth and autonomy. Rogers considered this actualizing tendency to be the only *basic* human motivation. A further key assumption was that optimal human functioning can occur only when the person is able to experience the sensory and emotional events currently taking place.

Roger's definitions of "perception" and "feelings" (1959) are especially important to his views on dysfunction, optimal functioning, and therapeutic change. Rogers viewed the process of accurate symbolization in awareness as involving a kind of hypothesis testing: "A perception is a hypothesis or prognosis for action which comes into being in awareness when stimuli impinge on the organism" (1959, p. 199). Thus, he saw perception as essentially transactional, involving both construction from one's experience and one's hypotheses for the future. Facilitating clients to access and explore feelings is a central focus of client-centered therapy. "A feeling denotes an emotionally tinged experience, together with its personal meaning. Thus it includes the emotion in its experiential context. It thus refers to the unity of emotion and cognition as they are experienced inseparably in the moment" (Rogers 1959, p. 198).

Rogers' theories concerning dysfunction center on the nature of the interference with accurate symbolization of feelings and other experience. He assumed that an almost inevitable split develops between the motivation toward healthy actualization and the *acquired* need to maintain and actualize the learned self-concept derived from relationships with parents and other early experiences. Rogers proposed that a need for receiving positive regard from significant others, and later from oneself, is central in the formation and maintenance of the self concept. When there is a potential *discrepancy between one's own organismic experience and one's own concept of self*, anxiety is aroused. The person experiences threat at some level, and the experience may be denied or distorted to be consistent with the self concept. When the person denies to awareness or distorts such potentially significant experiences, they are not integrated into the self structure. Rather than broadening the self structure to integrate the new awareness, this may increase the incongruence between one's self concept and one's organismic experience.

The goal of therapy is to facilitate fuller and more accurate perception including the experience of feelings in ways that will serve to develop a self structure that is more consistent with actual experience. Optimal psychological adjustment is characterized by a concept of self that allows all experiences that are potentially available to human awareness to be assimilated into the self concept. This diminishes the split between actualizing the total person or actualizing the self concept. Thus one can develop one's own life in ways that are guided by the basic actualizing tendency from moment-to-moment and over the long range.

Although this discrepancy between the person's learned self concept and his or her organismic experience was a central aspect of Rogers' explicit theoretical statement, the actual practice of client-centered therapy did not focus on this discrepancy. Rather, it was assumed that, if the therapist responded in an empathically attuned manner in an atmosphere of unconditional positive regard, the client would increasingly be able to tolerate the threat of inconsistency with the self concept. This would increase the client's motivation to move more and more deeply and accurately into his or her own perceptions and feelings. A process theory therefore began to be developed to capture the reality of client-centered practice.

Rogers (1961) described the process of change a client goes through during the actual therapeutic process. The overall process was broken down into seven stages in which the client was seen as moving from a position of remoteness from experience, to one of acceptance of experience. The seven stages in achieving "constructive personality change" are summarized below.

In Stage 1 the individual is at first unwilling to communicate about the self. Feelings and their subjective meanings are neither recognized nor owned. Personal constructs are rigid and problems are not recognized. Close and communicative relationships are perceived as threatening and/or painful. In Stage 2 expression begins to flow more freely but problems are perceived as external to the self and feelings are not owned. The individual is not in touch with subjective experience and may contradict him or herself, without being aware of doing so. Conflicts and problems may be recognized at this stage but they are external to the self. No sense of personal responsibility for the problems exist at this stage. In Stage 3, situations, feelings, and their subjective meaning are expressed more freely but they are talked about in the past tense and are often viewed as bad or unacceptable. Personal constructs are still inflexible but the individual may begin questioning their validity. There is a beginning recognition of contradictions in experience and that problems may be more internal than external: however, choices that are made are often seen as ineffectual.

Stage 4 represents a shift. The individual describes feelings and meanings as present and as owned by the self. More intense feelings, however, are not experienced in the present but are only described. There is still not a full and open acceptance of currently felt feelings, although the process is beginning. Contradictions in experience are seen more clearly at this stage and the individual usually voices concern over them. There are some discoveries of personal constructs as constructs, and a questioning of their validity. The individual is definitely starting to own problems, recognize incongruence between experience and self, and may be willing to express feelings to others.

In Stage 5 many feelings are freely expressed in the present. They are owned and accepted. Previously denied feelings are experienced although still feared. The individual starts to recognize that paying attention to feelings when they occur is important for wellbeing and involves attending to an inner referent. Contradictions are recognized as attitudes existing in different parts of the personality. There is an increasing ownership of feelings and a desire to be true to one's self. There is increasing acceptance of responsibility for problems and also more concern regarding self-contribution to problems.

In the sixth stage feeings are now experienced with immediacy and acceptance and flow to completion. Expression of these feared/painful feelings is usually accompanied by physiological changes including tears, sighs, and muscular relaxation. Experiencing takes on a real process quality. The individual can now fully accept experiences and use them as a clear referent for meaning and to make better personal choices. Internal communication is free and unblocked. In the final stage, Stage 7, the individual experiences new feelings with immediacy and richness. The person develops a trust in his or her own process and this experiencing becomes a clear guide for behavior. Personal constructs are held loosely and remain flexible and open to information from new experiences. The individual is rarely incongruent and internal communication is clear.

This process view, in combination with Gendlin's (1962) view of experiencing as an ongoing process of symbolizing internal referents that can become blocked, came to represent the client-centered view of function and dysfunction far more accurately than did the self concept/organism incongruence model.

The relationship conditions of empathic understanding of the client's internal frame of reference, unconditional positive regard, and genuineness were still viewed as the crucial change agents. It is the client's exploration of feelings, leading to their fuller and deeper owning and integration into the self, that is central to client-centered exploration and discovery. Rogers emphasized a process in which the therapist did not attempt to lead the client in a particular direction but, rather, responded to clients' expressions in order to help to deepen their exploration. This was done by paying particular attention to the uniqueness of each person's feelings and meanings.

Gestalt Therapy

Perls' primary motivational construct was also an actualizing tendency. In his view, this involved a self-regulatory organism meeting its needs, moving toward growth, and thereby establishing its own identity. Perls assumed that the well-functioning person engaged in organismic self-regulation, thereby achieving (through action) the realization of his or her most urgent needs at any given moment. The goal was to maintain equilibrium within the self and between the self and the environment. The assumption is that the ideally well-functioning person experiences clear gestalts, in which the awareness of a need and the object relevant to the need become clearly figural. In this view, awareness of both internal and external information is viewed as highly significant in healthy functioning and need satisfaction. This process of awareness or gestalt formation was called the contact cycle. In this cycle, *awareness* leads to the mobilization of *excitement*. This in turn leads to *action*, oriented toward *contacting* the environment, need satisfaction, and *completion* of the cycle. Thus the person is continually organizing him- or herself to make contact with the environment to meet the need. When the need is met, then this particular figure/background gestalt is dissolved, and the person returns to equilibrium.

In Perl's view, awareness of emotion was particularly important to help people orient in the environment and to provide them with information about objects appropriate to their needs. This is exemplified in the following statement:

> It is only through the recognition of your emotions that you can be aware, as a biological organism, either of what you are up against in the environment, or of what special opportunities are at the moment presented. It is only if you acknowledge and accept your longing for someone or something . . . that you obtain orientation for appropriate action." (Perls et al., 1951, pp. 98–99)

Awareness of emotion was thus central in healthy functioning.

On the other hand, dysfunction involved lack of awareness and the alienation of aspects of the forming self. Organizing the self in such a way that awareness and need satisfaction were chronically interrupted or blocked led to pathology. Dysfunctional self-regulation was seen as occurring in a variety of different ways at different points along the need-satisfaction cycle. One general and pervasive kind of interference involves the restriction of awareness. Restriction of inner awareness reduces accurate symbolization of one's emotions and needs. The restriction of outer awareness at the contact boundary with the environment reduces one's ability to identify objects to meet needs. In dysfunction, the person's attentional focus is thought to be primarily in a middle zone of intellectualized abstraction rather than being in contact with the self and the present situation. This limits the potential for healthy, organismic self-regulation. Healthy regulation occurs when focal attention is integrated with automatically occurring, organismic aware-ness.

A number of specific kinds of processes interfere with healthy functioning and become obstacles to completion of the need satisfaction or contact cycle. These include:

1. Operating in terms of introjected learned rules or "shoulds" that are alien to organismic concerns or needs.
2. Dysfunctional perceptual processes, involving attributions of one's own thoughts and feelings to others.
3. Automatic self-controlling actions, which interrupt experience or stop expression without the recognition that this is being done or how it is being done.
4. The intrusion into the present of unresolved emotional reactions from the past.

Especially important obstacles to free functioning are the habitual disowning of experience and the disclaiming of action tendencies leading to the formation of "splits" in the personality. It is assumed that polarities and their differentiation and integration are natural aspects of human functioning. Thus strength and weakness, kindness and cruelty, selfless-ness and selfishness integrate into a balanced capacity to act adaptively. If, however, polarities become warring dichotomies, where one part dominates or criticizes another part, what we term "splits," or if one part such as weakness is isolated or disowned, then adaptive or creative adjustment is impeded. The Gestalt view of dysfunction was both less clear and more complex than that stated by Rogers, but essentially involved the disowning of experience when there was a clash between self-actualization and self-image actualization (Perls, 1969). This made it highly similar to Roger's view of an incongruence between organismic experience and self concept.

Therapeutic work in Gestalt is aimed at promoting identification with disowned aspects of self and the differentiation and integration of opposing parts into a harmonious union. A central assumption in Gestalt work is that direct expression of present emotional experience and needs will both increase people's awareness of themselves and lead to a reowning of aspects of their experience. The direct expression of experience is viewed as more productive than a description of the experience. Expression increases the sense of identification with, and owning of, the experience. Furthermore, spontaneous nonverbal expression, such as fist clenching or jaw tightening, is viewed as the expression of automatic unconscious processing. Deliberate expression of these is seen as a way of turning them into controlled conscious processing and thereby owning the experience (Greenberg & Safran, 1981).

Therapeutic work is often facilitated by means of an experimentation process using Active Expression. These experiments are designed either to discover experience or to raise to awareness how experiences are being interrupted or dysfunctionally regulated. According to Perls et al. (1951), therapy involves "experiments of deliberate awareness" to promote "identification of the ego with the forming self" until the person has the experience that "it is me who is feeling, thinking, or doing this." Thus, Gestalt work emphasized both client discovery and reowning as well as the bringing to awareness of specific dysfunctional interruptive processes.

General Tenets of Experiential Theory

Two major common themes of practice can be extracted from the writings of Rogers and Perls on therapy, and they may be viewed as the central tenets of an Experiential Approach to therapy. First, both approaches are discovery oriented and consider clients as experts on their own experience (Rice & Greenberg 1992). Clients are viewed as having priviledged access to their unique inner experience and therefore are continually encouraged in therapy to check their own experience. Newness comes from clients attending more fully to their experience and, by this process, becoming aware of, symbolizing and further developing some aspect of experience. The clients active role in the process of identifying and symbolising their inner experience for themselves is therefore valued over the therapist's provision of meanings to help clients in making sense of their experience.

Second, both Rogers and Perls believed in a fundamental motivation toward growth and development, and this is central in an Experiential Approach to treatment (Rice & Greenberg, 1992). The individual's search for ways to maintain and enhance him- or herself is seen as a never-ending process, and therapy is viewed as a way of facilitating people's access to their growth possibilities. Choice and self-determination are viewed as key aspects of this functioning. Human beings are viewed as being influenced by a vision of the future and not totally determined by past experience. The potential for growth and choice is seen as being maximally enhanced when people are aware of their feelings and needs.

In addition to the above two central themes of the importance of discovery and growth and development, the curative role of the genuine relationship between participants in therapy is also seen as central. In Client-Centered therapy, experiencing the therapist as empathic and genuinely respectful is viewed as helping clients to free themselves from their constraining internal conditions of worth. In Gestalt, the I–Thou relationship (Buber, 1958) is seen as key, and therapy is focused on promoting genuine contact between client and therapist. A facilitatively genuine empathic relationship is thus seen as inherently curative and is viewed as leading to the self becoming stronger and more able to be authentic.

PERSPECTIVES FROM MODERN PSYCHOLOGY

Many of the humanistic assumptions about human functioning that characterize the Client-Centered theory of Rogers and the Gestalt approach of Perls that are summarized above are basic to the approach described in the present volume. But over the past decade, developments within psychology (particularly in cognitive science and emotion theory) make possible the development of more differentiated theories of functioning and change than those proposed in the explicit original models of Rogers or Perls. The experiential views suggested in their explicit structural models, that dysfunction in essence, was caused by the incongruence between self concept and organismic experience and by the disowning of experience. Incongruence or disowning was seen as being caused by the introjection of conditions of worth. Change was viewed as occurring by the undoing of these conditions, in a variety of ways, to allow for the integration of organismic experience into awareness.

However, this view, which essentially construes pathology as occurring because of denial and distortion, does not fully encompass the practice of these therapies (Wexler & Rice, 1974; Greenberg & Safran, 1987). Experiential therapies have developed much more of a process conception of functioning, dysfunction, and change. In this view the therapist's focus is not on bringing what is denied or distorted into awareness, but rather it is on facilitating the synthesis of new meaning from bodily felt experience (Rogers, 1958, 1961; Gendlin, 1968, 1981,

1984; Perls, 1969; Polster & Polster, 1973). In fact Gendlin (1962), attempting to deal with problems in the structural theory, first offered a process conception in his book on *Experiencing and the Creation of Meaning*, whereas Rogers (1958, 1961) began to develop the process strands to explain how change actually occurred. Some of the developments in cognitive science and emotion theory that have direct implications for a *process* view of both human functioning and change in therapy, in which the creation of new meaning is central, are reviewed briefly below.

COGNITIVE SCIENCE

Since the 1970s, there has been a shift toward a cognitive and, more recently, a constructivist "cognitive/affective" perspective on human functioning (Mahoney, 1991). There now exists an extensive and increasing literature in cognitive experimental psychology concerning the mental processes people use to go beyond the simple processing of information in order to create meaning. There have been many studies on encoding and retrieval in memory that address the role of expectation in construal, and the role of language and symbolization in knowing. This literature demonstrates that individuals are active creators of meaning. Four major strands of modern cognitive science are summarized below:

1. *Attention* has become a topic of central concern in cognitive psychology (Pascual-Leone, 1976a, 1976b, 1976c 1983, 1987; Posner & Snyder, 1975; Shiffrin & Schneider, 1977). It is viewed as a limited mental resource that is involved in all conscious and partially conscious processes. Attention is viewed as being selectively allocated and as constraining the number of separate processes that can occur simultaneously. Consciously controlled processes are thought to require attentional allocation, whereas automatic processes require little if any of a person's attentional resources. Attention is thus a limited resource, allocated selectively where selectivity can be under internal control. In addition, attention is central in determining what people experience and in generating truly novel experience and performance (Pascual-Leone, 1987; James, 1890/1950). For example, at any given moment a client can only be aware of a limited number of things, be it the meaning of the story she is telling, the hollowness in her stomach, or the therapist's expression. Attending to new features will produce new awareness and new meanings.

2. A useful distinction has been drawn between cognitive processes that are *automatic* or incapable of flexibility and those that are controlled

or can be directed by the person (Schneider & Shiffrin, 1977; Shiffrin & Schneider, 1977). Automatic processes involve a sequence of operations that are activated without the need for conscious effort. Once activated, these proceed independently from controlled processes. Thus, even though people may try to feel or respond in some particular fashion, they are generally unable to prevent the occurrence of their automatic responses. Whereas controlled processes cannot easily modify automatic processes, the reverse is not true. Once an automatic process has been activated this can direct a person's attention and conscious experience. It has been argued by Zajonc (1980) that the evaluation of the emotional quality of a stimulus is an automatic process occurring out of awareness and little affected by controlled processing. Automatic or unconscious processing of information has thus been shown clearly to have a marked influence on conscious experience, thought, and behavior (Kihlstrom, 1990). Therefore, people may find themselves feeling sad or uneasy or even depressed without being aware of elicitors or the internal processes generating this experience.

3. One of the early important developments in the cognitive area was the view of the organism as both a parallel as well as serial processor of information. *Parallel processing* helped to explain how information was processed out of awareness or automatically (Broadbent, 1977; Kihlstrom, 1990). Serial processing was viewed as occurring consciously in real time, with mental operations occurring in sequential order—one ending before the next could begin. Parallel processing, and more recently parallel distributed processing, are seen as allowing the organism to process a large amount of information simultaneously, without having to allocate valuable attentional resources to these essentially automatic activities (Rummelhart & McClelland, 1986). This type of preattentional parallel processing has also been seen as constituting the field from which attention selects material for serial processing (Broadbent, 1977). Thus clients in life are automatically processing much material that influences their conscious experience. In the therapeutic situation, for example, they process the manner and vocal quality of the therapist's responses without being aware of, or directly attending to these features, and this effects their interpretation and experience of what the therapist says.

4. It has become clear that *memory* is a highly dynamic and reconstructive process rather than a simple system of storage and retrieval of inputs. Long-term memory has been viewed alternately as a network consisting of a set of nodes connected by links, as a parallel-process system consisting of episodic traces activated in parallel, or as involving composite/distributed processes in which a trace is not a distinct localized entity but rather part of a combination of all traces put into the system

(Raaijmakers & Shiffrin, 1992). Recently Anderson (1990) has suggested that memory may possibly be dynamically organized so as to solve the memorizers current problem in an optimum fashion.

Breakdowns in memory have been explored as possibly occurring at many points in the process. Thus memory impoverishment can be caused by a variety of processes such as overgeneralized encoding, interference with retrieval processes, or lack of effort or distraction at the time of retrieval. Different categories of memory have been delineated. Episodic memory has been distinguished from semantic memory, whereas autobiographical memory has been distinguished from general memory. Better recall has been shown for material when it is related to the self, and this effect is even stronger for material imbued with emotion (Bock & Klinger, 1986; Kuiper & Rogers, 1979). Recently specificity of autobiographical memory has been related to problem solving and solution effectiveness (Williams, 1992). Thus more specific detailed memories of concrete features of actual autobiographical events such as "I stood in line next to my boss's secretary waiting for a movie yesterday after work" act to provide more alternatives for further processing than general abstract memories such as "meeting a co-worker after work." The more features brought into awareness, the more a differentiated view of experience is developed. This in turn generates more alternatives for viewing the situation, and for responding.

Explicit, consciously retrievable, memory has also been shown to be only one form of memory. Implicit memory, memory of events that cannot be consciously remembered, has been shown to influence current processing. Relearning and priming effects clearly show that task performance can be affected by available memories of prior experience even though these experiences are not accessible to conscious recall. Implicit memory occurs when the events contributing to memory are clearly detectable by the person at the time they occurred, attention is devoted to them, and they are at least momentarily represented in awareness but then are lost to conscious explicit recollection. It has also been demonstrated that conscious recollection of an event occurs best when the representation of the self as agent or experiencer of the event is retrieved along with the representation of the context of the event and the event itself (Kihlstrom, 1990). Thus both self and context representations need to be linked to the event for the construction of a full-fledged retrieval of what occurred.

The implications for therapy are clear. Memories of experience do reside out of awareness, and their retrieval for therapeutic purposes can be facilitated by therapists focusing clients on memories of specific features of the event and by focusing on the self as the experiencer of the event. In addition by posing the right exploratory problem as a retrieval context in therapy, new information might possibly be made more accessible.

With the above developments, cognitive science has provided us with a view of human functioning in which, the ability to process a large amount of information automatically requires different mental processes occurring in parallel, out of awareness. In addition, with the advent of the notion of parallel distributed processing, mental functioning increasingly is being seen as operating in separate modules operating in parallel (Fodor, 1983; Johnson-Laird, 1988), each module concerned with a particular type of information and transformation. This modular arrangement is seen as offering speed, reliability, and specialization as evolutionary advantages. Consciousness then, is viewed as a higher-level processor that monitors and regulates the operation of other lower-level modular processors that are not necessarily in awareness. This lower-level processing of information influences one's experience and behavior and, to differing degrees, can be brought into awareness by attentional allocation.

In addition to the modern views of attentional allocation, automatic processing, parallel modular functioning, and reconstructive memory in human information processing, a *schematic processing view* has emerged in attempting to understand human performance on complex tasks. We will draw strongly on the role of schematic processing in human experience to understand change in therapy. In this view, the individual is seen as organizing information into molar units (schemas) that guide processing (Bartlett, 1932; Piaget, 1970, 1985; Neisser, 1976). Once activated, schemas are seen as automatically directing attention, providing a framework to preserve information, combining generic and specific information to deal with concrete events, and as active in retrieving and editing material from memory (Brewer & Nakamura, 1984).

The term schema has been used by different researchers and theorists in different contexts with different degrees of precision. This has led to considerable confusion and lack of specificity in the use of the term. However, some common specific criteria are emerging (Williams, Watts, McLeod, & Matthews, 1988). These are that a schema: (1) is a stored body of knowledge with which incoming information interacts; (2) has a consistent internal structure that organizes incoming information in a particular fashion; (3) embodies generic prototypical information such that specific instances are processed using the appropriate schematic prototype to impose structure; (4) and finally that it is modular in nature such that the activation of any part will tend to produce activation of the whole.

The basic contribution of the schema concept is that it recognizes that humans internally represent objects or events by a configuration of features. Schemas include but go beyond purely propositional representations to encode regularities in categories that are both perceptual and conceptual. Schemas are abstract in that they extract regularity to encode what is generally true, rather than concretely encoding what occurred in a particular instance. They encode what experiences have in common. Schemas are also thought of as being hierarchically organized, with higher-level schemata being overarching generalization structures and more specific schemas being applied in a more context-specific manner (Anderson, 1990). Thus a person may have a high-level schema for dating, or for applying for a job, and more specific ones for making a phone call in these different contexts. Schemas of this sort have more of the character of goals or intentions and sets of procedures for attaining them, rather than being purely a representation of an event. Schemas also function in essence as prototypes, allowing variations in the instances that fit a particular schema but also providing constraints on what fits. Representations of an event or sequences of procedures therefore include both elements from the specific event and elements from the generic prototype.

In cognitive science, schemas are thus viewed as complex information networks or mental models that operate out of awareness to guide perception memory and experience. They represent our knowledge about how features fit together and how events are sequenced. This knowledge about what tends to occur together is very important in our ability to predict what we encounter in the environment. This view of schema theory will be discussed further in the next chapter (Chapter 4) highlighting certain problems with the view of schemas as providing only *representations* as opposed to emotionally experienced embodied *actions*. We will use the word *scheme* (as opposed to schema) for embodied cognitive/affective/action structures (Pascual-Leone, 1983, 1988, 1990a, 1990b, 1991; Pascual-Leone & Johnson, 1991).

In addition to the schematic nature of mental functioning, cognitive science has described a number of other features of mental functioning relevant to therapy. A useful distinction has been drawn between "data-driven" and "conceptually driven" processing—alternately referred to as "bottom-up" and "top-down" processing. A data-driven process relies predominantly on stimulus information and is assisted very little by already known information. It is therefore oriented to picking up new information. Conceptually driven processes on the other hand are those that rely much more on information in memory and expectations about the situation, and therefore, guide processing anticipatorily. Thus, human beings can be more attentive to the actual sensory data of experience, thereby increasing their discovery of new information, or they can be more guided by their anticipations of what they expect to find, thereby increasing their selective capacity to construct or perceive particular patterns. For example, in therapy it is often useful to help clients direct their attention to the specific details of a past scene (memory) or to present sensory experience, as opposed to attending to clients' expectations or beliefs about past or present experience.

Different types of knowing have also been discriminated. A key distinction has been made between declarative and procedural knowledge, or explicit knowledge of things that we know and implicit knowledge of how to do things (Anderson, 1990). In addition, tacit knowledge of patterns or rules has been shown to influence comprehension, demonstrating that we clearly "know more than we can say." Thus, in addition to explicit conceptual knowledge, people possess: (1) implicit procedural knowledge, (such as how to ride a bicycle), which associatively guides performance out of awareness and (2) tacit knowledge of rules and patterns (such as how to speak a language), which guides understanding out of awareness. The problematic experience and behavior that bring people into therapy are often governed by these implicit and tacit levels of processing.

Finally, thinking about our thinking, or metacognition, has also been shown to be a source of plans and strategies for improving memory performance, indicating the truly self-referential and active nature of the human information processor (Flavell, 1985). Thus, in addition to being guided by tacit knowledge, people also actively reflect on their own perceptions and thoughts, thereby creating new meaning. Clients in life and in therapy reflect on their experience, and this is important in self-understanding.

In summary, the constructive processing of information involves perception, attention, memory, thought, and language, and is facilitated by complex organized internal modules or schemas that automatically act on and organize incoming information and outgoing responses. Human beings clearly process information automatically out of awareness and organize information into internal modular structures or schemes that are the starting point of expectational or "top-down" processing of incoming information. In addition, people possess different ways of knowing, and have a capacity to be guided by things they know but cannot say. Automatic processing can draw on procedural modules that automatically guide motor behaviors, such as how to drive or dance. They also draw on knowledge of tacit rules or patterns that guide the organism's comprehension of the world and thereby their behavior. Thus, clients come into therapy with a complex set of internal schemes that guide their processing of information about self, other, and the world, and, once activated, these generate experience and reactions.

This view of constructive information processing from cognitive science provides support for the humanistic view of humans as aware agents who are "intuitively" guided by automatic or nonconscious schematic processing of complex information. In addition, humans are also capable of bringing this internal material into awareness, symbolizing, and using it as a basis for reflection, choice, and action. All this processing of information amounts to a description, in the language of modern cognitive psychology, of the substance of experiential therapy: that is *awareness* and *experiencing* (Gendlin, 1962, 1981; Bohart, (in press); Perls, 1969, 1973) or what we later discuss as *experiential processing*.

EMOTION THEORY AND RESEARCH

Cognitive science, as described above concerns itself with how knowledge is acquired, represented, and used. Although cognitive processes are of crucial importance in understanding human information processing and meaning construction, the emotions are crucial in understanding human action. Emotions arise in the course of human action, especially interpersonal interaction, and appear to provide biologically based solutions to human problems that cannot be managed by cognition alone (Oatley, 1992). A better understanding of human functioning results when emotion is incorporated into cognitive science. A focus on emotion has thus recently begun to emerge in modern psychology. Emotion is beginning to be seen as central in understanding both interaction and cognition, in that emotion is: first, attentional, influencing the salience of information; second, motivational, influencing goal setting; and, third, communicational, regulating interaction with others. Emotion has been investigated both in terms of emotional expression and emotional experience and will be reviewed below in these terms.

Emotional Expression and Action Tendencies

Emotions are best viewed as involving *action tendencies* that arise as a function of *automatic appraisals* of the relevance of situations to our *basic concerns* (Arnold, 1960; Frijda, 1987; Lazarus, 1991a). Emotions start with the detection of some notable change that acts as a signal to continue processing the input for its personal significance (Scherer, 1984). The continued processing involves first appraising the event in relation to one's concerns and then to one's ability to cope with the event.

In addition, emotions are seen as being adaptive. They govern goal priorities within people and communicate intentions between people in survival-promoting ways (Greenberg & Safran, 1984a, 1987, 1989; Greenberg & Johnson, 1988; Oatley & Jenkins, 1992; Safran &

Greenberg, 1991). Emotion expression and communication has also been shown to be both a primary self regulator, organizing infants' responses to environmental stimuli, and a primary regulator of the behavior of others by providing affective signals to caretakers to guide their actions (Stern, 1985; Tronick, 1989). Emotion expression is thus fundamentally communicative and serves to regulate social interaction. Emotions are best understood as complex syntheses of elements including primary affect (in the form of sensation and physiology), motivation (in the form of needs and concerns), and cognition (in the form of appraisals).

Discrete primary emotions such as surprise, happiness, anger, sadness, fear, and disgust are innate (Ekman & Friesen, 1975; Izard, 1977; Tomkins, 1962) action dispositions (Arnold, 1970; Frijda, 1987; Lang, 1984) biologically related to survival and adaptation. These basic primary affects have been shown to be universal, with associated characteristic facial expressions, neuroendocrine patterns, and brain sites.

It presently appears from psychobiological evidence (Panksepp, 1989) that the basic emotions are constituted by primitive genetically prewired circuits of the visceral brain, which influence information processing in higher cognitive areas of the cortex. By comparison, the higher cognitive areas have only modest control over the underlying emotive circuits, although it is clear that thinking can and does have some effect on everyday feelings. Panksepp (1989) in his review of the neuropsychological research, argues there is presently adequate neuropsychological evidence for the existence of four or five emotive command circuits in the brain. To overcome the semantic difficulties of labeling with these connotative affective terms, he uses multiple terms to identify these systems. They are: (1) the foraging–expectancy–curiosity–investigatory system, (2) the anger–rage circuit, (3) the anxiety–fear circuit, (4) the separation–distress–sorrow–anguish–panic network and, possibly, (5) a social–play system. Although these differ in some respects from the primary emotions based on facial expression evidence, there is sufficient overlap to confirm the neurological base of interest/surprise, fear, anger, sadness, and happiness.

Basic or primary affects such as these appear to have a distinct nonsymbolic neurophysiological manner of internal signaling that differs from the manner of processing cognitive information (Le Doux, 1989). Each affect signal is discrete, direct and, when clear or intense, does not need to be interpreted to understand its meaning. Rather, it automatically provides meaning and organizes action. The organism is thus provided with innate signals and innate knowledge of the significance of each signal. The interpretation of the signal is not semantic but involves direct appraisal. These emotion-based signals are specifically adaptive because they can rapidly influence behavior without relying on conceptual processing.

A complex organism has bodily sensations and affects, and these act as a means, independent of conscious cognition, of guiding behavior. They prepare the organism for a general course of appropriate action in relation to the environment rather than serving either as a *specific* innate response or requiring complex *symbolic* processing. Affects are thus a nonsymbolic way of guiding action that do not require complex inferential process. They are in fact, an evolutionarily older method of controlling action, with rapid and often effective results. They operate automatically and our perceptual system can therefore automatically, register information but signal to consciousness only an emotion toward the object, resulting in a person feeling something toward a person/ situation (e.g., anger) without knowing the reason. Therefore, primary affects appear to be in-wired and to be tied to information processing in that they help the person adapt and survive by helping the individual to select and respond quickly to information that would take too long to process without an emotional action tendency. It is from these primary affects that complex emotions evolve (Pascal-Leone, 1992).

Emotional Experience

Beyond organizing adaptive action, affects, with lived experience, become integrated with cognition to provide emotional experience. Emotional experience is seen as involving an integration of many different levels of information (Lazarus, 1984; Leventhal, 1979; Lang, 1983). Consciously experienced feelings are thus a complex synthesis of a variety of types and sources of information. These feelings are comprised of at least three measurable systems: a physiologically based, expressive-motor system; a semantically based, emotional memory system; and a verbally based conceptual system (Lang, 1984, Leventhal, 1984). Thus emotional experience is a multicomponent process including bodily changes, meaning, and action tendencies. This complex information-processing emotion system is seen as providing us with a rich source of complex meaning and with feedback about our reactions to situations in the form of feelings (Greenberg & Safran, 1984a, 1987, 1989).

In this view, each level of processing contributes different aspects to emotional experience. The lowest, sensory/expressive motor level provides nonpropositional sensory information and expressive action tendencies and operates without volitional control. Thus, an infant reacts with fear to a looming shadow or with anger to violation. The intermediate schematic memory level contains concrete representations of prior emotional experiences, initially encoding sensorimotor experience along with eliciting conditions. For example, one's emotional reactions to being comforted or frustrated by a primary caretaker are initially represented internally along with cues of the caretaker's expressions and actions in these situations. These representations are eventually expanded to include beliefs or expectations that the person associates with the experience such as "When I'm needy I am lovable" or "It's easier not to need." These emotion schemas then form the basis of much emotional life. They are activated automatically and influence the processing of current events. The final level of processing occurs through the conceptual system based on its capacity for conscious, volitional, propositional thinking about emotional events. This level, which incorporates and forms rules and beliefs, feeds back into schematic memory, as described above, so that both sensorimotor and conceptual levels are internally schematically synthesized. Emotional experience results from the complex integration of these levels of processing.

An additional way in which emotions affect experience is by their effect on cognition. Emotions have been shown to influence cognition in a variety of ways. The effects of mood on memory have been investigated (Blaney, 1986), and a mood-congruent memory effect has been reliably found demonstrating that people's moods affect what they recall and what they encode. Thus happy mood produces happy recall, and sad mood produces sad memories (Gilligan & Bower, 1984), whereas a positive mood at time of learning possibly enhances learning of positive content. Emotion clearly affects cognition and does so in a complex and differentiated fashion that researchers have only recently begun to investigate. It is clear however that once an emotional state has been elicited—by whatever means chemical, physiological, or cognitive—the person's subsequent cognition is immediately affected. First, the organism's current goal is altered in response to the newly emerging affective state. Second, the person's train of thought is altered in a manner related to the ongoing affective state.

In addition to the biologically based view of a basically adaptive emotion-reaction system governing expression, a more social/constructive view of a cognitively mediated complex emotional-experience system has emerged. In this view, it becomes clear that our cognitive and emotion systems are so closely linked that they are hard to separate. Complex emotions such as resentment or remorse, although based on basic emotions such as anger or sadness, also include more learned cognitive evaluations of self in relation to society and therefore are evoked differently in different cultures. These complex emotions, such as pride and jealously, are schematically based and clearly possess more cognitive elaboration and are more culturally dependent than basic emotions.

These emotions are in part constituted by language in that they need to be verbally symbolized in awareness to be experienced.

The emotional states of adults are produced predominantly by the activation of complex-emotion schemes. These states, or self organizations, serve to organize the individual for action and influence cognitive processing. Emotions are automatically *produced* by the organism, but to be *experienced* by the person, they need to be symbolized in awareness. Whether or not these states are experienced thus depends on whether they are attended to and symbolized. Emotional states may be in differing degrees of awareness: present but currently out of awareness; present but only partially or peripherally in awareness; present and experienced but not symbolized verbally; experienced and clearly symbolized; and, finally, experienced, symbolized, and understood fully in terms of precepitators, meanings, and the associated action tendencies, needs, or desires.

This view of different levels of processing and awareness suggests that emotions cannot be separated from cognition and that, rather than focusing on whether emotion and cognition are independent, it is important to focus on how cognition is involved in different aspects of emotion and how schemes complexly integrate information from a variety of sources to form feelings (Piaget, 1981). Our thoughts are thus always steeped in feelings, and affect and cognition can be separated only for theoretical purposes or only in extreme cases of lived experiences, such as when affect is chemically or electrically stimulated. Personal meaning, then, essentially depends on affect.

Recent advances in the study of *affective development* (Case, Hayward, Lewis, & Hurst, 1988; Campos, Campos, & Barrett, 1989; Lewis, 1990; Lewis & Michalson, 1983; Pascual-Leone, 1987, 1991; Stern, 1985) have begun to add to our understanding of how the simpler, early, core affects are transformed step-wise into the later more complex feelings and emotions by the addition of more complex cognitions made possible by the level of cognitive development. The role of affect in the development of the infant's sense of self, other, and reality has been studied, and emotion has been found to be far more organized than previously thought (Stern, 1985; Fischer, Shaver, & Carnochan, 1990; Pascual-Leone, 1991; Tronick, 1989; Cichetti & Sroufe, 1978), developing in a stage-wise fashion (Izard, 1984) and combining with cognition at particular points to form more complex self-conscious feelings such as embarrassment (Lewis, 1990; Lewis & Michalson, 1983). Complex emotions appear to relate to the self and involve self-evaluations.

To summarize, empirical and conceptual developments in the view of emotion provide support for the existence and the universality of certain discrete primary affects that are generated by automatically appraising situations in relation to needs. In addition, the schematic emotion system organizes and synthesizes complex high-level incoming information at multiple levels, to provide us both with complex meanings and with feedback about our responses to situations as well as producing rapid emotional response tendencies that are fundamentally adaptive. It is also clear that affective processes influence attentional allocation and information processing. In addition affect has been shown to be the infant's primary means of self- regulation and communication.

Affect is thus a core constituent of the human self and establishes links between self and the environment and organizes self-experience. In a sense, feelings are ultimately the meeting place of mind, body, environment, culture, and behavior. They can bring together in conscious experience various physiological and hormonal changes, appraisals of the self and situation, memories, cultural rules, and characteristic expressions and behaviors. Awareness of these complex integrations, in the form of feelings and action tendencies, is of crucial importance in therapeutic change because they give us information about our reactions to situations that are related to our biological and social survival and well-being (Greenberg & Safran, 1987, 1989). In addition it is no longer possible to think of cognition and emotion as distinct and separate. In general much thought is steeped in feeling, and thoughts only have personally relevant meanings for us if they are accompanied by feelings. Feelings, on the other hand (Greenberg & Safran, 1987), are laden with cognition, involving among other processes attentional allocation and automatic evaluation.

The above views on cognition and emotion will allow us to look at human functioning in a manner that transcends the false dichotomy between reason and emotion yet retains a perspective on the difference in nature and function between emotion and cognition. It is clear that cognition is not inherently rational (Kahneman, Slovic, & Tversky, 1982), nor is emotion inherently irrational (Frijda, 1986; Oatley, 1992). Instead the two processes are intertwined in complex ways to enhance human functioning. Human beings thus need to utilize both their rapid action emotion processes and their slower cognitive knowing processes to guide adaptive action in complex interpersonal environments. Rather than a model that dichotomizes thinking and feeling, we propose a model in which thinking and feeling encounter one another in a dialectical process that leads to their synthesis, integrating knowing and acting into a unified sense of self and situation.

A DIALECTICAL CONSTRUCTIVIST SYNTHESIS

The above theoretical developments in cognitive science and emotion theory provide the building blocks needed to integrate and expand

Experiential Therapy theory and practice in two ways. In the first place, this permits us to explicate more clearly the phenomena that Rogers and Perls and other humanists recognized and built into their experiential approaches. In the second place, it provides a more rigorous, dialectical constructivist process theory (Pascual-Leone, 1976a, 1976b, 1976c, 1984, 1987, 1991) with which to understand dysfunction and the process of intervention and change.

A more complex theory of functioning based on an integration of an Experiential Therapy view of functioning and the developments in cognitive science and emotion theory will provide a theory that recognizes the reality of both the client's inner experience and the client's capacity to construct meaning and develop concepts. This integration will include a view of human beings as multiple-level processors of different types of propositional (symbolic/logical) and nonpropositional (sensory/perceptual) information, who construct their conscious views of self and reality in a moment-by-moment fashion depending on what they attend to. In this view, experience depends on both the controlled, conscious, serial, conceptual processing of information and on the automatic, parallel processing of self-relevant information which occurs out of awareness. An adequate theory must recognize two major sources of experience, a conscious, deliberate, reflexive conceptual process (thinking) and an automatic, direct, schematic emotional process (feeling), and the constructive, dialectical relationship between them. In this framework, a view of the bringing of previously denied material into awareness is replaced by a view of the dialectical construction of new meaning.

The Epistemology

In this book we therefore adopt a dialectical constructivist epistemology (Pascual-Leone, 1984, 1987, 1990a, 1990b, 1991) in which we see clients engaged in a dialectically constructive exploration process that leads to the construction of a new view of self and world. Dialectics in its most essential form is the splitting of a single whole into its contradictory parts. The polar parts when brought into contact interact to produce transformation. Novelty then emerges from a dialectical synthesis. The dialectic with which we are most concerned is that which constitutes consciousness—the dialectic between concept and experience, between reflexive explaining and direct being, between mediated and immediate experience (Greenberg & Safran, 1981, 1987; Guidano, 1991; Mahoney, 1991; Rennie, 1990; Toukmanian, 1986; Wexler & Rice, 1974). From a dialectical constructivist view, people are seen as continually engaged in a process of reflexively constructing reality from the dialectical synthesis of these two sources of experience. The person's experience of internal and external reality is viewed fundamentally as a process of constructing views of self and world from constituents that actually exist as constraints on one's constructions.

In therapy this dialectical constructive process involves constructing meaning from immediate experience and conceptually held views of how one expects that experience to be. Contradictions between one's reflexive or acquired concepts or explanations about how things are, or ought to be, and one's immediate experience of how things *actually* are constitute a great source of emotional distress. Reflexive conceptual knowing processes provide explanations, whereas emotion schemes provide immediate reactions. It is the dialectical synthesis of these different and sometimes contradictory sources of experience, of what is often referred to as thought and emotion, or the "head" and the "heart," that ultimately determines wholistic lived experience.

A dialectical constructive view thus goes beyond a purely descriptive phenomenological approach which, in claiming that experience is simply given, leaves unexplained the constructive process by which "what is," is brought forth into conscious experience and symbolized. In addition, a dialectical constructive position does not fall into the deterministic position of presupposing the existence of theoretically specified psychic contents that determine existence as do some dynamic approaches, but it assumes only the operation of a certain set of processes that can generate any realities. This results in respecting clients as experts on the contents of their own experience. Finally, a dialectical constructive position does not assume that behavior is lawfully governed by stimuli or by thought alone as do behavioral and cognitive approaches but, rather, that behavior is determined by the dialectical synthesis of concept and experience.

In a dialectical constructivist view, therapeutic exploration and change therefore are primarily generated by a dialectical process of synthesizing, or actively exploring contradictions between, concept and experience and by constructing new meaning through a process of differentiation and integration of experience. A dialectical constructivist view does justice both to the reality of immediate subjective emotionally based experience and to the active constructive cognitive processes by which people create meaning from immediate experience. Becoming aware is neither a purely passive process of simply perceiving sense experience nor a purely constructive one of radically constructing reality by imposing categories on experience to create meaning. Rather, experience is simultaneously discovered and created in a dialectical manner in which the dialectic is between the immediately sensed and the conceptually mediated, between people's emerging experience and their previously constructed views. Thought and emotions both play a role in experience, and experience and behavior are generated ultimately out of the dialectical interplay between two systems, one a conceptual, reasoning system, the other the rapid, adaptive-reaction emotion system.

Construction of Meaning

In this view, conscious, controlled processing acts to create meaning by attending to and symbolizing what is occurring both internally and externally. Conscious emotional experience comes from attending to a symbolizing, an automatically generated emotional state. An emotional state comes from the activation of schematic processors that are activated by internal or external patterns of information or events. Schematic processors automatically generate internal reactions, action tendencies, and bodily based experience, which may or may not be attended to or consciously symbolized.

Construction of personal meaning then involves a process of continuously synthesizing information from a variety of different sources and consciously symbolizing these to form a subjective reality. This is a dialectically constructive process that requires simultaneously attending to embodied felt experience and constructing a particular current representation of it. This dialectical process of symbolization of experience in awareness leads to the construction of new views of self and reality. It is here that language plays an important role in constituting our emotional experience. Our feelings are influenced by how we formulate them. Our linguistic description influences our experience while experience influences and constrains our possible descriptions. In addition, once we have represented our experience we also examine our representations and work out new possibilities and select alternatives for action.

Within this view, it is high-level schematic structures—what we have called emotion schemes—that generate the complex internal emotional reactions and experience. It is important to recognize that these emotion schematic modules do not simply generate primitive passions but rather complex responses. These complex emotional reactions and experiences are available to consciousness if attended to, but at any moment they may or may not be symbolized or incorporated into a person's construction of reality. Thus, rather than being actively denied to awareness, emotional states may not be attended to and synthesized in awareness. Once symbolized in awareness, however, they provide the basis for our subjective sense of reality and evaluation of the significance of events to us.

Conscious self experience, which does incorporate this emotion-based information, is created by the process of attending inwardly to and symbolizing one's emotional responses to situations. This process involves the conscious dialectical interaction of our conceptualising activities with our immediate emotionally toned experiences to aid problem solving and adaptive responding. Consciousness of our self-in-the-world occurs by the creation of meaning from immediate experience, in order to survive and grow. This occurs through a moment-by-moment process of synthesizing and symbolizing tacitly generated experience in awareness. In this process, newly created meaning in turn generates new experience in the symbolic domain, which in turn leads to new immediate tacit responses. We thus continuously both discover and create meaning (Greenberg & Safran, 1987) in a dialectical process of meaning construction.

Thus, to construct personal meaning a person guided in some situation by an emotion scheme may automatically react to an experience as rejecting or threatening and pull back in fear. In order to behave adaptively, the person must: first, attend to the response tendency; second, symbolize it accurately as feeling afraid; third, construct a complex situational meaning such as feeling threatened because one sense of one's worth is diminished; and fourth, generate an adaptive response such as (whichever is appropriate) to say one is feeling afraid, or to withdraw to protect oneself from further attack.

Our view therefore is one of an agent who is engaged in an ongoing constructive *process* of *synthesizing* information from a variety of sources into a conscious experience of self and creating meanings from this synthesis. This view can be seen as elucidating the *process* conception of functioning and as extending the classical structural incongruence theory of Rogers (1958) and Perls (1969) into a more complete *process* theory (Whitehead, 1929), a theory more consistent with their practice.

In a process-constructive view, the idea of a structural, unitary self concept, which denies or distorts experience, is replaced by a conscious, cognitive synthesizing function that draws on a variety of sources of information in its construction of experience and can construct a variety of different "selves" at different times or even at the same time (Hermans, Kempen, & Van Loon, 1992). Therefore rather than *having* a single, self concept, people are seen as being constantly engaged in actively representing themselves to others and themselves in images and narratives. Thus people *construct* views of themselves in an ongoing fashion.

In addition, in a process-constructive view, Rogers and Perls' idea of *organismic experience* is explicated as being the result of a set of automatic emotion schemes, which generate experience. Now, rather than a simple dichotomous view of an organism and a self concept, the person is seen as a multilevel, modularly organized, agentic processing system. Consciousness is able to receive and synthesize messages into unified wholes out of a variety of different lower-level schematic modules that process information out of awareness.

Within this perspective, tacit emotion schemes are seen as being particularly important automatic processors that generate people's emotionally toned reactions and experience and their wholistic sense of who they are. These emotion modules can be thought of as context-specific processors relevant to certain domains of experience. As we have said, emotion schemes are unique in that they represent innate as well as learned experience and provide crucial nonpropositional, noncognitive, sensory information to consciousness. With experience and learning, these emotion schemes also come to incorporate cognitive and propositional information about the self to form integrated cognitive/affective modules. These are our highest-level integrations of all our experience. They give us our "feeling" or "sense" of our self and of things ("felt sense") (Gendlin, 1981). They produce experiences such as global feelings of being worthwhile or worthless, as well as more specific senses, for example, of feeling small or of feeling valued in a particular situation.

Experience is thus created by the dialectical interactions of an organism within itself and with the environment (Pascual-Leone, 1980, 1983, 1990a, 1990b, 1991). The organism is viewed as a complex, modularly organized, multilevel information-processing being. Organismic, emotionally toned experience and reactions are continually generated both by immediate sensorimotor responses and by automatic schematic levels of processing of external and internal information. These levels of processing proceed automatically and produce responses that may or may not be attended to in the creation of one's conscious sense of oneself. People's conscious views of themselves at any moment thus may or may not incorporate their automatic organismic responses.

To restate our argument, we have two major sources of information dialectically interacting in the creation of meaning and self experience. The first source is the set of processors that automatically generate emotional experience and reactions. Of these processors, two levels are most important in generating emotional experience. One is our immediate sensorimotor emotional response in the moment. This most basic level of ongoing sensory experience and expressive-motor responding generates primary affects such as anger at violation or fear in response to threat. The other and vastly more complex source, is the set of schematic emotion modules that provide us with complex felt meaning and with information about our reaction to situations based on our past emotional experience in similar situations. These may often be only weak or attenuated signals, ones that require deliberate attentional allocation in order to be raised to awareness (Pascual-Leone, 1987, 1991; Perls, 1947).

The second major source of self experience and meaning is our conscious synthesizing construction process. This later process, which is oriented toward problem solving and adaptation, is highly dependent on attentional allocation and on the symbolic, linguistic-reflexive capacities available to us. The conscious synthesizing of one's self in the moment can to greater or lesser degrees rely on schematic and sensorimotor processing for its information. It can also be guided by such other sources as cultural and social learning, learned conditions of worth or introjects obtained from others, or from views or beliefs about the self obtained from others or inferred from past experience. People actively construct meaning in consciousness with the option of top-down or bottom-up processing, either attending to experience or imposing patterns on it. Conscious views of one's self can be influenced as much by purely reflexive views of the self and expectations and values learned from others as by self experience, and it is not totally controlled by either of these. In terms of self-knowledge, consciousness can create descriptions and explanations of self by attending to and symbolizing different aspects of actual self experience or it can define the self in terms of "shoulds" and "oughts" or reflexive views of the self obtained from others' views. It can symbolize the organismic automatic responses, or it can utilize constructed or externally derived beliefs, rules, values, or ideals for describing the self.

Consciousness is the final arbiter of meaning, both by selecting what source of information to attend to and what interpretation to generate. This conscious process involves components of will and choice, in that an individual can guide his or her attention at will, under the control of an internal executive-like process. However, consciousness is multidetermined (Pascual-Leone, 1980, 1987, 1990a, 1990b). It is influenced by deliberate, controlled processing as well as such features as the salience of certain external stimuli, the views and attitudes of others toward the self, and past responses of the self in similar situations (Pascual-Leone, 1980, 1990a, 1990b). Consciousness is thus the arena for the dialectical synthesis of the different sources of information about the self as the person encounters and resolves felt contradictions between aspects of self, and between self and the world.

The process of being conscious involves a constant synthesizing of information into awareness. In this process, automatically generated self experience is, to differing degrees, consciously symbolized. This synthesizing and symbolization process creates meaning, which generates new self experience, which, in turn, is further symbolized. Thus we have an ongoing process in which people continually create their conscious experience of themselves and by so doing provide material for a reflective narrative view of themselves. Self-representations are thus multiply determined constructions, and we can at any one time construct a number of different views of ourselves. In healthy functioning, this process is oriented toward problem solving to enhance survival and growth.

Attentional allocation is the central processing activity determining awareness and our constructions of ourselves. What is important for therapeutic purposes is that *attention is under both deliberate and automatic control* and thereby provides a medium for change. People can utilize attention and conscious capacities to alter their focus of attention and to accurately symbolize their inner experience. Personal change can be achieved in many ways, including: (1) by attending to one's ongoing flow of automatic experience; (2) by symbolizing information from sensorimotor and schematic processors into higher-level conscious meaning (no longer dissociating them from consciousness); (3) by making the schematic structures that generate automatic experience accessible to new experience; (4) by reflecting on experience and creating new meaning.

Contributions of a Dialectical Constructive View

This dialectically constructive view of the creation of meaning provides us with a new, more dynamic view of human functioning than that provided by Rogers' or Perls' early theorizing and explicit structural models, a view that is more consistent with the later views of these authors (Rogers, 1961, 1975; Perls, 1973). A number of differences between the process and the classic views result. First, in this new view, conscious emotional meaning is created by the dynamic and circular interaction between our conscious synthesizing capacities and our tacit immediate emotional experience in a dialectical process (see Gendlin, 1962). Rather than a structural view of a stable self concept, we have a more complex view of an ongoing *dialectical process*. This process constantly constructs meaning and a self narrative by synthesizing information from a variety of sources. Therapy thus needs to facilitate the meaning construction by facilitating both the process of attending to inner experience and its symbolization.

Second, organismic emotional experience is seen as being largely created automatically by modular emotion schemes and by sensorimotor responses in order to guide action. The organism or *self is modular*, contains many levels of processing and is not purely biologically based. Instead, it is constituted of both innate expressive sensorimotor and experience-based schematic emotional processing. Therapy thus needs to intervene differentially in ways most suited to the processing difficulties related to different modular aspects of experience.

Third, the organism and the meaning-construction process are not in a relationship of congruence or incongruence, nor is denial or distortion operating; rather the person is an *active agent* in a *dialectical synthesis* creating meaning from immediate experience. This dialectical construction occurs by the conscious symbolization of automatic emotional experiencing and examination of the symbol. Neither immediate organismic experience nor construction of meaning predominate in this conception. Instead, we propose the operation of a truly *dialectical synthesis* involving both discovery and creation in which concept and experience interact to produce meaning. Human nature is in part given but in part creates itself. We create a sense of ourselves by symbolizing what we discover in ourselves. Therapy thus needs to be viewed as a meaning-construction process involving both emotion and cognition.

The fourth and final point of difference with the classical model, a difference highly significant for therapy, suggests that when *structural* change occurs, it occurs, not through a self concept changing to incorporate experiencing, but through *change in the modular self*, constituted by a specific emotion scheme or set of schemes. Therapy thus needs to access emotion schemes in order to make them amenable to restructuring.

This dialectical constructivist model of functioning (Pascual-Leone, 1976a, 1976b, 1976c, 1980, 1983, 1987, 1991) is derived from an integration of modern cognitive psychology and emotion theory with Experiential Therapy theory; it serves to explain the clinical observations of experiential therapists that people are both wiser than their intellects alone and active agents in their construal of reality. On this basis we proceed in the chapters that follow to develop a therapeutically oriented view of functioning and dysfunction to guide therapeutic practice. This view will be based on the importance of emotion-schematic functioning in determining experience and of attentional allocation and symbolization in experience and the creation of new meaning. The model focuses on the emotion-based, constructive information-processing activities that generate performance and experience in the session. Using this model, we will be better able to understand and explain how change occurs in ways that promise to make therapy more effective. In addition, the model suggests optimal methods of facilitating different types of cognitive/affective processing at different times for different modular aspects of functioning to help clients reorganize the tacit schematic structures that govern their emotional experience. The result will be a view of therapy that is process-oriented. It will focus on facilitating the client's moment-by-moment attentional allocation and symbolization in order to help clients construct new emotional meanings and to reorganize schematically based experience.

CHAPTER 4

TOWARD AN EXPERIENTIAL THEORY OF FUNCTIONING

T HE DEVELOPMENTS in our own thinking about therapy and psychological processes described in the previous chapters make it possible to begin to elaborate a schematically based theory of emotional functioning more differentiated than those proposed by Rogers and Perls. These developments also illuminate clinical practice by suggesting ways of thinking about different kinds of attentionally based interventions and change processes that are needed for remedying schematic dysfunction.

Below we sketch a multifaceted, emotion-schematic view of functioning. This view allows for greater complexity than the view of congruence/incongruence between organismic experience and self concept originally posited by both Rogers and Perls. In essence, we suggest that individuals are engaged in a dynamic, dialectical synthesis of information to construct conscious meaning. In this process tacit emotion schemes automatically *organize* people's experience of self-in-the-world and *generate* their emotional meanings and reactions. However, these meanings and reactions may or may not be symbolized in consciousness. Therapy involves symbolizing these emotional meanings and facilitating change in emotion schemes where necessary.

Clinical experience has demonstrated that intellectual knowledge about the self, although it has a certain appeal to clients, does not effect very deep or lasting change. Such knowledge does not affect behavior-determining emotion structures. Therefore, we argue that a person's core, self-relevant emotion schemes are the key to change. These schemes are formed around affect-laden interactions with the environment and are at the center of organismic function and dysfunction. Emotion structures are central in guiding and creating our lived experience. We will, in addition, argue that dysfunction occurs as a function of problems in the meaning-creation process, when the constructive process does not attend sufficiently to information generated by affective processes and by tacit emotion schemes or is guided by emotion schemes that are themselves dysfunctional. Therefore, if therapy is to make a difference, it needs to access these affective/emotional structures and operate at the level of change in emotional meaning. Experience generated by these schemes needs to be brought into awareness and symbolized to help orient and guide the person. Alternately, those emotion schemes that result in maladaptive functioning need to be reorganized and restructured by the client's emotional processing *in the session.*

In addition to suggesting the centrality of emotion schemes in human functioning, and the value of working with emotional meaning in therapy, we also suggest that growth motivation is important in understanding therapeutic change. We will argue that a modern view of emotion is important in understanding the experiential view of a growth motivation. Experiential theory initially proposed an overarching tendency toward adaptive functioning, referred to alternately as an actualizing or growth tendency. This portrayed the organism as being oriented toward psychological survival, growth, and enhancement of the self. However, the notion of an actualizing tendency also implies that if one can be "who one truly is" then this will be growth- and esteem-producing. Rather than offering a mystical notion of becoming who one truly is, we further suggest that it is biologically adaptive to attend to one's emotional reactions because they provide us with access to our evaluations of the significance to us of events. We will, therefore, embed the humanistic view of an actualizing tendency within the growing body of evidence on the biologically adaptive role of emotion in human functioning. This will help support the contention that experiential information is essentially trustworthy and can be used to guide adaptive choice and action. In addition it will help illuminate why clients in an experientially oriented therapy are encouraged to attend to their own affectively toned experience—even when this is painful—why this focus facilitates growth, and how empathic attunement and the symbolization of meaning are crucial factors in helping therapeutic growth to occur.

We suggest as well that emotional experience arises from an appraisal of situations relevant to our needs for well-being and provides us with a constant readout of our automatic reactions to situations that matter to us. Given this precept, it is clear that emotions must be attended to and symbolized with accuracy and immediacy if they are to serve their biologically adaptive function.

In our view, the growth tendency relies on awareness and symbolization of the emotional meaning of experience in order to operate effectively. People are constructive-information processors continually creating emotional meaning by symbolizing inner experience. Attending to inner experience is most helpful in guiding people in an adaptive, self-enhancing fashion. This is because the emotion system that forms the base of internal experience is fundamentally adaptive. It provides individuals with information about their current response to their appraisals of the situation in relation to their needs. Thus, becoming "who one is" does not involve the actualization of a biogenetic blueprint, rather it involves attending to our automatic emotional evaluations of the significance of events to us and creating meaning by consciously symbolizing experience generated by emotion schemes. Attending inward and symbolizing one's emotional experience is essentially adaptive and self-enhancing, because self-awareness is necessary for any self-regulatory process. Being aware of internal experience helps people identify how they are reacting thereby both respecting their tempera-ments as well as attending to their automatic emotional evaluations of what is significant to them. In addition, a consistent focus on problematic experience, so as to expand awareness of experience, helps people identify what about their own reactions is dysfunctional or may need to change. Attending inward is thus a necessary first step in an experiential change process.

SCHEMATIC FUNCTIONING

Internal schemes of our self-in-the-world functioning appear to us to be crucial in understanding human functioning and in generating emotional meaning. Bartlett (1932) defined a schema as "an active organization of past reactions or of past experiences operating in any well-adapted organismic response" (p. 201). In addition he stated that "schemata are active without any awareness at all" (p. 200) and are not available to introspection. Schemas are complex, nonconscious knowledge structures, which result in the active processing of information. Schemas, as we discussed in the previous chapter, can be viewed as containing higher-level rules for processing information and involve anticipations of what to expect. These anticipations guide processing. It is this active anticipatory processing that is the medium by which the past affects the future (Neisser, 1976).

The above view of schemas emphasizes their pattern representation aspect and offers a view of a schema as a blueprint. Piaget used the term *scheme* rather than schema to define these internal structures, and he emphasized the action-oriented aspect of schematic processing (Piaget & Morf, 1958; Pascual-Leone & Johnson, 1991). He defined a scheme as the common structure of all the interchangeable *actions* that a subject uses to attain the same goal (Pascual-Leone, Goodman, Ammon, & Subin, 1978). In this view, it is the schematization of the motoric functional aspects of a scheme that is emphasized. He defined a scheme as an "organized set of reactions" that one transferred from one situation to another by assimilation of the second situation into the first (Piaget & Morf, 1958, p. 86). Piagetian schemes are intentional structures that actively attempt to apply and produce responses (Pascual-Leone, 1990a, 1990b, 1991). Neisser (1976) has also emphasized the active motoric nature of schemes in perception. According to him a scheme is not only a plan but also the executor of the plan. Schemes provide not only plans *of* action but also plans *for* action. They are much more like action plans than schematic diagrams or scripts of what to expect.

We will use the term emotional *scheme* rather than emotional *schema*. This emphasizes the goal-directed, action-oriented embodied nature of our view of emotion. The best representation of this view is Pascual-Leone & Johnsons' (1991) neo-Piagetian notion of schemes. They define them as goal-directed, functional units, ultimately addressed to the environment to negotiate the meeting of some need. According to them, schemes possess both a releasing component and an effecting component, providing a set of conditions for cuing the scheme to apply and the set of desired performance effects of the scheme, respectively. In this view, schemes are activated by appropriate cues, and this leads to their application.

As well as guiding what is perceived and done, adaptive schemes are also open to accommodation or change. They both direct experience and are changed by it as they actively interact with incoming information. At output, schemes interact with new incoming information to allow a variety of appropriate responses to a variety of new situations. The person acts flexibly but according to a plan. Thus, schemes are nonconscious mental structures or modules that interact with incoming information to determine both what is perceived and experienced and to provide the framework for our responses to the world. They are our core means of organizing both our experience and our responses, and they change by accommodating to new experience.

Schemes that affect people's psychological well-being (and therefore are the focus of therapy) are those that represent self-in-the-world emotional experience. It is these self-in-the-world integrative cognitive/affective/motivational/relational action structures that we henceforth refer to as emotion schemes. They are the targets of our therapeutic work. In our view what is crucial about emotion schemes is that although they involve cognition, they go beyond purely representational cognition to include emotion, motivation, and relational action as well. They are not simply conceptual and classifactory in nature, but rather, they are embodied organizations of sets of anticipations and reactions. Thus a client enters therapy with a nonconscious emotion scheme that, when activated, generates a feeling of, say, inadequacy. The client may not be aware that a situation has activated the inadequacy producing scheme and may say "I just feel bad" or "I don't know why I reacted in that way." Or a client may anticipatorily feel inadequate in imagining situations that do not necessarily call for such a response. The inadequacy emotion scheme is either activated out of awareness or is overly accessible and anticipatorily guides behavior. It is schemes like this that need to be accessed and restructured in therapy. Self-in-the-world emotion schemes that generate feelings such as feelings of being inadequate, or of being unlovable or insignificant are all highly affectively laden structures, which, when evoked, result in feelings of sadness, shame and disappointment. They also involve action tendencies to withdraw and give up, and they produce behaviors and thoughts that are dysfunctional and exacerbate the person's negative experience.

The point of therapy is not to use reason or evidence to change purely cognitive schemes (Beck, 1976; Ellis, 1962). Rather, it is to change the complex cognitive, affective, motivation, and relational action components of emotion schemes. Thus, an emotion scheme that generates, for example, disappointment in relation to lack of support, involves not only the expectational belief that "no one will be there for me." It also involves an action tendency such as to withdraw and curl up into a self-protective ball, a feeling such as emptiness in the pit of the stomach, and a desire to be comforted. This whole response complex is activated when the scheme is activated. Emotion schemes essentially contain internal representations of our need-related, action tendencies to appraised situations in a form that produces a response when applied. They lead us to anticipate experience and to react in line with past experience. Once activated, they are the cognitive/affective/motivational structures that produce our relational actions. These internal structures come to form our core sense of experienced self. Once activated, they provide the referent for our conscious mental state. They produce what it is like to be oneself, providing a sense of an embodied self that can or cannot be attended to and consciously represented.

The foundation of the self lies in the affectively toned expressive and sensorimotor patterns of early life that are represented internally in these emotion schemes and begin the process of ordering experience (Stern, 1985). These emotion schemes ultimately come to involve a representa- tion of the lived situation, including a representation of the stimulus, its appraisal in relation to a need, the belief or attribution about the self in the situation, and the affective response to the appraised situation. In our view the organism has a strong tendency to construct these emotion schemes from affect-laden experiences involving need satisfaction or frustration. According to emotion theory, emotion emerges as a function of appraisals of match/mismatch between situations and need, goals or concerns, and our appraisal of our ability to cope with the situation. Emotions are thus most strongly evoked when we are unable to meet our needs or when we succeed in doing so. Thus emotion schemes are constructed in relation to situations that frustrate or satisfy needs, goals, and concerns. Emotion schemes that are central in personal and interpersonal functioning, as we have suggested, go beyond purely cognitive schemes that contain only conceptual propositions and beliefs. They are instead complex cognitive/affective/motivational internal organizations that guide constructive information processing and produce relational action. They provide the referent for self-awareness and are the basis of our conscious experience of ourself.

Stern's (1985) work on the development of the self has been most influential on our thinking and has similarly influenced modern dynamic views that are giving greater significance to affect and internal representations than to drives (Greenberg & Mitchell, 1983; Eagle, 1984; Kohut, 1977, 1984; Kernberg, 1976, 1982; Sandler & Sandler, 1978; Basch, 1976, 1983, 1988). This is leading to an interesting convergence between experiential and some object relations (Sandler & Sandler, 1978), self-psychological (Kohut, 1977), and interpersonal (Mitchell, 1988) views of functioning. In addition, Kohut's (1977) views of a coherent agentic self, although not explictly connected by him to Rogers' (1951) and Perls et al.'s (1951) views of the self, are highly compatible with them (Kahn, 1985; Tobin, 1990, 1991) and lead to a growing convergence between experiential views and self-psychological views of human functioning. Despite possible convergence in views of human *functioning*, experiential and psychodynamic theories of *treatment* are still somewhat divergent. Dynamic views appear still to emphasize interpreta- tion and understanding of the transference as fundamentally curative, although Kohut in addition certainly promotes the use of empathy making his approach highly similar in some ways to that of Rogers (Kahn, 1985). Our process-experiential view, in contrast to focusing on transference, emphasizes empathy and differential experiential processing as curative and sees these as leading to the construction of new representations of self, other, and the world.

SCHEMATIC EMOTIONAL MEMORY

The relationship between schemes and affect has only recently begun to be elucidated and to be applied to psychotherapeutic change. We discuss below the formation and development of emotion schemes. Initially, human beings possess innate expressive motor programs for certain primary affects that are evoked by particular stimuli (Tomkins, 1970; Izard, 1977; Ekman & Friesen, 1975; Ekman, 1984). Children rapidly begin to represent their affective experience in internal models. As we have said, these models or self-in-the-world emotion schemes include representations of aspects of the evoking situations as well as the organism's sensory and expressive motor responses to the situation (Leventhal, 1984; Greenberg & Safran, 1987). When the child develops more advanced conceptual capacities, the beliefs and meanings associated with or generated during any lived experience are also coded into their schemes as a part of that lived experience. The schemes essentially exist as emotional memories of experience that influence future experience and responses by producing emotional experience when activated (Leventhal, 1984).

Emotions play a key role in the development and organization of schematic emotion memory. Experiences and perceptions registered during states of emotional arousal, because of the increased sensory experience and attentional allocation brought on by the intensity, are more likely to be stored in memory than material registered in affectively neutral states. In addition, because of the salience of emotion as a cue, those experiences that evoke certain affects appear to be linked in associative networks with other experiences that evoked the same affect. Therefore, emotion binds together elements in memory that are related because they evoke the same emotion. We develop schematic emotional memories related to fear and threat, sadness and loss, or anger and violation. These schemes contain an integration of common features from a variety of different instances and situations that involved one of these emotional experiences. Therefore, emotional schemes form the core of a person's memory of lived emotional self-experience.

The situations or events that evoke affective responses are encoded in internal models because human beings are designed so that subjective, affective experience is salient for them. Because affect is motivational and relational, providing biologically adaptive response tendencies, those human beings who were more sensitive and able to symbolize their affective responses to situations were endowed with an evolutionary advantage in the struggle for survival. Humans have become in-wired to learn from and build schemes of their need-related emotional responses to situations. We therefore are suggesting that core self-related schemes are built around affect-laden responses to situations in which the state of the self is enhanced or diminished by the meeting of or the failure to meet of needs.

Emotion schemes are developed from birth to organize the infant's experience. Initially, the infant's primary responses to the world and its own inner experience are affective. Affect as noted previously provides us with a primary self-organizing system as well as with a primary communication system. For example, fear of a looming shadow leads to the self being organized for flight, and/or to the expression and communication of fear and distress that is aimed at obtaining security and protection from the other. Repeated affective experiences of a particular kind lead to the internal representation of the sequences of events involved in the experience and to the formation of a set of rules for predicting, interpreting, responding to, and controlling these experiences. This is the cognitive/affective/motivational/relational action, "emotion" scheme that governs a person's experience of self-in-the-world. As the infant develops both the cognitive and affective capacity to represent the object and its absence, the feeling associated with this experience develops. With the increase in life experience, the scheme eventually comes to contain a representation of the organismic need and the person's affective responses to the situation. Ultimately, with further cognitive development, the scheme also incorporates beliefs about the situation, and rules learned, for regulating these experiences. The beliefs and rules are both learned from others and constructed by the person.

Within this perspective, one does not think of therapeutic intervention in terms of accessing or interpreting unconscious or repressed emotion or even warded off or disavowed emotions. It is seen in terms of accessing schemes that contain "potential" emotion. Emotions are not stored, but are reconstructed. This reconstruction depends on how information is currently appraised and organized and whether or not emotion schemes are currently activated. For example, the emotion associated with painful memories is not itself stored or conserved in memory. Instead, it is reconstructed or resynthesized in the present by the application of the scheme as the memory comes into awareness. Thus, emotion is not conserved in the unconscious. It is the emotion scheme that is conserved. Therefore, emotion schemes represent "potential" emotions, emotions which come into existence depending on whether or not they are actually evoked. An important therapeutic focus becomes one of activating emotion schemes and helping people attend to the emotional experiences generated and their emotional meanings. Clients in therapy need to become aware of any emotions and action tendencies that have been evoked and the specific adaptational meaning connected with them. Where necessary, they need to reorganize emotion schemes that are leading to current maladaptive responses and to construct new emotional meanings that can led to more adaptive responding.

In summary, emotion schemes operate automatically at a tacit level, governing the person's experience of the world by both encoding the world and producing responses to it. In this view the emotion scheme is: (1) a complex biosocial integration of cognition, affect, motivation, and relational action; (2) operates automatically out of awareness to produce felt meanings and action tendencies; (3) produces affective responses by an appraisal of a situation in relation to a need or concern; and (4) reconstructs emotional experience in the present.

THE GROWTH TENDENCY

In addition to the importance of emotion schemes in the creation of human experience, we also see the organism as possessing a growth tendency and regard this ever-present developmental tendency as important in understanding therapeutic change. As noted in the previous chapter, in our view the tendency to survive and grow is a fundamental organizing principle of all life.

The growth tendency is a formative, developmental tendency that is oriented toward maintaining a sense of system coherence or organismic balance while the organism is in a continual process of exploration and development (Goldstein, 1939; Maslow, 1954, 1971; Rogers, 1958, 1961; Perls et al., 1951). Thus growth involves change and adaptation to the ever-changing situation in order to maintain and enhance the self. The organism is oriented toward maintaining a sense of coherence and well-being while consistently assimilating new input. Growth and development consist of the differentiation of internal structures and their integration (Werner, 1948, 1957). This involves a continual process of reorganizing at higher and higher levels of complexity in order to maintain and enhance the self and to attain maximum creative flexibility in whatever environment the organism finds itself. Thus, self-coherence and self-enhancement through adaptive flexibility are the aims and the effects of the growth tendency. Affect serves the growth tendency by informing the organism of its progress toward organismic goals and organizes it for actions that serve the tendency to self-preservation and -enhancement. Affects and emotions are thus essential in the operation of the growth tendency. In order to protect and enhance the self, they inform the organism of its current state, they keep the organism on the track of relevant biosocial goals, and they provide social signals to others of inner states.

This view of a growth tendency is not a naive view of humans as "natural savages," nor is it a value judgment that people are intrinsicly good. Growth is not in the domain of morality; it is about development and adaptation, not about good and evil. The growth tendency thus is essentially a biological tendency to survive and meet one's needs in a complex social environment. It operates as part of a dialectical process of constantly reestablishing balance between the ever-changing organism and its ever-changing environment, and by so doing, it enhances the organism's well-being. Humans, in addition to being growth oriented, have the capacity for choice, and it is this that ultimately determines whether their actions are good or bad. Thus, in an organism oriented toward maintenance and growth, choice ulitmately determines *how* an individual sets about attaining his or her goals of survival and enhancement. People in the final analysis are thus nondeterministic systems. The final action is determined by choice, and *will* plays a central role in determining what will be done. Subjective choice, personal agency, and responsibility are thus at the center of who we are. It is will that finally determines action. The growth tendency sets the *end goal*, and choice selects the *means* whereby the goal is attained (Perls, 1969).

This tendency toward growth and development exists in every human individual, but it requires a "good enough" relational environment in order to be realized. One of the goals of this approach is to evoke and support the tendency toward growth and development. Safety is the evolutionarily most ideal environment for facilitating growth because it promotes exploration. Exploration increases the probability of the discovery and generation of variation and novelty. Exploration is therefore evolutionarily adaptive and enhances survival and growth. Therapy that provides the safety that is optimal for exploration will thereby facilitate psychological growth. Psychological safety is best provided by a warm, empathic, nonjudgmental environment.

In addition to promoting exploration and growth by the provision of safety, therapists can help maximize the growth process by focusing their responses on the novel edges of the clients' exploratory thrusts. This both recognizes and confirms the developmental thrust in clients as it emerges and helps clients focus on their own inner emerging experience and on what is novel or interesting to them. The therapist's role in focusing on growth possibilities is like that of any facilitator of development, such as a parent encouraging a child to take a first step. If the facilitator encourages more than is developmentally possible, like walking too early, damage will be done; if the facilitator prevents the developmental potential from being actualized when it is ready, like discouraging the child from taking a first step, damage will also be done. What is needed is an attunement to and matching of the developmental capacity and the facilitation of an appropriate step (Stern, 1985). The therapist's role is thus one of providing safety and being attuned to and matching the client's developmental possibility as the client struggles towards growth. An important aspect of matching is providing security and safety by recognizing the fear and anxiety involved in the risk of change and the pain involved in the struggle to overcome difficulties. Thus responses such as "It feels really scary to speak up and risk being seen," in recognizing the fear of change, help people feel more confident and secure in themselves and thereby enhance their ability to change and grow.

We see the growth tendency as encompassing a variety of motivations including both the motivation to be attached to others, to grow to interdependence, to be curious, to master the social and physical environment and to satisfy basic needs. In addition to these motivations, we see the person as possessing certain resources that help the organism to grow. These resources are self awareness, a fundamentally adaptive emotion system, and internal strengths supported by knowledge and skills.

The first resource serving the growth tendency is consciousness and *self* awareness. With the advent in humans of self-reflective consciousness, the organismic tendency to survive and grow becomes a major impetus in human beings toward the search for and construction of meanings that foster survival and growth. What most distinguishes growth in humans from growth in most other biological organisms is the unique human capacity for self-reflective consciousness and ultimately the *capacity* for meaning, choice, self-determination, and freedom. Consciousness thus operates to aid the organism in its survival and growth. This combination of a growth tendency with the capacity for meaning then provided beings who were motivated to maintain and enhance the self both at the physical level of the organism and at the psychological level of the meaning system. Because people's psychological sense of themselves are so strongly guided by the emotionally based meanings they generate, empathic understanding of the person's emotional meaning thereby becomes a crucial aspect of a facilitative environment to support human psychological growth. As air is needed to support breathing, so empathic attunement to feelings is needed to promote development of the affectively based self (Kohut, 1984).

A second crucial resource serving the growth tendency is the emotion system. We see the organism as possessing certain inherent biologically adaptive emotion tendencies that need to be acknowledged in order for the growth principle to operate most effectively. At the core of the organism is a biologically adaptive emotion/motivation system. There are two major points here. The first is that the human organism has inherited a fundamentally adaptive emotion/motivation system that provides essentially adaptive information that facilitates orientation in the environment and also aids problem solving. The second is that this resource can be made use of by directing attention toward emotional experience. This allows the adaptive information to be clearly symbolized and used to guide choice and action.

Essentially, we are arguing that it is important to attend inwardly to the information generated by the emotional response system both because emotion is fundamentally adaptive and because organisms are by nature designed to be sensitive to this rapid appraisal system in order to survive and enhance themselves. Positive emotions such as joy, excitement, and interest are also crucial in the organism being proactive. Neglect of all this emotion information robs the organism of important orienting information crucial to well-being. As noted in the previous chapter, emotions are generated when the organism is concerned about the situation. Emotion involves an appraisal of the significance of what is occurring for one's personal well-being and therefore is fundamentally tied to survival and growth. Attending to the emotional response system provides crucial information related to one's well-being, information that needs to be used to aid problem solving and informed choice, decision and action. Having significant others empathically attuned to one's emotional responses, particularly at times of crisis and new development, when new experience is generated, is crucially helpful in supporting one to be attuned to one's own internal experience.

Another resource that supports the growth tendency is the people's lifetime of learning and experience, experience that they can access as strengths to help them change. Clients come to therapy with a vast storehouse of such strengths and resources. Therapy is the process of helping clients access these resources to aid them in solving therapeutic tasks and psychological problems. In this approach to therapy we are not primarily dealing with people who lack skills or who have a deficiency but, rather, with people who seek out therapy because they are not using their internal resources to achieve some type of desired psychological or behavioral change. Thus, clients are strengthened by attending inwardly to their inner resources, and it is the therapist's function to facilitate this inner attending and utilization of these resources.

Trusting in one's organism, as implied in a belief in the growth tendency, is a complex concept. We use this concept to acknowledge both that it is important to access and utilize one's internal resources, and that it is important to attend to internal feelings as a guide to what one is experiencing. Attending inwardly helps people accept their own temperamentally based responses. Rather than being guided by images of *how to be*, people need to attend to how they actually *are* and to respect this. For example, people differ temperamentally in their sensitivity and reactivity to stimuli, in their responsiveness to change, in their degree of

extroversion, and on a variety of other nontemperamental characteristics. They need to respect their own way of being rather than try to be other
than who they are. Attention to their own temperamentally based bodily responses as well as to their feelings of what is significant to them is the best way of staying true to themselves.

By saying that a person needs to trust his or her feelings, we are not, however, suggesting that the individual can rely purely on personal feelings or impulses to guide behavior. Emotional responses need to be used as a *guide* to choice or action, not as their *determinant*. Once we are aware of our emotional responses, we possess information relevant to our well-being that enhances orientation and problem solving, but this response-related information still requires further reflection and integration with other aspects of our experience before translation into action. Once we have attended to our internal response, we need to incorporate this information into our decisional process both because it is our reaction and because it is potentially adaptive. Given that we are aware of our emotional responses we also need to consciously appraise the situation for opportunities and evaluate our skills and resources for dealing with the situation. We then need to integrate our emotional response into our overall system and act in terms of all the sources of information. Thus choice is a crucial determinant of behavior.

Clearly not all our emotional responses are primary biologically adaptive responses. Distinctions between primary, secondary, and instrumental emotional responses and between primary adaptive and maladaptive emotions have been offered as an initial means of distinguishing different types of affective responses (Greenberg & Safran, 1984a, 1884b, 1987, 1989). These are described below.

Primary emotions are here-and-now, immediate, and direct responses to situations. *Secondary emotions* are secondary responses to more primary emotions or thoughts. They often obscure the primary generating process. Thus, secondary anger is often expressed when the primary feeling is fear, or people may cry or express sadness when the primary emotion is anger. *Instrumental emotions* are those expressions that are used in order to achieve an aim, such as expressing sadness to elicit comfort or anger in order to intimidate. Of importance here is that in dysfunction it is often the primary organismic emotional response that has not been acknowledged and that must be searched for and incorporated. Often this requires the facilitation of a highly attuned, empathic environment.

In addition to the three-part classification of primary, secondary, and instrumental emotions, primary emotions can also be divided into primary, adaptive, and maladaptive, responses. Primary emotion as well as being adaptive can, in certain instances, such as panic become maladaptive through a process of learning. In panic, the fear is a primary emotion, but it has become a maladaptive response.

Primary emotional responses themselves are however generally fundamentally adaptive. Though emotions have often been viewed as not "rational" they are inherently neither rational nor irrational, merely adaptive (Oatley, 1992). For example, a response of feeling angry at being criticized or "put down" is not necessarily irrational or dysfunctional. Rather it is a response based on an appraisal of the situation in relation to a need. It may be that the intensity with which the person reacts, the type of action taken, or the sequence of feelings and thoughts that follow the anger are dysfunctional. The anger itself may be adaptive. Thus it is often people's inability to accept that they feel angry, or the fear of what will happen if they express the anger, or the process of building from anger into a rage that may be dysfunctional, rather than the anger itself. Therefore, the initial response may not be inherently problematic. Instead the complex processes and meanings that follow the response are the phenomena that may lead to dysfunctional behavior and experience.

Schematic emotional memory can however produce primary emotional responses not appropriate to the current situation, and these maladaptive responses can both influence behavior and override more primary biologically adaptive responses (Greenberg & Safran, 1987, 1989). Once people have acknowledged their emotional experience, they need to become aware of whether their emotional responses to situations are primarily: adaptive ones and can help determine adaptive action; complex secondary or instrumental emotional responses that require further exploration to get at their primary responses; or primary emotions that are maladaptive in that they are not helping the person to enhance his or her well-being. Becoming aware of emotions and whether or not they are primary adaptive emotions is thus an important first step in therapy. However, in order for people to behave adaptively, they, in addition to becoming aware of their feelings, must also identify the need associated with the feelings, realize that this need has not been recognized or met, and utilize skills to meet the need appropriately. It is thus recognition of primary adaptive emotions, acknowledgement of the need with which they are associated, and the use of appropriate means to meet the need that are important in guiding adaptive action.

Once we attend to our emotional feedback, our survival/growth tendency ensures that we are constantly attempting to make the decision most advantageous to our well-being in terms of how we currently perceive ourselves and the situation. Thus the growth tendency is constantly pushing the organism toward adaptive flexibility and need satisfaction in a specific context. As will be noted later, therapy is a process of helping the client access and strengthen this tendency.

AN INTEGRATIVE OVERVIEW

In this book we operate within a developmental, dialectical constructivist framework as our broadest frame of reference (Mahoney, 1991; Pascual-Leone, 1976a, 1976b, 1976c, 1980, 1988, 1990a, 1990b, 1991). We are dialectical constructivists because we see the organism as actively organizing its view of reality based on experiential referents, and we may be considered developmental because we view the organism as fundamentally oriented toward interaction with the environment to develop so as to survive and grow. We see the organism as possessing reflective consciousness, which, in line with its thrust toward development, results in it being an active agent. The organism continuously organizes itself to meet the situation adaptively by differentiating and integrating internal structures to create new meaning. This creative adjustment leads to the development of greater organized complexity in the service of improved adaptation, need satisfaction, and self-enhancement.

Within this broader perspective of the adaptively self-organizing function of the growth tendency, two fundamentally adaptive motivational concerns appear crucial. These are relatedness and attachment to others (Bowlby, 1969/1982) (including the associated polar process of autonomy and separation) and exploration and mastery of the environment (White, 1959, 1966) (and the associated process of maximally utilizing one's potentials). With regard to other-relatedness, it is important to note first that affect is fundamentally relational. Second, that in our view, the infant comes into the world with the components of a ready-to-be-organized attachment-response system. These responses include the need to be attached to others and to seek contact/comfort, and a basic sense of security from others. With regard to mastery we view the infant as a fundamentally curious being designed to manipulate and assertively explore the world and its constituents to the utmost of its abilities in order to attain mastery of its environment. Thus, other-relatedness and interdependence, and competence and mastery are fundamental aspects of human nature. This is not to deny that other more drive-like aspects of functioning, such as, hunger, sex, and avoidance of harm, do not operate. Nor does this imply that more complex higher level "being" needs (Maslow, 1971) such as the need for truth, beauty, and justice are not also ultimately important determinants of behavior and development. Drives and being needs, plus cognitive factors such as expectancy and goals, and extrinsic motivators such as reward and punishment, plus affect, are all influential in motivating different people's behavior at different times. Thus, when we refer to motivation, we consider a combination of all these influences and think in terms of an amalgam of needs/goals/concerns, thus recognizing the influences of biology, learning, and culture in motivation. However, we choose to emphasize attachment/interdependence and curiosity/mastery as well as the emotions as fundamental in understanding human motivational problems worked on in therapy because we believe these help shed the most light on how to effect change in treatment.

The organism is endowed with certain fundamental or in-wired propensities in the form of a motivational/emotional system. Whether motivations in the form of needs or fundamental concerns are independently provided for by nature, or whether they emerge from a complex interaction among a basic in-wired emotion system, cognition, and the environment (a view which we favor), is not too important for our purposes. What we emphasize is the fact that the organism possesses certain in-wired motivational/emotional characteristics. These systems, in interaction with the environment, soon develop into somewhat idiosyncratic motivational/emotional structures in each individual representing the individual's lived experience.

Therefore, rather than attempting to propose a definitive grand motivational theory in our approach, we suggest rather that it is therapeutically helpful to understand people's functioning in terms of their current needs, goals, and concerns as well as their own attempts to satisfy these. By the time a person reaches adulthood, there are probably hundreds or even thousands of needs, concerns, desires, goals, influencing experiences, and behaviors. Rather than attempting to fully specify basic human needs or fundamental human goals, we suggest that, although there probably are some more basic needs, human functioning is complex, idiosyncratic, and intentional. Although there probably exists some hierarchical structuring of needs (as suggested by Maslow) and some prioritizing principle such that survival needs generally take precedence over growth needs, it is most profitable for therapists not to work by a singular, potentially constricting view of the contents of basic human nature. Instead, it is important to both develop a process view of how motivation operates in dysfunction and change and to listen to clients to discern their idiosyncratic feelings and needs.

THE FORMATION OF SELF

The organism is thus an integrated cognitive/emotional/motivational/relational action system in which the perceiving and appraising of stimuli, the experience of affect, and the generating of action tendencies or motivational potentials are all part of a holistic dialectical relational system in operation.

Repeated need-related, affective responses to a situation form a self-in-the-world emotion scheme. Affect thus forms the bedrock of a relational self. Emotion schemes are however formed over life and related to different domains of experience. From the start these schemes then combine together to form the beginning units of the emerging sense of self. The relational self (Gilligan, 1982) is, however, modular in nature and is continually engaged in the process of dialectically constructing momentary self-organizations in reponse to situations (Greenberg & Johnson, 1988). It is this modularly organized, relational process-self that then becomes the center of initiative, that wants or needs something, and anticipates self and other's responses. It is then that these modular, dialectically related organizations become the targets of therapeutic intervention and that, because of their modular nature, call for differential intervention for different, modularly based processing difficulties.

The relational self is thus not an entity but, rather, is continually *constructing* itself as a center of initiative (Pascual-Leone, 1990a, 1990b; Varela, Rosch, & Thompson, 1991). As Stern (1985) has demonstrated, infants develop "an integrated sense of themselves as distinct and coherent bodies with control over their own actions, ownership of their own affectivity and a sense of continuity" (p. 69). The sense of an integrated self is thus constructed and, in our view, is an integration that is continually occurring and one that can at times break down. During development when a need is satisfied or met, the result is a sense of one's ability to regulate one's experience in relation to the environment. This sense of the ability to regulate is at the center of a competent sense of a relational self. This sense of a competent, coherent, and stable self is however continually being constructed. At any time a greater or lesser sense of integration and coherence can be attained. Our basic assumptions are that personal reality is continually constructed, and that self-experience and experience of self are created moment-by-moment through an interaction of consciousness with reality and with automatically cued emotion schemes.

DYSFUNCTION

IN OUR VIEW, pathology or dysfunction is not a product of currently operating unconscious motivation, nor are people seen as being driven to behave maladaptively by repressed emotions. Rather, it is people's present awareness or lack of it, their construals, and the *meaning* of their experience that determine much of their maladaptive behavior and dysfunction. Awareness of automatically generated emotional experience is particularly important in the creation of meaning and in adaptive problem solving in human environments (Greenberg & Safran, 1987, 1989). As we have already argued in this book, people essentially behave in a fashion they construe to be the best adaptive alternative given their current perceptions of themselves and the situation. If their constructions are not informed by their automatic emotional responses they are disoriented, and if the emotional responses that inform their constructions are dysfunctional, they behave maladaptively. Therefore, problems in the creation of emotional meaning are central in dysfunction.

In our view, problems related to emotional meaning and resultant dysfunction are created by two fundamental processes: (1) the ongoing conscious construction of meaning, a process in which meaning is created by synthesizing and symbolizing experience in awareness; and (2) the automatic activation of emotional schemes, a process in which experience is automatically generated for potential synthesis in awareness. The first process is a dialectically constructive one, involving a process of ongoing synthesis; the second is an automatic process involving scheme activation.

Dysfunction comes both from a failure in the constructive symbolizing process and from the activation of dysfunctional emotion schemes developed from life experience. On the one hand, *dysfunction in the symbolizing* of emotion leads to emotional response information not being utilized at all, or being restrictively or distortedly symbolized. Thus a woman may react automatically with certain physiological, sensory, and facial muscular patterns of anger to her automatic appraisal that her husband wishes her to "read his mind," or that her mother expects her not to "rock the boat." Whether her appraisals are or are not accurate is not our primary therapeutic concern here. What is of concern is whether, in her construction of her subjective reality, she is able to synthesize her affective response into her construction of self and situation. Often in circumstances like this, clients who are unable to synthesize their own anger into their construction are left feeling intimidated and insecure and end up being overly compliant or anxious.

On the other hand, *activation of dysfunctional emotion schemes* can lead to the production of maladaptive primary responses or maladaptive secondary responses. Thus the client described above may experience a primary maladaptive fear in response to getting too close to her mother or her husband. This comes from her schematic sense of herself as being unworthy and a continual disappointment. She thus may tend to react with maladaptive fear in response to genuine attempts by her husband to be intimate and may pull away from him for fear of being criticized. Clients in general may react with maladaptive fear to closeness or to other harmless stimuli or with maladaptive anger in response to being touched or to kindness. These maladaptive responses are generated by schemes in which these emotions were orginally evoked as adaptive responses to closeness or touching that was intrusive, to kindness that was manipulative or unreliable, or to harmless stimuli that were evaluated as being associated with threatening stimuli.

Schematic response *sequences* are often involved in the generation of maladaptive *secondary* emotions. Thus, clients often express secondary anger in response to underlying fear or express sadness by crying when their primary response was anger. In these situations the maladaptive response results from a chain of internal responses in which the primary responses such as threat or fear are so rapid that they escape awareness, and the secondary anger comes to govern behavior and experience. In addition, secondary emotion occurs when people have emotions about their primary emotions, that is, fear about anger or shame about sadness that are produced by these sequences.

Both of the above processes, problems in the symbolization of emotional meaning and schematic dysfunction, are described more fully below. We view these as providing a process perspective on dysfunction, more differentiated than those offered by the structural models of incongruence or of conflict between self-concept and experience proposed by Rogers (1951) and Perls et al. (1951).

PROBLEMS IN THE GENERATION OF EMOTIONAL MEANING

The developments in cognitive science and emotion theory reviewed in Chapter 3 allow us to view the person as essentially possessing the capacity for two different global and complex types of information processing or meaning generation, one deliberate and volitional, the other automatic and involuntary (Buck, 1985; Epstein, 1990). We will refer to these as conceptual, cognitive processing and experiential, emotional processing, respectively. Breakdown in the coordination of these two types of processing or levels of meaning is a generative source of dysfunction. The two types of processing and the breakdown are described below.

Conceptual processing involves sequential, propositional processing. It operates by means of causal reasoning, analytic thinking, and the development of narrative explanations, and it focuses on the relationship between semantic concepts. It is concerned with rational thinking and determining whether propositional meanings are true or false. In relation to self-knowledge, conceptual processing can provide a type of reflective, abstract, intellectual knowing "about" oneself, or a view or story about oneself.

Experiential processing puts a primary focus on the symbolization in consciousness of the nonconscious, preconceptual, or implicit level of meaning generation. On this level, we grasp the situation directly in terms of its emotional meaning for our well-being. This involves automatic appraisals of how things effect us, whether they are good or bad for us, safe or dangerous, enhancing or diminishing. This is not a cognitive appraisal of whether things are true or false, which is the function of rationality. Rather it is our wholistic sense of how things are. Experiential processing provides the *symbolization in awareness* of immediate, direct experiential knowing or nonconscious processing that represents lived experience (Gendlin, 1962, 1984). Using this system, a person in therapy views something freshly and might say in an emotionally poignant manner "I feel unsure" or "I feel so wounded inside—like a part of me has been ripped away." This reflects the symbolizing of a currently felt experience and is a dialectically constructive process in which one creates meaning in a dynamic manner from the given elements of one's experience.

In contrast, conceptual processing in therapy would offer a propositional statement about the self concerned with an intellectual abstraction about the self drawn from the self's or other's views of the self. This would be reflected in statements such as "My problem is I have not achieved my goals" or "I'm afraid of intimacy" said as rational propositions. Each type of processing engages the person in a different manner of processing information and generates different types of meaning. The conceptual system produces purely intellectual meaning, the experiential system, emotional meaning. However, it is not a simple distinction between cognition and emotion that distinguishes these two styles, for both involve cognition (Greenberg & Safran, 1987; Bohart, in press). Experiential processing involves synthesizing conceptual, propositional meaning with sensorimotor, procedural knowledge to provide a wholistic emotional meaning. Conceptual processing however provides only propositional, unembodied "descriptive knowledge" (James, 1890), knowledge about things and involves appraisals of truth and falsity of propositions. Experiential processing provides direct, wholistic embodied "knowledge by acquaintance" (James, 1890) integrating many levels of information processing including automatic evaluations of how good or bad something is for one. This later form of wholistic processing produces the emotional meaning of our lives.

When people's conceptual meanings predominate, contradict, override, distort, or ignore their emotional experience and felt meanings, the person is unable to function in an integrated manner, and the seeds of dysfunction are sown. Chronic reliance on conceptual processing produces dysfunction because people completely loose touch with their own experience. They are unable to rely on their fundamental orientation system and become "divided or false selves" (Laing, 1966). From a therapeutic vantage point, it is important in therapy to engage clients in dialectically constructive experiential processing, which synthesizes concept and experience, rather than in conceptual processing, which provides purely conceptual explanations.

Conceptual knowing does not draw on the integrative feelings and meanings synthesized by emotion schemes. Instead it is more deliberate, rational, analytical, and intellectually abstract. It is purely propositional and is more rooted in logical, cultural, and social bases of self-description. This system draws on sets of learned rules for how one "ought to be" (Rogers's conditions of worth, or Perls's introjects) as well as a set of learned values and ideals. These are often developed from others' expectations and not from personal experience. In addition, the conceptual system develops "self-" and "situation" narratives as ways of rationally comprehending and explaining ourselves and our experiences, both to ourselves and to others. Gazzaniga (1985) provides a clear demonstration of how split brain patients produce totally inaccurate reasons for their behavior in order to develop rational explanations of their behavior. Using this system, humans represent themselves to themselves, focusing reflexively on themselves as objects of their own and others' attention. This occurs when a person conceptualizes him- or herself in an abstract fashion as a person who is "sensitive to rejection" or as "shy," "confident," or "lazy." This is not a symbolizing of immediate emotional experience but, rather, an abstract concept or belief about oneself, condensing information from an overview of experience into an explanatory view of oneself. As we have said, this explanation of oneself or one's behavior is often guided by beliefs and expectations about how one should be, based on others' views.

On the other hand, experiential processing is characterized by the symbolization in awareness of automatic, preconceptual, bodily experience (Lakoff, 1987; Johnson, 1987). It represents our bodily lived experience of being in the situation. Experiential knowing integrates a variety of sources of information, drawing predominantly on the sensorimotor and schematic levels of emotional processing as discussed in the previous chapters. Whereas our sensorimotor system is prewired to respond adaptively to certain stimuli, our tacit emotion schemes function in terms of past experience and incoporate propositional learning. Emotion schemes automatically deploy attention in such a manner that we process information in terms of its relevance to ourselves. We apprehend immediately the meaning to us of the situations in which we are engaged. This processing system generates action tendencies and emotional responses to situations and felt meanings. To differing degrees people consciously attend to and symbolize their experience to themselves, thereby orienting themselves in the world and creating conscious emotional meaning. The awareness of this type of information provides explicit emotional or experiential meaning, which is necessary to help deal with "problems in living" and often enhances well-being.

Awareness of experiential or emotional meaning is required in therapy and needed for adequate functioning. It involves symbolizing in awareness some of the vast amount of automatic schematic processing of complex information that occurs out of awareness or preconsciously. In therapy this level of processing is facilitated by a process of attending inward toward one's experience or by becoming aware of one's expressive actions in the world. Bodily felt experience is an especially significant referent for the meaning-construction process (Gendlin, 1981) as well as serving as an organizing factor in our construal of events (Lakoff & Johnson, 1980). In addition, the promotion of specific concrete memories such as "I remember him glaring at me, and I felt this knot in my stomach," rather than a general memory such as "We argued," is an important way of facilitating experiential processing as opposed to conceptual processing.

The emotional meaning system provides the basis of our construction of lived reality and is also the channel for fundamentally adaptive emotional response information. It is based on our evolutionarily developed, biologically adaptive emotion system. One of our basic assumptions is that people need to attend to and consciously, linguistically symbolize the output of the tacit, rapid-processing experiential system in order to solve problems in living and be adaptively oriented in the world. As we have said, the emotional meaning system cannot serve its biologically adaptive function in the complex human environment if bodily felt, emotionally toned experience is not attended to and symbolized with accuracy and immediacy. If access to this emotionally based experiential information is blocked by learned processing of experiences in relation to self and environment, people's functioning will be hampered, and dysfunction will ultimately ensue. Thus, dysfunction is caused by problems in the constructive process, particularly by the inability to automatically synthesize one's generated experience. Rather than conflict between self-concept and experience, there are problems in the process of dialectical synthesis.

A crucial task of therapy is to facilitate experiential processing rather than conceptual processing, to enable the person to process wholistic, emotionally toned experience in more effective ways. Therapy needs to open people to more internal and external information and to stimulate and evoke the emotion schemes that generate the person's fundamental experience and that serve as the basis of emotional meaning. By exploring a *particular* situation as completely and fully as possible, people can access their fundamental, wholistic models of the world, the models responsible for their experience of self. It is these wholistic models, not conceptual meanings that need reorganizing. However, it is important to note that in this view it is not insight into abstract *patterns of behavior across situations* such as "rebelling against authority," or "pushing people away when they get close," that is searched for in therapy. Rather it is the reexperience of a concrete, particular instance that is sought after. It is the *full experience of a single instance* of an experience that will bring forth all the elements of the actual experience from memory. This evocation of the experience will make new information available to challenge a conceptual belief or construct one has about a situation and makes both the belief and/or the elements amenable to reorganization. Thus, it is the presently relived experience in awareness of, say, a desperate yearning, or a presently lived feeling, in awareness, of inferiority, inadequacy, or unlovableness (and the action tendencies associated with these) that needs to be accessed, attended to, and, when necessary, changed in therapy. It is *not* the intellectual concept of these emotions that needs to be addressed.

SCHEMATIC DYSFUNCTION

In our view, dysfunction stems from problems in people's meaning-synthesis process as described above. On the other hand, dysfunction also results from people's general manner of being-in-the-world. It is emotion schemes that govern their ways of being-in-the-world—the manner in which they perceive and act in the world. As schemes develop they come to be a mental model that influences the person's view of, and experience of, being-in-the-world. These views become the primary mode through which people experience themselves in the world.

When a scheme is activated, it guides both preattentive and attentive processing and produces anticipations and responses that have been forged from past learnings. What people experience and how they respond now are generated by their schemes. First, as described above, if the information generated by these schemes is not attended to and synthesized, the organism, unaware of its own reactions, is ungrounded by its own experience and is disoriented. However, the schemes themselves can generate dysfunctional responses as a function of traumatic or damaging experience, or as a function of the construction of maladaptive or imbalanced, internal representations of self, other, and world. For example, a schematic representation that views the world as threatening and the self as vulnerable, when activated, will generate experience and behavior consistent with this view. If the scheme generates shame, this experience will govern the person's behavior. Thus, schemes based on traumatic or negative learning histories can produce primary emotional responses that are dysfunctional in new contexts. Thus, currently feeling shame or fear at exposing one's feelings or views to others results from a history of having been shamed or threatened for having revealed one's feelings or views. Therapists need to help clients evoke and symbolize maladaptive affective responses in therapy, and once these responses are in awareness, they need to help clients restructure these schemes. It is these schemes that need to be restructured not specific thoughts or beliefs.

However in this view, it is not generally a person's primary needs or emotions that are dysfunctional, for they are viewed as essentially adaptive. Often, it is other aspects of the schematic modules or the complex schematic system that generate needs and emotions in specific contexts that are faulty and are in need of change. Thus, emotions such as love or anger, or needs such as need for attachment or autonomy, are never maladaptive in themselves. Rather, dysfunction results from learning and from the experience and expression of anxiety related to primary needs and emotions.

Anxiety, depression, and other dis-ease often results from people anticipating that a need will not be met or that their emotion or need is unacceptable because it will have a negative impact on others. In addition, people often have dysfunctional responses to these perceptions, becoming anxious, enraged, or despondent in response to their own anticipations. Thus the intense, dysfunctional despair and clinginess found in certain states come from the anticipation of abandonment and disappointment. In these schemes, it is the expectation of abandonment or disappointment and the response to this that is dysfunctional, not the attachment need. All the complex processing and the meaning of the experience involved in these situations come from the scheme. If the scheme or schematic sequence is dysfunctional, then the individual's behavior and experience will be dysfunctional.

As we have said, it is often not the emotions or needs per se, embedded in the scheme, that are pathological. Rather, it is the secondary feelings and thoughts about the basic emotions and needs that are a major source of dysfunction. For example, an often-observed dysfunctional response sequence involves disappointment followed by rage. The rage typically occurs because the person is unable to articulate the primary disappointment, is terrified at the prospect of doing so, and instead reacts with secondary rage. What has occurred is that the automatic activation of the disappointment scheme results in a rapid experience of hurt. This may pull with it the emotional memory of earlier disappointment and hurt. When this schematic emotional memory includes feelings of danger associated with it and beliefs such as "I won't survive the hurt and violation," another scheme associated with memories of being violated is activated. This in turn produces rage at being violated. In this case, the rage response is a secondary response to thoughts and feelings about the more primary emotions and needs and to the complex meanings involved in loss, abandonment, and disappointment.

A further major problem of schematic dysfunction occurs by the emotional splitting that occurs in relation to childhood abuse. Any strong recurring emotional experience will shape the development of a scheme. If, during childhood, a child experiences from the same caretaker affection and care at some time producing positive emotions, and abuse and neglect at other times producing negative emotions, the child will probably construct separate modular schemes representing each type of experience, thereby splitting the self in relation to the primary caretaker into two distinct self-organizations. When modular self-organizations of this type are formed around different dominant emotions, they result in dissociative disorders in which different distinct organizations related to the abuse are activated by different cues. Either the good or the bad are strongly separated, or the reciprocal roles of victim and victimizer, seducer, and seduced are formed and are activated in strongly independent fashion or people dissociate totally from their emotional experience.

Psychopathology, in many instances is thus related to people's inability to integrate, accept, and deal with their primary feelings and needs over the course of their development. Rather than being related to neurotic "infantile" needs, dysfunction, especially of the neurotic type, is related more to people's feelings that their primary adult feelings and needs are unacceptable and to the manner in which they have come to construe themselves and their world in order to deal with this. It is how people have organized themselves to deal with their feelings and needs that is problematic rather than the feelings and needs themselves. It is the sense of unentitlement to these feelings and needs (Horney, 1966; Perls, 1969), and all the processes involved in the disowning and disallowing of these feelings and needs, that results in dysfunction. The emotion/ motivation response system is the original biologically adaptive given. How people handle these responses over life and the schematic development that occurs in relation to them determine adjustment and maladjustment.

DEVELOPMENT OF DYSFUNCTIONAL SCHEMES

Emotion schemes have been developed from infancy and lead either to functional or dysfunctional responses, depending on what internal representations related to need satisfaction have been developed. For example, when an infant's physiological state, such as thirst or discomfort, is translated into an expression and is met by an appropriate need-satisfying response by a caretaker, the sequence of occurrences is recorded in memory. Repetition of these experiences leads the sequences to be represented in an internal model that becomes part of the schematic structure of the self. Repeated frustration of the need leads to a representation of a core self-structure that involves a particular view of the world and a mode of being-in-the-world. This might include negative affect and negative beliefs about self and the world as nonresponsive. Consequently, a dysfunctional response occurs when the scheme involving this need is evoked. These schemes can change and continue to develop throughout life. They can be changed by new life experience and by reflection, but the initial scheme can and often does exert a marked influence on how information is processed and how the world is viewed. Thus pathology emerges from the way people have come to view themselves and their world from their mode of being-in-the-world.

Healthy development on the other hand occurs through the empathic attunement of the caretaker to the infant, involving the accurate recognition by the caretaker of the infant's emotional expression and related need. This confirms the infant's sense of directly experienced self and helps the infant build a secure and confident sense of self and of being-in-the-world. Repeated disconfirming responses or chronic failure in responsiveness, overresponsiveness, or inconsistent attunement, however, will all lead to the construction of an anxious, insecure general sense of self-in-relation in which the infant begins to learn that it cannot rely on others for need satisfaction and affect regulation. The inability of the self to achieve regulation for whatever reason, be it internally or externally caused, eventually becomes an inability to self-regulate. This produces potentially dysfunctional emotion schemes, laden not only with faulty cognitions but with negative affective responses such as anxiety on frustration. This scheme then determines a predominant mode of being-in-the-world.

It is important to note that in emotion schemes—those schemes that go beyond cognition to encode affective, motivational, and relational response information—it is the repeated sensorimotor and affective experiences associated with needs, represented in the schematic module, that require change in therapy, in addition to the beliefs associated with the experience. For example, in a scheme that generates intense disappointment when a need for support is not met, many things need to change. These may be the inner swirling sensations in the head, the tightness in the chest, and the wounded hurt sensations. The include the tendency to curl into a ball, the yearning for comfort, plus the tacit belief that "I'll never get what I need, and if I don't get it, I won't be able to survive." All these affective aspects associated with the disappointment need to be changed, indeed, a total mode of being-in-the-world, not merely a belief. The dysfunctional belief, although an important part of the emotion scheme related to intimacy and dependency, is only a part of the scheme. It is the entire affective/cognitive/motivational/relational action scheme, not the single belief alone, that is the source of dysfunction and that needs to be reorganized.

A MULTIFACETED VIEW OF DYSFUNCTION

In our view dysfunction thus occurs in two major ways. First, it occurs when the dialectical meaning-construction system fails to attend to the fullness of the information from the emotional scheme system, or cannot process this information in conscious awareness because of some processing limitation or interference. Thus, when an aspect of emotional meaning is not assimilated into the person's more conceptually derived self-image, beliefs, or explanatory narrative, a split results, and the organism is no longer unified. The conceptual meanings are now no longer grounded in emotional experience and may involve all forms of distortions. Breakdown in the operation of this system that governs conscious behaviors and experience results in dysfunction.

Secondly, dysfunction occurs when the emotion schemes themselves that generate a person's being-in-the-world are dysfunctional such as when a scheme repetitively organizes incoming information in distorted or maladaptive ways, resulting in recurrent dysfunctional emotional meanings and inappropriate reactions. Many types of dysfunctional schematic processing exist in addition to the above encoding problem: overrigid schematic processing producing an inability to assimilate change or challenge; a response problem, involving the activation of a scheme in which a dysfunctional emotional response is coded; a systems problem involving faulty schematic sequences in which two incompatible schemes are simultaneously activated or the activation of one scheme leads to the activation of another in a chain that may be dysfunctional. One of our basic assumptions is that much dysfunctional experience, attitude, and behavior stem from certain schematic processing problems. The faulty processing results from the content, structure, and organization of the cognitive/affective schematic systems. This affects the means by which emotional information about self, others, and the world is processed. In Part III of this volume we identify at least six types of recurrent, complex schematic processing difficulties for which we have developed specific interventions.

A crucial aspect of a schematic view of dysfunction is that there is not a single core self that is involved in dysfunction, nor a single mechanism of dysfunction. Instead, the self is modularly organized into many partial selves, and there are many different core self-related emotion schemes related to different domains of experience. An important implication of this is that different types of modularly based dysfunction will ideally require different types of intervention, as we discuss in the *Treatment Manual* section of this volume.

In this view, schematic dysfunction occurs both by the activation of a particular dysfunctional schematic module (a partial self) and by dysfunctional sequences of and relationships between schematic modules (parts of the self). Experiential theory initially posited an incongruence between the self-concept and the organism as the sole cause of dysfunction. We suggest a pluralistic view of dysfunction in which dysfunction occurs both because a person is unable to attend to and synthesize the fullness of schematically generated emotion response and/or because of the activation of domain-specific dysfunctional emotion schemes or schematic processes. As we have said, the self-concept is replaced by a synthesis process and the organism by modularly organized schematic processors that can be synthesized into awareness. This pluralistic view provides a more differentiated, and in our view, more accurate, description of what actually occurs in dysfunction, and it thereby provides a basis for differential intervention in experiential therapy.

In addition to seeing dysfunction as being determined both by attending and symbolizing problems, and by schematic-processing difficulties, we also believe that *specific disorders* such as anxiety or depression are not uniformly or singularly caused. Rather, disorders have multiple and different determinants depending on the individual and situation involved. This results in a complex, multifaceted view of disorders in which there are a variety of attending and symbolizing, and schematic-processing difficulties in any disorder, and these are seen as being uniquely and specifically combined in particular ways in each person to result in a particular disorder. Therefore, although it is possible to distinguish different disorders such as depression and anxiety as somewhat homogeneous clinical phenomena, it is important to recognize that the various cognitive-affective processes underlying these and other disorders are heterogeneous in nature (Greenberg, Elliott, & Foerster, 1991; Lewinsohn, Hoberman, Teri, & Hautzinger, 1985; Safran & Greenberg, 1988).

It is our contention that affective and personality disorders are best viewed as complex clinical syndromes composed of a variety of different attending, symbolizing, and schematic processing difficulties. Anxious and depressive experience, as well as experience in other disorders, may then be fruitfully analyzed for the specific types of emotional processing difficulties involved for each individual (Greenberg & Safran, 1987; Safran & Greenberg, 1988; Foa & Kozak, 1986, 1991). Disorders then need to be addressed, by identifying and remedying the particular schematic processing determinants of the disorder (Goldfried, Greenberg, & Marmar, 1990).

The six processing difficulties we identify and elaborate on in Part II involve: (1) The automatic activation of self-relevant schemes not appropriate to one's conscious view of the situation resulting in the puzzling over a problematic reaction. (2) The activation of two opposing aspects of self resulting in self-evaluative and (3) self-interruptive splits in which the person is either self critical or suppresses the expression of emotion. (4) The automatic activation of schemes related to unresolved and traumatic experience with others leaving the person with a lingering bad feeling toward a significant other. (5) The inability to symbolize adequately one's schematically synthesized sense of things, leaving the person with an unclear felt sense. (6) The activation of a very private previously unrevealed partial self-scheme leaving the person feeling deeply vulnerable.

WHY EMOTION SCHEMES DO NOT CHANGE

An important feature of growth and change is the dialectical process involved between conservative and transformative processes. For example, schemes are constantly being pushed toward growth by accommodating to new features of the environment, resulting in an organism that is constantly in flux while simultaneously striving to survive and to maintain a sense of coherence. However, in certain circumstances the conservative tendency may predominate, resulting in schemes not being able to change or accommodate to new experience and, instead, remaining rigid. This causes a loss of adaptive flexibility and is a key source of dysfunction.

Emotion schemes are self-maintaining and somewhat resistant to change for a number of reasons and by virtue of a variety of mechanisms. Our self-in-the-world views provide an implicit structure to our experience: they provide order from possible chaos and make sense of our world. Without these anticipatory structures we would be overwhelmed and inefficient in our attempts to engage with the complex variety of situations that cross our paths. In addition, dysfunctional schemes that have been formed from traumatic experience generally contain protective elements and a tendency to prevent retraumatization. Schemes in general, and emotion schemes specifically, by their nature change slowly. However, when emotion schemes are dysfunctional, this conservative tendency to self-maintenance leads to problems. For example, a scheme that construes anger as destructive or intimacy as intrusive may contain responses to protect the self from the assumed dangers. The therapeutic issue is how to understand how schemes prevent new information from entering and how novelty, change, and newness do emerge.

Why certain emotion schemes are not changed by experience and why they cease to accommodate a number of processes seem important. First, *selective attending* in the automatic picking up of information leads to a self-reinforcing cycle in which the scheme is confirmed again and again. Given that schemes guide perception and are anticipatory and expectational in nature, there is a self-confirmatory bias inherent in them. Thus an individual who feels unlovable scans for cues of rejection.

Second, schemes assimilate information picked up into their existing structure and therefore *distort* information. If the schemes were constructed in highly anxious or trauma-inducing conditions, the distress-producing perceptions perpetuate in the face of disconfirming experience. This is because the disconfirming information is distorted to fit the scheme and is not actually perceived as disconfirming. Thus, when threatened, the insecure person can perceive intended support or neutrality as unsupportive or as criticism.

Third, *lack of exposure* to new information prevents change. First, proneness to abstract conceptual processing often prevents the core, preconceptual schemes from being brought into awareness and exposed to new, concrete, internal experience. Thus if a person "talks about" feeling untrusting but does not experience this in that moment, the untrusting scheme remains inaccessible to reorganization by new information. In order for schemes to change, they need to be activated and exposed to new information. If experience is not in awareness, it cannot be confronted with new reorganizing information. In addition, lack of exposure can occur by virtue of the fact that people are just not that often in situations that impinge on these aspects of self-experience. Thus, a successful businessman might seldom enter into situations in which he experiences the humiliation and powerlessness he felt as a child. In addition, people often do not classify certain disconfirming experiences as relevant to the scheme, that is, the scheme is isolated and is not activated in processing relevant new experience. Thus, successes at work or school may not be assimilated into one's sense of being unrecognized or unworthy. Also, people often use strategies to avoid situations that directly confront these areas of self-experience because they are so anxiety-provoking. Thus, avoidance of internal experience, such as anger, and of anything that will evoke this experience, is an important means of isolating schemes.

Fourth, when a situation does evoke a dysfunctional scheme, the scheme-governed *emotional response* can *interfere with processing new information*. The emotional response, such as feeling afraid or worthless, can be so salient that it is difficult for the person to make the processing capacity available to process new environmental information. People are fully occupied with processing and coping with their own responses. They are therefore unable to attend outward to any disconfirming information. In addition, their responses often lead to negative interactional consequences that serve to confirm rather than disconfirm their perceptions of self and others.

In our view, there are a variety of processes that prevent scheme changes. Some are idiosyncratic and others more general; some are momentary and some more lasting; some are simple and others more complex, and these processes also need attention in therapy.

CHANGING EMOTION SCHEMES

In our observation, a number of general factors are involved in helping people change their emotion schemes that are inherently oriented toward development by differentiation and integration. In the first place, it is the interpersonal safety of the relationship in therapy that leads to an overall reduction of intrapersonal anxiety. This then *increases processing capacity* and allows conscious schemes to change. Conscious schemes, according to Pascual-Leone (1987, 1990a, 1990b; 1991), are formed by attention simultaneously focusing on a number of facets of information and bringing them into consciousness for symbolization and synthesis into a new structure. In therapy, by reducing interpersonal anxiety through empathic prizing, the person has more attentional resources available with which to attend inward to new facets of experience. With the increased capacity available to attend to self-experience, the person is now able to attend to and process more internal experience and thereby expand or change his or her views.

In the second place, directing *attentional focus* to actual features of experience affords the client the opportunity to attend to new information that is available but that was not included in the narrative construction of that client's experience. Focusing attention to contact information experientially generates novel experience that is more likely to change existing schemes. Direct experience provides the strongest and most valid source of expectancy-changing information. In addition, changing the focus of attention always changes both the focal object of attention and the attending person's self-organization. This automatically produces some change of self-in-the-world experience.

Third, *stimulation and evocation* in therapy of schematic emotional memory and of episodic memory provide new information for symbolization. The engaging of nonverbal, motor, and kinesthetic memory constitutes an important aspect of this stimulation of tacit schemes. The actual experience of emotion by the client in therapy signals that the emotion scheme has been activated and is currently operating. This makes the tacit information that guides experience and behavior more available to awareness and also makes the scheme itself more amenable to the input of new information and to reorganization.

Fourth, encouraging people *to contact directly* that which is anxiety provoking and was previously avoided also leads to new experience being admitted to awareness. People need to experientially contact new and disconfirming information in order to actually have a new experience from which to learn.

Fifth, an active experimentally oriented therapy sets up a therapy situation designed to try out or experiment with doing certain things such as actively expressing what one is feeling. This *generates new experience.* Newness comes from both the new experience generated by the performance one has produced, for example, talking to a deceased parent and from the awareness of ways one prevents or interrupts one's experience. A therapy that involves enactments elicits new experience by the enactment itself and promotes awareness of interruptions of experience.

Sixth, new experience is also generated in the here-and-now interaction with the therapist in an I–Thou dialogue (Buber, 1958). *New interpersonal experiences* occur in therapy that are relevant to and can affect core structures.

New schemes are also *created* in therapy by synthesizing elements of existing schemes and by creating new conscious meaning. Therapy involves the production of new meaning and involves not only scheme change but scheme creation. New syntheses created in therapy become represented in a new scheme. Pascual-Leone (1980, 1987, 1991; Pascual-Leone & Goodman, 1979; Pascual-Leone & Johnson, 1991) has described the dynamic synthesis involved in the production of truly novel performances. He suggests the operation of at least four factors are involved in creating a new scheme. These are (1) the deliberate executive control or plan to engage in some cognitive operation, (2) the person's ability to attentionally "boost" or activate relevant schemes, (3) the person's ability to inhibit or interrupt the activation of irrelevant interfering schemes, and (4) the capacity to produce closure in consciousness of a single integrated whole from the set of activated schemes. In therapy, this involves deliberately guiding attention to particular features of experience, concentrating on them to activate relevant schemes, inhibiting irrelevant schemes that might interfere with experiencing relevant emotional meaning (e.g., self-image schemes), and integrating the elements in consciousness into new meaning. Emotion because of its wholistic implicational nature is also important in the creation of new schemes that are constructed not only by synthesizing new bits of information but also by integrating the affective qualities of experience.

In therapy, one creates an optimal environment for enhanced attentional allocation and for activation of emotion schemes so that the person can freshly experience, explore, and reexperience troublesome situations. Therapy, in fact, is a process of helping the client to attend to inner experience in a new way that will help the client reorganize his or her view of self and situation, and it provides an optimal low-threat environment for doing this. The process of generating and constructing new experience and meaning in the newly lived experience of the therapy hour is also important.

In summary, the combination of safety and process facilitation leads to a change in manner of processing for the therapy client. This includes broadening attentional allocation and perceptual structuring, facilitating memory reorganization and meaning construction, and providing new emotional and relational experience. Schematic change occurs by bringing the schematic modules into awareness. This makes them accessible to new information and reorganization, exposes them to new experience, and fosters the clients' awareness of how their own schematic structures guide their views, thereby helping them gain some control over their own construals.

THE MANUAL: BASIC PRINCIPLES AND TASK-GUIDED INTERVENTIONS

TREATMENT MANUAL: THE GENERAL APPROACH

I N THIS SECTION of the book, we turn from theoretical elaboration to a practical description of what client and therapist actually *do* using a process-experiential approach to facilitate emotional change. In our presentation, we emphasize specific therapeutic tasks and techniques (Part III, Section 2). However, we see it as particularly important that the facilitative therapeutic relationship not be given priority over any kind of "experiential technology of emotional facilitation." Therefore, it is important that therapists first absorb the underlying therapeutic principles and second, develop specific skills in implementing the basic process-experiential intentions and response modes that underlie the general approach and the specific tasks. These are the subject of the next two chapters, which comprise Section 1 of the *Treatment Manual* section of this volume.

TREATMENT PRINCIPLES FOR A PROCESS-EXPERIENTIAL APPROACH

IN THIS CHAPTER we introduce six basic treatment principles that guide the process-experiential approach to therapy. These principles offer a bridge between the theoretical and practical parts of this book. Our view is that therapists learning this approach need first to grasp and to absorb these guiding principles before they attempt to carry out the specific task procedures with clients.

For our purposes here, we have found it is useful to distinguish six fundamental principles, organized under two higher-order principles: Offer a Therapeutic Relationship, and Facilitate Therapeutic Work. These principles are shown in Table 6-1.

The two higher-order principles, Offer a Therapeutic Relationship, and Facilitate Therapeutic Work, represent the two general change processes operating in the therapy. As noted in Chapter 2, these higher-order principles define the two main sources of the therapeutic action in this approach. These are the therapeutic relationship, including genuine empathy and prizing; and the therapeutic work, including process directiveness to facilitate optimal experiential processing (versus purely conceptual processing). Together, the Relationship and Task principles define an essential creative tension or balance in the therapy.

Nevertheless, in our view, the Relationship principles are crucial and are to be given logical and temporal priority over the Task principles.

TABLE 6-1. Treatment Principles in a Process-Experiential Approach

---

A. Relationship Principles: Facilitate a Therapeutic Relationship
  1. Empathic Attunement: Contact and be Empathically Attuned to the Client's Internal Frame of Reference
  2. Therapeutic Bond: Communicate Empathy in a Genuine, Prizing Relationship
  3. Task Collaboration: Facilitate Mutual Involvement in Goals and Tasks of Therapy

B. Task Principles: Facilitate Therapeutic Work on Specific Therapeutic Tasks
  4. Experiential Processing: Facilitate Optimal, Differential Client Processes
  5. Growth/Choice: Foster Client Growth and Self-Determination
  6. Task Completion: Facilitate Completion of Specific Therapeutic Tasks

---

Note. A creative tension or balance exists among treatment principles, requiring adaptation to specific clients and situations within sessions.

Furthermore, as described in Chapter 2, the therapeutic relationship brings about client change in two ways: first, through interpersonal learning (e.g., by disconfirming the negative expectation that trust is followed by betrayal); and, second, indirectly, through establishing the safe working conditions needed for carrying out various therapeutic tasks (e.g., by helping the client to feel safe enough to express the full extent of previously suppressed hurt) (Greenberg, 1983; Rice, 1983). That is, we see the empathic, nonjudgmental relationship as providing optimal conditions for experiential processing and the accessing of underlying emotion schemes. Specifically, nonjudgmentalness reduces interpersonal anxiety, thereby increasing the client's capacity for facing intrapersonal pain and anxiety, whereas therapist empathy helps the client to turn his or her attention to internal experience.

Our position on the long-standing question of the role of therapist empathy, prizing and genuineness in facilitating client change may be stated succinctly. We believe that the therapeutic relationship is always *necessary* (for providing the basis for therapeutic work), generally *sufficient* in the long run (i.e., curative in itself), but not always *efficient* (i.e., can be enhanced by task-focused interventions) (A. Bohart, personal communication, April 20, 1992; cf. Patterson, 1990).

RELATIONSHIP PRINCIPLES: FACILITATE A THERAPEUTIC RELATIONSHIP

The Relationship principles provide a model of the type of therapeutic relationship viewed in this approach as being inherently curative. This relationship possesses three characteristics: *Empathic Attunement* to the client's immediate experience; a genuine, prizing, accepting *bond* with the client; and client *collaboration* in treatment. The first of these emphasizes the therapist's process of tuning in and making contact with the client; the second highlights the importance of communicating this to the client; and the third underscores how a mutual commitment to the therapeutic work is built on this base.

Principle 1: Empathic Attunement: Contact and Be Empathically Attuned to the Client's Internal Frame of Reference

We begin with Empathic Attunement because we regard it as the basis for all that follows. Specifically, the other relationship principles all build on Empathic Attunement. Also, Empathic Attunement is needed for carrying out therapeutic work, especially facilitating accessing underlying emotion schemes and moment-by-moment optimal experiential processing by clients.

Our Empathic Attunement principle is directly inherited from the Client-Centered therapeutic tradition. Our concept is synonymous with Rogers' (1957, 1975) view of accurate understanding, Barrett-Lennard's (1981, 1988) empathic resonance, and Gendlin's (1968) view of experiential listening. The therapist continually attempts to make contact with and to maintain a genuine understanding of the client's internal experience or frame of reference. As Rogers (1959) has said: " . . . being empathic, is to perceive the internal frame of reference of another with accuracy and with the emotional components and meanings . . . as if one were the person, but without ever losing the 'as if' condition." The therapeutic relationship begins with the therapist attempting to enter the client's frame of reference; it continues as the therapist tries to follow closely in the client's "footsteps," "tracking" what is most important to the client as it evolves through the session.

Note that here we are deliberately focusing on the therapist's empathic *attunement*, not his or her communication of that empathy to the client (that aspect is discussed below, under Principle 2). We wish to emphasize that the crucial issue here is one of the vantage point taken by the therapist. The therapist enters the client's frame of reference, tries to see the world from the client's subjective perspective, listens from the inside as if he or she were the client, and tracks the client's subjective experience moment-by-moment as it unfolds. This is different from taking an external realistic or expert vantage point. One does not take the client's message as something to be evaluated for truth, appropriateness, or psychopathology as occurs often in interpreting patterns, drives, or defenses, or in challenging irrational beliefs.

From the therapist's point of view, Empathic Attunement is an experience that is unmistakable, but difficult to describe. This inner experience can be summarized as taking place in the following order (cf. Vanaerschot, 1990). First, the therapist lets go of or sets aside his or her previously formed ideas or formulations about the client. Second, he or she actively enters into and makes contact with the client's world. Third, the therapist resonates with the client's experience, experiencing it for him or herself. Fourth, the therapist "grasps" what is most crucial, poignant, or touching for the client.

In Empathic Attunement, one tries to respond to the client's perception of reality at that moment, as opposed to one's own or some "objective" or external view of what is real. Instead of agreeing or disagreeing, one tries simply to sense the client's experience. The therapist takes in and tastes the client's intentions, feelings, and perceptions, developing a feel of what it is like to be the client at that moment. At the same time, he or she retains a sense of self, as opposed to being swamped by or "fusing" with the client's experience.

In putting the Empathic Attunement principle into practice, the therapist becomes attuned to the client's experience by first making contact with the client's internal experience (empathic entry), next attending to what is most poignant, and then tracking the client's evolving moment-by-moment experience.

First, to achieve this, the therapist begins each session or topic by empathically *entering* the other's internal frame of reference. As each session or new topic begins, the therapist tries to clear his or her mind of external concerns or diagnoses, waiting in a state of expectant openness (letting go of preconceptions) for what the client brings to the session. It is often useful for the therapist to leave him- or herself a few minutes of "quiet time" before entering the session, in order to foster readiness for this openness. The therapist may begin by focusing on the client's experience, using inquiries such as: "What would you like to focus on or talk about?" or, "Where would you like to start?"

As the client begins to talk, the therapist maintains this attitude of openness, while trying to enter into the client's world and be attuned to the client's feelings. In the same way, when the client introduces a new subject, the therapist attempts to clear him- or herself for what will come next. The therapist attempts to absorb whatever the client is communicating in whatever channel, as this fosters entry into the client's internal frame of reference. For example, empathic entry is greatly facilitated by being attuned to the client's nonverbal expression.

Second, Empathic Attunement involves *tracking* the client's evolving moment-by-moment experience. The client's experiencing develops and changes from one moment to the next in the therapy session, requiring the therapist to listen carefully and respond to these small changes. For example, the therapist may follow a client's experience as it moves from memories of adolescent rebellion, to fear of her father's rejection, to her disappointment and frustration with herself at that moment in the session.

Finally, the therapist attends to what is currently most alive or poignant for the client. What clients experience and what they say about their experiencing is complex and ever-changing, requiring the therapist to select what to attend to. This *"empathic selection"* process typically involves tuning in most strongly to parts of the message that seem live and important to the client, usually feelings, the "edges" of experience, and idiosyncratic meanings. As we discuss later, however, what is selected varies according to the type of work being carried out, making this a difficult skill to master. Nevertheless, the therapist's "baseline" form of empathic contact is toward whatever is most immediately important, alive, powerful, pointed, or touching for the client.

Principle 2: Therapeutic Bond: Communicate Empathy in a Genuine, Prizing Relationship

Our second treatment principle, Therapeutic Bond, follows Rogers (1957, 1959, 1961, 1975) in suggesting that it is vitally important for the therapist to foster the therapeutic relationship through communicating to the client genuinely founded empathy and positive regard.

Over the course of therapy, the therapist communicates to the client the Empathic Attunement described directly above, as well as genuine nonintrusive acceptance, tolerance, openness, and above all prizing or valuing of the client and his or her inner experience. As the client "receives" (cf. Barrett-Lennard, 1962, 1986) this attitude, he or she begins to internalize it, gradually replacing conditions of worth (Rogers, 1959) and hostile self-criticism (Greenberg, Elliott & Foerster, 1991) with acceptance and support of self. Thus, the therapeutic relationship is a key curative element in a process-experiential approach, whose consistency provides the basis for work on therapeutic tasks. In keeping with this, the therapist responds from an internal attitude characterized by empathy and acceptance/prizing, both genuinely founded in the therapist's experience and beliefs.

Empathy

In addition to becoming empathically attuned to the client (Principle 1), the therapist communicates this understanding to the client and attempts at all times to foster a relationship in which the client feels deeply understood. The therapist does this by regularly communicating to the client his or her understanding of what the client is experiencing. The therapist's accurate understanding implies acceptance, and the therapist's "presence" or involvement is confirmed through communicated empathy. In fact, clients typically experience communicated therapist empathy as a supportive relationship message, indicating that the therapist is "on my side" (cf. Elliott, 1985).

In addition to the traditional reflection response, therapists use a very broad range of responses to convey empathy. These include: "back channels" (head nods, "Uh-huh," "Yeah"); matching or appropriately reactive nonverbals and facial expression; well-timed questions; and even tactful disclosure of lack of understanding (e.g., "I didn't quite get that last part, something about being unappreciated. . . "). In fact, clients are often quite satisfied simply with the sense that their therapist is *trying* to understand, perceiving many inaccurate reflections as empathic because of their intent.

Prizing

If one really gets a feeling of what it is like to be the other person, acceptance and warmth almost always follow automatically. The therapist experiences and communicates warm, unconditional acceptance of the client; a positive sense is thus communicated, of the client as a worthwhile person whose value does not depend on performing certain behaviors or having particular feelings. The term *prizing* (versus appraising) (Butler, 1952) seems best to capture this stance. The therapist prizes the client, valuing and honoring the client just as he or she is now, because of being human, not simply because he or she is entertaining, hard-working, or in pain. Each person is unique and interesting, someone whose world one has the privilege of entering for a time.

Thus, in addition to being empathic, it is also essential that the therapist foster the therapeutic bond through developing and communicating a sense of warmth and respect for the client. We distinguish two subordinate aspects to this attitude: acceptance (i.e., unconditionality or consistency) and warmth (cf. Barrett-Lennard, 1962).

Acceptance refers to a "baseline" attitude of consistent, genuine, noncritical interest, and tolerance for all aspects of the client (Rogers, 1957, 1959). In other words, prizing is not felt as contingent on being a good client. Accepting the client unconditionally requires an act of "letting go," not only of preconceptions and expectations for the client, but also of the therapist's personal values, preferences, and standards ("conditions of worth," Rogers, 1959). Where a person might typically "rush to judgment" in other situations or relationships, the therapist in this situation waits with a genuine attitude of interest, without any impulse to evaluate. For example, the therapist accepts the client's reluctance to engage in exploration of a particular area, or his or her anger, or disappointment with the therapist.

The internal act of consistent acceptance on the part of the therapist is made easier if one believes that clients, like all people, are intrinsically motivated toward coping, mastery, or growth. Unconditional acceptance comes easier if one has "unconditional confidence" in the human potential for self-understanding and change (Harman, 1990).

The second aspect of prizing, *warmth*, is a stronger, more active state that the therapist may experience at times in therapy. At particular times, the therapist experiences an immediate, active sense of caring, appreciating, feeling privileged, and valuing the client in the moment. Warmth also refers to desiring the best for the client, or valuing, or wishing him or her well, but without a sense of feeling responsible for "fixing" how the client is.

It is important to point out that prizing is not the same as offering reassurance, although it may have this effect on the client. Prizing is seldom expressed directly in words, but it can nonetheless be pervasively felt in a good process-experiential relationship. It comes through indirectly and nonverbally in voice (Rice & Kerr, 1986), manner, and perhaps most important, consistency. Occasional, brief reactions of shared excitement and caring may also be appropriate; however, the therapist generally refrains from direct reassurance, as this steps outside of the client's experience and may set the therapist up as a judge, expert or caretaker, violating the client's autonomy.

Genuineness

If the therapist's communicated empathy and prizing are not based on genuine understanding and caring for the client, they are very likely to be seen as phony and to breed distrust in the client. Thus, the final aspect of the Principle of Therapeutic Bond is genuineness, expressed in the idea that the therapist is appropriately congruent, whole, open, "real," or authentic in the relationship. In the literature, this has also been variously described as openness or congruence (Rogers, 1961), transparency (Jourard, 1971; Lietaer, 1992), authenticity (Lietaer, 1991; Trilling, 1972), and the "I–Thou" (Buber, 1958). Genuineness is also related to, but not synonymous with, therapist responses whose subtask is making personal contact with the client (e.g., self-disclosure). We will follow Lietaer (in press) in distinguishing between two aspects of genuineness, congruence and transparency.

It is important to keep in mind that genuineness itself cannot be "put on." First and foremost, genuineness consists of what Rogers (1959) calls *congruence*, that is, the therapist's self-awareness, wholeness or integrity in him- or herself (versus being at odds with oneself). This means that one is in touch with and accurately symbolizing one's own experience during the therapy hour and is thus able to interact with the client from a base of self-awareness. *Transparency* is a second, outer aspect of genuineness, which complements congruence (Jourard, 1971; Lietaer, 1991). The transparent therapist is appropriately open or present in the relationship (versus closed or secretive). That is, he or she responds to the client as openly and spontaneously as is appropriate or therapeutic.

Consistent with this, the therapeutic relationship is viewed as a real, *human* relationship, in which the therapist avoids playing roles or hiding behind the "expert role." Such a genuine relationship between client and therapist may at times be experienced as "risky" by both therapist and client. However, therapist genuineness models and encourages client openness and risk-taking and helps to break down the client's sense of isolation.

The condition of genuineness has a direct impact in itself, but in a very real sense, it makes the other two conditions effective. Without genuineness, communicated empathy and prizing would be perceived as phony, or even dangerous, manipulations. At the same time, on those occasions when genuineness is expressed (in the form of transparency), it is always offered in the context of Empathic Attunement and prizing of the client.

On the other hand, the concept of genuineness is often mistakenly assumed to mean blurting out whatever is on one's mind, often inappropriately burdening the client with having to deal with the therapist's reactions. Thus, we are not advocating impulsive therapist openness or "promiscuous self-disclosure" (Goodman & Esterley, 1990) but are, instead, suggesting *facilitative* genuineness. This is a form of *disciplined* spontaneity based on the therapist's *accurate* self-awareness of his or her deeper levels of experience and shared in a facilitative manner at a therapeutically *appropriate* moment.

For example, upon finding in herself a rising sense of criticism or annoyance toward the client's "controllingness," the therapist would not blurt out these perceptions or feelings. In most cases, it would not be therapeutic to disclose this annoyance. More to the point, such feelings are almost always secondary to more primary feelings, such as helplessness; that is to say, they are not internally congruent. Therefore, it is generally more helpful for the therapist to direct, in a disciplined manner, some attention inward to these feelings (sometimes between sessions) in order to discover the underlying feelings (cf. Gendlin, 1967). These might be expressed transparently as,

T: You know, as we go on, sometimes I feel I'd like to find a way of being more helpful to you, but often I feel unable to do so, sort of helpless or unable to break through to you. I worry that I'm not helping you explore more deeply, and I wonder how you feel.

Although transparency, the communicated state of internal genuineness or congruence, is typically conveyed through the therapist's manner, it may also be communicated directly through therapist disclosure, as above. It is worth emphasizing that it requires discipline and training to know one's essential experience and to communicate it to clients in a nonexploitive, nonmanipulative manner.

Finally, in more complex treatments, particularly with people with personality disorders, the genuine relationship becomes central. It is in the relational working through of the client's hurt, rage, and disappointment and in the therapist's ongoing awareness of his or her feelings in the therapeutic interaction that the therapy takes place. The therapist needs to be aware of how what the client does affects the therapist and to use this to help understand what is occurring in the client. In addition, therapists need to be aware when they have reached their own limits or feel they need to protect their own personal boundaries, and they need to be able to genuinely communicate these limits or boundaries to their client. It is from encountering another real human being who both cares for him or her and who is able to be authentically present, that a client grows.

Principle 3. Task Collaboration: Facilitate Mutual Involvement in Goals and Tasks of Therapy

Following Bordin (1979), we distinguish between Bond, Task, and Goal aspects of the therapeutic relationship or alliance. We have described how the therapist fosters an emotional bond with the client through experienced and communicated empathy, prizing, and genuineness. However, an effective therapeutic relationship also entails commitment and involvement by both client and therapist in the long-term and immediate goals of treatment (Goal aspect). It also involves commitment to the specific therapeutic activities carried out within sessions in order to realize these goals (Task aspect). In this section, we take the position that it is very important for the therapist to foster the closely linked Task and Goal aspects of the relationship (here combined under the heading of Task Collaboration).

Goal Agreement

First, the therapist needs to establish agreement on the general goals of treatment, those problems on which the client wishes to work in therapy. In this approach, the therapist works to understand the client's view of his or her goals and problems and accepts the client's goals rather than imposing goals on the client.

Thus, in order to avoid misunderstanding and to provide clarification, it is important that the therapist first explore and communicate understanding of client goals. The therapist then explicitly or implicitly agrees to work with the client on the presented problems; these may be specific problems such as dealing with procrastination or a decision about a relationship, or general goals such as feeling better, becoming less depressed, or the gaining of a greater sense of being in control of one's life.

As treatment continues, the client will typically refine and develop a particular goal, requiring the therapist to be attuned to its evolving nature. The goal that the client and therapist are working toward must at all times fit the client's current state, or else the treatment will founder. Active participation by the client in the treatment is the *sine qua non* of success; correctly understanding the client's goals and proposing tasks to help achieve these goals is a major factor in whether the treatment will succeed (Bordin, 1979; Horvath & Greenberg, 1986, 1989).

Global Task Agreement

Because treatment is based on the general or global task of experiencing and exploring feelings, therapy will only succeed if clients at least provisionally accept these tasks. Although these tasks sound general enough to be agreeable to most clients, in actual practice, a small group of clients find them unacceptable. This usually occurs because they perceive themselves as helpless and in need of guidance from a powerful authority who will provide them with guidance, self-understanding, and support, or because they seek specific behavioral interventions.

Specific Task Agreement

In order for clients to work on the specific therapeutic tasks, they must be both willing and able to carry out the various forms of therapeutic activity or "modes of engagement," such as attending and active expression. For example, in order to perform the therapeutic task of resolving an internal "split" or conflict, the client needs to engage in the task activity of actively expressing different partial aspects of self. Thus, the therapist informs the client of the specific proposed task and works to foster the client's collaboration and agreement to engage in it.

Empathic Attunement and the Therapeutic Bond go a long way toward establishing the "safety conditions" needed for clients to be willing to attempt novel or unusual therapeutic activities. In addition, orienting information can be provided as appropriate or necessary, when questions, ambiguity, or problems arise during the course of therapy. The therapist shares information, as needed, about the rationale or basis for specific therapeutic tasks or activities (e.g., talking to the "empty chair"), discussing and negotiating engagement in a task when this is called for.

Collaborative Tone and Client Task Abilities

Certain additional task-related relationship factors are necessary for motivating and enabling clients to engage in the activities of therapy. Generally, the therapist believes in the equality of therapist and client in cocreating the therapeutic relationship, and he or she acts in accord with this attitude, thereby helping to create an egalitarian and collaborative atmosphere. Typically, this attitude is communicated by using a collaborative, nonimposing style and avoiding an overly definitive or "expert" manner. It is engendered by a willingness to consider alternatives, to admit error or misunderstanding, and to negotiate disagreements. All of this is intended to foster a coexploration alliance, in which both participants are working together to explore and promote reorganization of the client's experience. The client's active participation is central.

In addition, the therapist sometimes needs to help the client to develop specific task abilities. As noted in Chapter 3, many individuals have difficulties with how they process their own experience, particularly their feelings. As a result, some clients beginning treatment will be unable to carry out some therapeutic activities, even though they are willing to do so. For example, some clients may not know that unclear feelings can be clarified by attending to an internally felt sense, or some may find it too embarrassing or anxiety provoking to express internal conflicts as arguments between aspects of oneself.

In summary, the three relationship principles (Empathic Attunement, Therapeutic Bond, and Task Collaboration) provide a model of the optimal client–therapist relationship in a Process-Experiential approach. The therapist begins by attuning him- or herself to the client's immediate experience, realizing and communicating an attitude of empathy, acceptance, warmth, congruence, and transparency, which attitude itself fosters the development of a positive emotional bond. For some clients this may be all that is needed to produce therapeutic benefit. Beyond this, the therapist also discusses the treatment rationale as needed and negotiates with the client in order to help him or her to become engaged with the global and specific tasks of treatment.

TASK PRINCIPLES: FACILITATE WORK ON SPECIFIC THERAPEUTIC TASKS

The three relationship principles discussed above describe the type of therapeutic relationship offered in this approach. We now turn to three treatment principles that specifically govern the pursuit of therapeutic tasks, keeping in mind, of course, that successful completion of therapeutic tasks also contributes to the further development and deepening of the relationship. The Task principles are based generally on the assumption that human beings are active, purposeful organisms, with an innate need for exploration and mastery of their environment (see Chapter 4). This is specifically expressed in attempts to achieve personal goals and solve internal problems. The therapist engages with clients to facilitate their resolution of their problems.

We will distinguish three task-oriented treatment principles. It is useful to think of these Task principles as providing a set of overall tasks for therapy. These are: the therapist facilitates productive experiential processing (Principle 4); the therapist fosters client growth and self-determination (Principle 5); and the therapist helps clients complete the therapeutic tasks they present (Principle 6).

Principle 4: Experiential Processing: Facilitate Optimal, Differential Client Processes

As noted in earlier chapters, it is important to engage the client in experiential as opposed to purely conceptual processing; furthermore, optimal client therapy performance is not limited to a single type of in-session experiential processing. Therefore, in helping the client to work on specific therapeutic tasks, the therapist facilitates the kind of client experiential processing that is most likely to be productive for that moment in the session and for that client.

In fact, everything that the therapist says has bearing on the client's experiential processing. A good proportion of what the therapist does in this approach is aimed directly at facilitating optimal experiential processing for that moment. On the other hand, some of what the therapist says is only indirectly intended to facilitate client experiential processing because its major intent is to provide a safe, understanding, receptive relationship.

We have delineated four different client modes of engagement (attending, experiential search, active expression, and interpersonal contact) that are valuable in different in-session contexts. Which of these is productive or optimal will vary between and within therapeutic tasks and can be differentially facilitated by the therapist. Furthermore, at different times, within any of these processes and more generally, the therapist will be attempting to facilitate different internal client processes in order to enhance the client's experiential processing. Consequently, the therapist continually uses "micromarkers" to make momentary "microprocess diagnoses" of what is likely to be optimal at given moments in therapy. The therapist then intervenes differentially to best stimulate the client's experiential processing.

Given Empathic Attunement and a good therapeutic bond and task collaboration, the therapist has a number of options available at any moment for helping the client to work optimally in the session, including helping the client to direct attentional focus in particular ways at particular times, to modulate affective intensity, to explore experiences with particularity and concreteness, to own experience, and to symbolize ongoing experiencing.

Thus, when an opportunity for exploring internally appears, the therapist can facilitate the client's process by suggesting that the client focus attention on a specific domain of current experience, such as a bodily sensation, a feeling, or a need. This is particularly appropriate for tasks where the attending mode of engagement is important.

At other times, when an increase in the client's level of arousal would help bring the material alive for the client, the therapist can help the client to intensify, heighten, or evoke experiencing. This is most consistent with the active expression mode of engagement, but it may be relevant at other times as well. Alternatively, there are times when feelings are experienced as being overwhelming, and the client expresses a desire to set aside these feelings. At such times the therapist may try to help the client regulate his or her level of arousal (e.g., by breathing or "coming back to the present").

The therapist at other times may help the client to explore an experience, particularly in tasks where the experiential search mode of engagement is central. In promoting exploration, the therapist may encourage the client to explore the "edges" of experience by attending to what the client is groping toward, to what is unclear, emerging, poignant, idiosyncratic, or possibility oriented (Bohart et al., in press; Martin, 1983; Rice, 1974). At times, the therapist may work toward helping the client to differentiate experience, encouraging the client to describe experience in more detail or to elaborate further meanings implicit in his or her experience.

Further, at appropriate moments the therapist may help clients to identify with their experience and internal processes by speaking in the first person or by "becoming" some aspect of themselves.

Finally, there are times when it is valuable for the therapist to help the client to create meaning from experiencing, often moving them from bodily experiences to symbolizing what is experienced. Especially near the end of a session, or after some unit of therapeutic work has been accomplished, the therapist may help the client "process" any therapeutic impacts that may be emerging in order to develop a "meaning perspective" on what has happened. This is done by asking the client what has happened for him or her or how he or she understands what has occurred.

Principle 5: Foster Client Growth and Self-determination (Growth/ Choice)

Working within a humanistic framework with existential roots, this approach emphasizes the importance of the client's internal agency. This is manifested in the twin tendencies toward growth/mastery and self-determination/choice. Thus, the therapist emphasizes and values the client's potential for both development and self-ownership on the one hand, and for freedom, choice, and mature interdependence, on the other hand.

In this approach, helping clients to realize their potential for growth and self-determination is an overall treatment task. It is one of the few instances in which the therapist pursues a therapeutic aim that may sometimes differ from the client's, for example, when the client tries to get the therapist to make decisions for him or her. However, this goal or principle is not pursued in isolation or imposed on the client. Instead, the Growth/Choice principle is typically reflected in the manner in which the therapist carries out other tasks and principles.

Like the other treatment principles, Growth/Choice is based on a set of attitudes held by the therapist. In order to realize this principle, the therapist views the client as capable of growth, mastery, and active positive coping, as having genuine rights, as truly free, and as the expert on the content of his or her experiencing.

Listening for Growth

One way for the therapist to encourage client growth and self-determination is by listening carefully for, and encouraging ownership of, the client's "growing edge." The major method for doing this is "empathic selection." That is, the therapist reflects aspects of client experience that involve emerging experience, or ownership; strengths, progress or active coping; desire for change, mastery, or contact with others; personal rights, mature interdependence and mutuality; positive aspects of self; and plans or projects for the future.

Sometimes the client's mode of expression communicates that this is "new ground" that is possibly being lightly tread upon for the first time. At other times, the client may express something verbally or nonverbally but without full awareness of it. For example, the client may briefly express anger, through a facial expression, a kicking movement, or an inflection in the voice. In either case, the therapist offers the client an opportunity to attend to the emerging new experience, indirectly encouraging the client to "own" it.

Active Participation and Self-determination

Engaging the client in an active role in the change process is central to our approach. Allowing the client freedom or choice about the goals and tasks in therapy is an important aspect of this principle and a basic stance for the therapist. At times, the therapist explicitly offers the client choices about what happens in therapy. This includes the tasks and topics for each session, whether to approach or avoid a particular painful topic, whether to try a particular method (e.g., Two-Chair Dialogue) for working on a task, and even when to stop working. In addition, the therapist implicitly supports client choice in a variety of ways, such as listening carefully for task markers (which are indirect signs of client interest in working on particular in-session tasks) and treating the client as the final judge of his or her experience.

It should be noted that the process of choosing described here is not primarily an intellectual one of weighing alternatives, or a deliberate process of forcing oneself to choose (cf. Yalom, 1980). In the experiential approach, choice is viewed as coming out of an open, patient, intuitive consideration of the range of one's current experiencing.

It is important to recognize that, even though the Growth/Choice principle is generally consistent with Empathic Attunement and Therapeutic Bond, there are situations in which these do conflict with one another. Such a case would occur when the therapist's desire to foster client growth and self-determination creates the risk of misunderstanding or not accepting the client. The most striking of these situations occurs when the therapist believes that the client is free and capable of overcoming his or her difficulties, while the client feels utterly trapped or undeserving. In this situation, the therapist tries to balance the two values, understanding and accepting the client's view while disclosing his or her sincere personal belief that change is possible.

Principle 6. Task Completion: Facilitate Completion of Specific Therapeutic Tasks

Many therapeutic tasks are not completed, at least not the first time they are introduced! Thus, the last process-experiential treatment principle is helping the client to finish therapeutic tasks. Because there are so many ways to *not* finish things, the therapist needs a number of different strategies to help resolve therapeutic tasks.

First, the therapist trains him- or herself to think in terms of therapeutic tasks. The therapeutic task is an important element of the client's immediate experiencing, and it is vital for the therapist to track the client's task as it moves forward and evolves. However, neophyte therapists are often so caught up in listening to the client's content and with practicing skills that they "lose the thread" of the task!

Second, each therapeutic task has its own unique set of steps and pitfalls. The successful resolution of therapeutic tasks involves a natural sequence. By knowing these steps, the therapist can help the client avoid getting stuck or "dead-ended" and can facilitate the client's movement to the next step when he or she is ready to do so. In Chapters 8–13, we describe the steps followed by clients in successfully resolving each of six different major therapeutic tasks. Thus, it is very useful for the therapist to be able accurately to recognize the steps within each task as well as the therapist interventions likely to facilitate work within each step.

Third, it is important for the therapist to develop an attitude of patient, gentle persistence when working on therapeutic tasks. The therapist stays focused on the session task, gently returning to it when the client wanders into other issues. The therapist also knows that a task often needs to be focused on a number of times in order to achieve resolution and that if the task is important, the client will bring it up again in a later session.

Fourth, the therapist evaluates when to switch tasks or continue to focus on the same therapeutic task. Overall, it is best to minimize most kinds of task interruption, especially the initiation of another task. On the other hand, it is sometimes useful to encourage the client to move to a task that is currently more alive and that may in fact be more likely to be resolved. At other times, it might be better to move back to empathic exploration when a specific task "goes dead" or is currently not alive or central.

Thus, there are times when the therapist is uncertain about whether to stay with the original task (Task Completion) or whether to switch to a new, apparently more compelling task (Experiential Processing). If the therapist routinely encourages switching whenever something new comes along, sessions may end up feeling scattered, and few therapeutic tasks will be finished. On the other hand, rigid adherence to a particular current task is counterproductive, especially in situations where the client is not ready to resolve, or where an emerging task is clearly more alive for the client. This is obviously a clinical judgment requiring sensitivity, experience, negotiation, and, most important, following the client's lead.

Finally, it is important to maintain a balance between task-focusedness (exemplified by the Task Completion principle) and the therapeutic relationship. At times, the therapist's efforts to identify and persist on the task focus, even though gentle, may be experienced by the client as a threatening pressure to stay with experiences that are painful or frustrating. This may strain the relationship, requiring efforts to evaluate and repair possible damage. Anticipating this possibility, the therapist listens carefully and is prepared to offer the client the choice to back off or move to a different task. Empathic Attunement to the client's experience is the ultimate guide in such situations.

SUMMARY

In this chapter we have presented the six basic principles followed by therapists who use a process-experiential approach for facilitating emotional change. These principles are the basis for the therapist's specific interventions (see Chapter 7) and the major therapeutic tasks (Chapters 8–13). The principles include three Relationship principles (Empathic Attunement, Therapeutic Bond, Task Collaboration) and three Task principles, (Experiential Processing, Growth/Choice, and Task Completion). These principles are understood not as absolutes but as a set of values that must be combined and balanced with one another in particular situations.

In the next chapter, we describe the fundamental therapist intentions and types of therapist responses used to realize the treatment principles in the process-experiential approach for facilitating emotional change.

C H A P T E R 7

WHAT THE THERAPIST DOES: EXPERIENTIAL RESPONSE INTENTIONS AND MODES

I N THE PREVIOUS CHAPTER, we gave an account of the essence of the process-experiential approach, those principles that guide the therapist. In this chapter, we describe what the therapist actually *does* in order to carry out those principles. In doing so, we will use the concept of different basic *experiential response intentions* to organize the different classes of therapist response according to their primary functions in Process-Experiential treatment. Response intentions are not exactly the same as response modes (Elliott et al., 1987); instead, they provide the basis for the response modes and are a more fundamental way of describing therapist behavior (Goodman & Dooley, 1976; Stiles, 1986). This chapter is organized according to experiential response intentions, with response modes used to define the most common means used to carry out each intention.

We divide the experiential response intentions into three groups, essential, additional, and out-of-mode intentions (see Table 7-1). These three sets of therapist intentions provide an initial view of exactly what the therapist does and does *not* do. First, the therapist relies most heavily on a set of specialized experiential response intentions. These "essential experiential intentions" include Empathic Understanding, Empathic Exploration, Process Directing, and Experiential Presence. Second, the therapist also sometimes carries out supplementary intentions, including Experiential Teaching, Process Observation, and Revealing Self to the client. Finally, the therapist tries to avoid the "out of mode" intentions of

TABLE 7-1. Therapist Experiential Response Intentions and Response Modes

A. Essential Experiential Intentions

1. Empathic Understanding: Responses intended primarily to communicate understanding of immediate client feelings and emotionally-tinged meanings:
   a. Empathic Reflection: Reflections of central, poignant or vivid in client feelings or meanings (including evocative or growth reflections)
   b. Following responses ("Uh-huhs")

2. Empathic Exploration: Responses intended to encourage client exploration while maintaining empathic attunement:
   a. Exploratory Reflection: Evocative, "open edge," and growth reflections
   b. Exploratory Question: Experiencing, "fill-in," and "fit" questions
   c. Empathic Conjecture: Tentatively reflecting what is unexpressed but likely to be in the client's immediate experience

3. Process Directing: Responses intended to direct in-session process, i.e., process suggestions:
   a. Attention suggestions
   b. Action suggestions
   c. Structuring tasks
   d. Awareness homework

4. Experiential Presence: Stylistic aspects of therapist action intended to manifest the therapist's attitude, state or manner of being with the client:
   a. Silence
   b. Vocal quality
   c. Appropriate nonverbal communication

B. Additional Experiential Intentions

1. Experiential Teaching: Responses intended to provide information about treatment processes or tasks

2. Process Observation: Responses intended to point out nonverbal and verbal communication

3. Revealing Self: Responses explicitly intended to disclose the therapist to the client:
   a. Process Disclosure (immediacy responses for repair, limit-setting)
   b. Personal Disclosure (facilitative, responsive to client)

C. Generally "Out-of-Mode" Nonexperiential Intentions

1. Giving News: Responses intended to tell the client something new about self or others; i.e., interpretations (explaining, linking, or belief-modifying responses)

2. Providing Solutions: Responses intended to modify client behavior; i.e., general advisements (telling client what to do outside session; except awareness homework)

3. Offering Expert Reassurance: Responses directly intended to make the client feel good; i.e., content reassurances (praising, agreeing with client, etc. from an "expert" position)

4. Directing Content: Responses intended to direct the topic of the session; i.e., content suggestions

5. Disagreeing/Confronting: Responses intended to differ with the client or to point out discrepancies

Giving News, Providing Solutions, Offering Expert Reassurance, Directing Content, and Disagreeing/Confronting.

The experiential response intentions and associated response modes describe only one aspect of what the therapist does in therapy. It is vital that they not be implemented mechanically or as a substitute for the underlying attitudes or principles described in the previous chapter. The current overall task in the session guides the therapist's response intentions and modes. In addition to summarizing the response intentions under the three general headings, we will attempt to describe how and when they are best carried out.

ESSENTIAL EXPERIENTIAL RESPONSE INTENTIONS

We begin with the therapist experiential intentions that are most consistent with the treatment principles described in the previous chapter. These account for most of what the therapist does in the process-experiential approach. The major experiential tasks described in later chapters are generally built out of these intentions, and they are central to other experiential tasks as well (e.g., creation of meaning; Clarke, 1989, 1991). Previous versions of essential therapist actions and intentions have been developed and tested (Goldman, 1991; Greenberg & Goldman, 1988). This version represents an updated description of therapist intentions and responses, developed for the purposes of this book.

Empathic Understanding

A key intention of the process-experiential approach is Empathic Understanding, carried out by therapist responses that seek simply to communicate understanding of the client's message. These responses include simple reflections and related responses ("Uh-huh's") made famous by Carl Rogers (1951). In addition to communicating empathy, such responses commonly serve to enhance the client–therapist relationship, to offer prizing and support to the client (through understanding), and to underline emerging issues. Thus, Empathic Understanding responses are a major means by which the therapist realizes the Empathic Attunement and Therapeutic Bond principles described in the previous chapter.

In our discussion, we are drawing a distinction between Empathic Understanding and another key response intention, that of Empathic Exploration, which will be defined as facilitating client exploration within an empathic frame. Empathic Exploration responses seek to communicate understanding and to help clients to enter into their experiencing more intensely, or to move toward the unclear or emerging edges of their experience; they thus combine both understanding and exploration intentions. In contrast, Empathic Understanding responses simply attempt to provide the client with "solid" empathy, without trying to "do" anything but understand.

Understanding versus Giving News: Reflection and Interpretation

Another very important distinction is between both kinds of empathic intention (Empathic Understanding and Empathic Exploration) and a very different, out-of-mode intention, Giving News. In terms of therapist responses, this distinction comes down to the difference between the responses traditionally referred to as reflections and interpretations (Elliott et al., 1987).

Thus, in the process-experiential approach, it is essential for the therapist to be able to distinguish between reflections and interpretations. When the therapist reflects, the primary intention is either to communicate understanding of the client's immediate experience or to help the client explore, or both. When the therapist interprets, the intention is to give the client "news," something new about self, generally in the form of motivational explanation or linking across domains. For example, the client might say,

C: My mother had high blood pressure and a bad heart, but I think she was a hypochondriac. And once us girls got old enough, she didn't do hardly anything, and it was left up to us. I had to do it or else it didn't get done.

In response, the therapist might reflect with:

T: Uh-huh, so it was either you did it or it didn't get done, just a sense of "I have to do it!"

Here the therapist intends to convey her understanding of what it felt like for the client.

On the other hand, an interpretation of the same content might go as follows:

T: So perhaps this connects with why it's difficult now to get things done at home when it's all left to you, because it makes you feel like you did then.

The second response intends to shed new light rather than to communicate understanding of client experience in the belief that if the client sees the connection or the pattern, this will lead to greater self-understanding. This response is *not* a reflection and is *not* an appropriate response in this approach (see discussion on "Out-of-mode" responses, later in this chapter).

The definitions of reflection and interpretation, and particularly the distinction between the two kinds of therapist responses, have long been the subject of debate. For the purpose of this book and for the sake of promoting clarity in describing what the therapist does, we believe that it is more useful to define reflections as responses intended to communicate understanding of the client's immediate experience and to define interpretations as responses intended to offer the client something new, outside his or her current experience or frame of reference. This distinction holds, in spite of the fact that empathic responses, including reflection, involve a perceptual "act of interpretation," in the broad or hermeneutic sense of finding the client's meaning in what he or she says. By the same token, therapist news-giving or interpretive responses often may be experienced by clients as empathic when they are perceived as accurately respresenting some aspect of the client's experience. Modern self and interpersonally oriented psychodynamic therapists may in fact offer interpretations that are experienced as empathic and may also reflect. It remains true, in our view, however, that interpretations are often implicitly disempowering or sometimes even punitive or critical (Piper, Debanne, Blenvenu, Carufel, & Garant, 1986) and that empathic responses rarely if ever are viewed this way. This is a further reason for us emphasizing the importance of empathy and empathic intentions in this approach and attempting to maintain rather than blur the distinction between empathy and interpretation.

We will describe two types of Empathic Understanding response empathic reflection and following responses:

1. *Empathic Reflection.* Empathic reflections convey understanding and prizing most successfully when they focus on the most central, poignant, or vivid aspect of the client's feelings, subjective meanings, and inner reactions, for example:

C: . . . I had a lot of difficulties with my parents. They were so controlling. Like when I was little, my parents used to make me eat every last piece of food on my plate, they stood over me watching, and I couldn't *stand* it! I felt so helpless.

T: Being forced like that was almost more than you could bear.

Therapists often oversimplify the idea of reflecting feelings, thinking that responses such as "You really feel angry" or "You feel very unhappy," are generally sufficient. However, Rogers' (1959) definition of *experiencing a feeling* suggests that something more is often needed: "It denotes an emotionally tinged experience, together with its personal meaning. Thus it includes the emotion but also the cognitive content or the meaning of the emotion in its experiential context" (p. 198). This definition makes it clear that it is not just "emotion" to which the therapist responds but the whole experience, including its meaning for the client. A good reflection usually has quite a different flavor from a response that simply parrots the emotion. This does not mean giving a lengthy summary, but it suggests instead that the therapist pay careful attention to the particular nuance and flavor of the particular experience, for example:

C: And after he made fun of me for feeling pleased with how I'd done, my sense of accomplishment just disappeared!
T: The sparkle just vanished, and it left you feeling so robbed.

The goal is to capture what it was really like for the person, not merely to capture some theme of dysfunctional process. Good empathic reflection is difficult to master. It requires careful attunement to the nature, quality, and intensity of ever-changing client experiencing. In any client statement there are typically a number of different things for the therapist to reflect back to the client. This requires that the therapist use "empathic selection" to identify what is to be reflected, usually based on an intuitive sense of the "core" or most poignant aspect of the client's message. Good empathic reflections require extensive practice, close listening, and full absorption within the session.

2. *Following Responses.* In addition, it is important to mention the role of following responses, those small signs of understanding also known as "acknowledgments," "minimal encouragers," and "following responses." These responses include

- Uh-huh, Mm-hmm.
- I see; I understand.
- Yes; OK.
- Head nods; smiles.

Here is an example that illustrates the role of following responses and empathic reflection:

C: It's like a new part of me, that I never really accepted before, is starting to come out. [T: (*quietly*) yes] And (*pause*) and I feel a bit afraid of it, [T: Mm-hmm] but as I start to let it out, (*silence*) [T: Yes] There's an anger.
T: Yes, you're a bit scared of it, but there is an anger there.

Following responses, such as these, serve largely to communicate the therapist's understanding, enabling the client to continue and elaborate.

Empathic Exploration

In our description of what the therapist does in the Process-Experiential approach, we have taken the step of distinguishing between Empathic Understanding and Empathic Exploration responses. In our view, many therapist responses in this therapy are intended to do more than communicate therapist understanding and maintain the relationship. These responses provide another way of facilitating the client, in which empathy is present but is accompanied by important intentions—those of fostering client self-exploration (the Experiential Processing principle) and of creating a coexploratory alliance. These key responses take a number of different forms, including exploratory reflection, exploratory question, process observation, and empathic conjecture, with a number of variant subtypes under the first two forms.

Exploratory Reflections

Exploratory reflections are defined as therapist responses that intend to create a coexploratory set and to guide or stimulate client self-exploration through communicating partial, tentative or "in-process" understandings. They are expressed as the therapist's own attempt to follow the client. These responses often focus on the edges, emerging or unclear aspects of client experiencing, and as a result, they typically have a tentative quality, for example:

T: (*said with a questioning quality in the voice*) I'm not sure . . . , sounds like you felt kind of put down when he said that.

In addition to communicating in-process partial understanding and stimulating the exploration process, exploratory reflections have several related uses, expressed in a number of closely related and sometimes overlapping subtypes.

First, *evocative reflections* attempt to "open up" the client's meaning with fresh language, vivid imagery, expressive manner, or tentative, exploratory manner (Rice, 1974; Martin, 1983). Consider again the client example used earlier:

C: My mother had high blood pressure and a bad heart, but I think she was a hypochondriac. And once us girls got old enough, she didn't do hardly anything, and it was left up to us. I had to do it or else it didn't get done.

Here are several alternate evocative reflections for this response:

T: Almost like she would say, "Oh my *heart!*—*You* do it!" and you would just feel this tremendous sense of responsibility.

T: And so I guess you were handed this real burden to carry; and you just gritted your teeth and carried it.

In addition to using metaphor, these responses are also sometimes done in the first person, with the therapist speaking as the client. Thus, in response to a client statement about feeling cheated the therapist might say.

T: So it's like you want to say, "You weasel! It wasn't fair!"

Second, an *"open-edge" reflection* leaves the focus of the response on the open or "leading" edge of the client's experience, usually that aspect of experience that is most alive or poignant in the client presentation. Thus, in using exploratory reflections, the therapist does not respond in a way that packages the client statement and hands it back in a "finished" or closed form; instead the therapist offers an open response that leaves its emphasis on the most poignant aspect in a manner that promotes further exploration. Closed empathic responses stop client exploration, as when the client responds "Yes, that's just what I feel!" then waits for the therapist to say something else. Take, for instance, responses to the following client statement:

C: I'd like to be able to speak up more in class, I really would, but when I think of something to say, I get scared, and I just clam up.

If the therapist's reflection balances both sides of the conflicted feelings, this is likely to have a packaging effect:

T: So you really want to speak in class, but at the same time you're too scared to.

In an "open edge" response, the therapist leaves the focus on one side or the other. For instance, the open edge might be left on the desire to speak up:

T: Even though it scares you, it sounds like what you really long for is to be able to speak up, give a voice to your thoughts.

Another exploratory reflection might pick up the fear, if that is most poignant or seems to be the leading edge of the client's experience:

T: So, when you even think of speaking up, there's a kind of scared feeling, sort of tightening up like, I dunno, it's just so risky to open up.

Third, *growth-oriented reflections* pick up on the client's growth edge or new possibilities and are useful for focusing clients on their developmental trajectory when it emerges, even to the slightest degree (cf. Bohart et al., 1991). This follows the Growth/Choice principle discussed in Chapter 6. The following example of a growth-oriented reflection is also evocative and leaves an open edge:

C: I feel like I'm stuck at the bottom of a big black pit. It's so lonely and I'm stuck. I keep struggling to get out but I can't seem to make it.
T: It's so dark and deep down, it's hard to get out, you can't quite make it, but you keep trying desperately to get out, to make contact.

This type of response, which leaves the focus on the sense of struggle rather than the sense of failure, accurately reflects that the client is more in touch with struggling to survive than with failing to do so, and serves a crucial function in helping access clients' growth possibilities. A balance is needed between appropriately attuned possibility-oriented responses and those that are focused more on *what is* rather than what is sensed but not yet achieved. Nevertheless, the ability to focus on a growth edge is an important aspect of the Process-Experiential approach.

Exploratory Question

Open-ended, exploratory questions play an important role in the Process-Experiential approach, where questions are rarely asked for purely information-gathering purposes. Exploratory questions, together with process suggestions (described below), reflect the influence of Gestalt therapy on this approach. The major purpose of exploratory questions is to encourage client exploration of experience.

The most important form of exploratory question is the *experiencing question*, an inquiry about various aspects of the client's present or past experiencing, including:

- Emotional feelings.
- Perceptions of situations.
- Bodily sensations.
- Meanings.
- Wishes or desires.
- Intentions.

Particular versions of this question are not to be over-used, lest they become therapy cliches. Responses such as, "How does that make you feel?" seem particularly vulnerable to becoming cliched and may also be asking the client for information that is not in his or her immediate awareness. Therefore, such questions are generally to be avoided. Alternative versions of the experiencing question can be used, and the particular form varied, including:

T: What are you experiencing right now?
T: What were you aware of right then?
T: What do you want from her?
T: What does that feel like?

Other variant subtypes of exploratory question are collaborative questions and "fit" questions. In *collaborative questions*, the therapist stops in the middle of a sentence and leaves a definite blank or open edge intended to help the client to fill in or elaborate. Client and therapist are therefore collaborating on constructing the sentence:

C: Up until this week it's been OK.
T: And now you're feeling . . .
C: . . . very uptight about seeing him again.

Collaborative questions are useful for modeling a joint therapeutic exploration process, but it is best not to overuse them.

"Fit" questions (short for "Does that fit?") seek confirmation of a therapist or client statement, and they are important for helping the therapist to maintain responsiveness and avoid imposing on the client. Although they are used with a variety of other responses, fit questions are most commonly combined with exploratory reflections, for example,

T: (*tentative manner*): So, it's like you're worrying that you're losing a friend, is that how it feels?

or:

T: Almost a "gnarled up" feeling? Is that what it's like?

Empathic Conjecture

Another, deeper form of empathic exploratory response is empathic conjecture, in which the therapist empathically guesses at what the client may be currently feeling but has not yet said out loud. Typically, but not always, the client may have been expressing this nonverbally or may have been hinting at something or saying it "between the lines." These responses are about current inner experience (rather than psychogenetic causes or patterns) and are intended to help capture the client's current experience rather than to interpret an unacknowledged experience. They attempt to promote client experiencing, not to help the client to see something in a new way. However, because they are speculative, the therapist delivers them in a tentative manner, typically as a reflection–question hybrid or combined with a "fit" question, thus encouraging the client to check the empathic conjecture against what he or she actually experiences. For example,

C: I don't know, somehow I just can't seem to get up the extra energy to do it, and so I'm just going to kiss it goodbye (*sighs*).

T: I guess I hear some real sadness there. Is that what you feel?

Here is another example:

C: (*voice shaky*) Gee, I don't know if this is a good thing to talk about. I'm not sure.

T: Maybe it's a bit scary right now.

Process Directing

"Direct process not content." This simple slogan sums up our position on therapist advisement or directive responses (e.g., guidance, suggestions). It is "out of mode" to tell the client what to do to solve problems outside the therapy session, but it is "in mode" to suggest in a nonimposing way that the client try certain things within the session, in order to facilitate here-and-now exploration and problem resolution.

Process-directing responses offer in-session suggestions about process, in keeping with the Experiential Processing principle (discussed in Chapter 6). They correspond to the response mode, process suggestion. The therapist attempts to facilitate optimal client experiencing, most commonly by guiding client attention or action in the session. The process-directing response intention includes setting up or structuring new tasks and "stage-managing" ongoing tasks (e.g., Chair Work).

It should be noted that the therapist's manner in process-guiding responses is warm, gentle, and tentative. This type of response does not include imposing, pressuring, or manipulating the client. The client should get the feeling that what is suggested is just something that might possibly be useful to try right now, but if he or she does not care to do it, that is perfectly all right with the therapist. In addition, process-guiding responses are only made when they are clearly appropriate to the current task and the client's level of perceived safety with the therapist.

Attention suggestions direct the client to attend to some aspect of his or her current experiencing, for example,

T: See if you can stay with the heavy feeling a bit longer.

T: Can you pay attention to your breathing as you tell me this?

T: Turn you attention inward and see what comes to you.

Action suggestions, on the other hand, seek to facilitate productive client experiencing by directing the client to take specific actions in the session, most commonly:

- Enacting an aspect of self.
- Experiencing something in an enactment.
- Carrying out some mental action, such as asking oneself a question, waiting patiently for a feeling, or pushing away an experience that is too painful.

For example:

T: Will you change chairs and tell her how you react to her criticisms.

T: The next thing is take a minute and ask yourself, "What is this feeling all about?"

Structuring tasks is another form of process-directing response, in which the therapist suggests or sets up an in-session experiment, often accompanied by an explanation of what it is and how it works.

T: OK, I am going to suggest that we put these two sides in different chairs. Presumably you have never bounced around in chairs before and there may be some self-consciousness about it, but let's just set it up and see where we go, OK?

Awareness Homework is a variant form of process suggestion in which the therapist suggests a method for carrying the therapeutic process beyond the confines of the session. Thus, the therapist may suggest that the client attend to certain kinds of experiences outside of the session. For example, if the topic of the session has been how a client criticizes himself, the therapist might say at the end of the session,

T: During the week, it might be useful for you to become aware of when and how you do this to yourself.

It is important to note that Awareness Homework is not intended to provide "answers" to the client's problems (which would violate the Growth/Choice principle), but merely to carry the therapeutic process beyond the confines of the session.

Experiential Presence

As we have been attempting to stress, it is not only *what* the therapist does, but *how* the therapist does it that is important. In addition to describing intentions and response modes, manner and style are an important aspect of what the therapist does. We have therefore emphasized the importance of a therapist manner that is genuinely patient, warm, gentle, and involved. In helping the client pursue the "work" of therapy, the relational attitudes involved in fostering the

Therapeutic Bond (Principle 2) are largely communicated through the therapist's "presence" or manner of being with the client. This "Experiential Presence" can be described concretely in terms of paralinguistic and nonverbal behaviors, including silence, vocal quality, and appropriate posture and expression.

Silence

Because silence seems to facilitate inner exploration and the emergence of new experience (Gendlin, 1981; Goodman & Esterly, 1990), it has an important role in this approach. However, once again, the attitude is more important than the action: the therapist's attitude of patience and respect for the client's inner processes is more vital than the behavior of allowing silence to occur. Thus, the therapist waits for the client to finish what he or she was trying to say, avoiding interruption or overtalk. At the same time, the therapist does not impose silence on a client who is uncomfortable with it, and he or she notes the client's reactions to and use of silence.

Vocal quality is another important aspect of the therapist's Experiential Presence, especially because it is tightly linked to the therapist's own immediate experience and attitude toward the client, and it communicates much of the therapist's prizing, empathy, and genuineness with the client (Rice & Kerr, 1986). In fact, therapists can use their own vocal quality as an indicator of their immediate attitude toward the client. For example, if a therapist becomes aware that she is speaking in a "definite" or "patterned" (i.e., lecturing) voice, this probably means that she has departed from a genuinely prizing, empathic, or collaborative stance.

On the other hand, it may be productive for the therapist to try to develop in him- or herself the attitude that goes with an irregular, inwardly focused voice of exploration, or a softened or "prizing" voice signaling warmth, gentleness, and caring. The latter, prizing voice is particularly important when the therapist is suggesting exercises or when new or painful client experience is emerging. Finally, the therapist should remember that vocal quality cannot be "faked"; in fact, therapists who try to "put on" a prizing voice may end up sounding merely distanced or uninterested (Rice & Kerr, 1986). Therapist vocal quality has to be regarded as a genuine expression of the therapist's immediate experience of the relationship.

Nonverbal Behavior

In addition to vocal quality, various aspects of the therapist's nonverbal behavior are also important, including appropriate physical posture and distance, speech gestures, eye contact or gaze, and facial expression. This can take a wide variety of forms at different moments in therapy. For example, the therapist typically sits comfortably and naturally but in a way that indicates genuine involvement with the client and gestures naturally while speaking. He or she makes appropriate eye contact with the client to communicate genuine interest and involvement but does not stare at the client or intrude upon the client when the client's attention is turned inward. The therapist also allows him- or herself to express genuine concern, caring, or surprise through facial expression and shares in laughter with the client.

ADDITIONAL EXPERIENTIAL INTENTIONS

A number of other experiential response intentions are also used in the process-experiential approach, including Experiential Teaching, Process Observation, and Revealing Self. These intentions are less common than the essential experiential intentions described in the previous section, and they are typically restricted to special therapeutic contexts or tasks, where they are employed in support of one or more of the Treatment Principles.

Experiential Teaching

The most important additional experiential intention is providing the client with general information about the treatment and the nature of the experiencing process (e.g., the importance of exploring feelings). Experiential Teaching responses typically only occur in one of two specific contexts: First, they may be used in discussing the treatment rationale or process or when introducing a new therapeutic task to the client, for example,

T: In our work together, I attempt to understand what you feel and make suggestions to help you explore your feelings.

T: It's helpful to try and listen inside to what you're experiencing in the moment and to speak from that feeling.

T: It sounds like you're experiencing a kind of argument between two different parts of you. The purpose of putting the two parts in different chairs is to bring this inner dialogue out into the open.

Second, Experiential Teaching may be used when there is some form of disruption in the task aspect of the alliance (Principle 3). This might involve client complaints about the process or client difficulties in carrying out therapeutic tasks. For example, if a client complains about the therapist not giving advice, the therapist might say something like:

T: I understand it's hard to have me not tell you what to do, but I feel I just

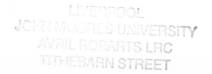

couldn't possibly know what is the best solution for you. I would like to help you to find your *own* answer to your problem.

As can be seen, Experiential Teaching is often best combined with disclosure (see below) and empathy. The therapist should be careful to avoid using a lecturing or critical tone.

Process Observation

Therapists in the process-experiential approach need to be particularly tuned into the manner of their clients' verbal and nonverbal expression. Brief, nonconfrontational comments calling the client's attention to these may facilitate awareness and exploration of as yet unspoken aspects of client experiencing and tacit emotion schemes. Thus, the therapist may make note of a facial expression, bodily movement, vocal quality, or style of speech in the session:

T: I'm aware that you're kicking your leg right now.
T: When you say this, you have a pained look on your face.
T: As you talk, your attention seems to be focused on other people rather than yourself.

These responses are often accompanied by a process suggestion to attend to or do something with what has been observed. It is very important that such responses be done in a warm, nonjudgmental manner, with no sense of "pouncing on" or trying to "catch" the client in conscious or unconscious "slips." Similarly, Process Observations are not used to point out discrepancies or contradictions between verbal and nonverbal expression.

Revealing Self

A final supplemental experiential intention is Revealing Self, which typically involves the therapist response mode of self-disclosure. In keeping with the notion of genuineness or transparency (described under the Therapeutic Bond principle), Revealing Self responses are primarily used to maintain a genuine relationship in which the therapist encounters the client as one human being to another in whatever way is felt to be important to help the client grow. In doing so, the therapist may share either an immediate, within-session experience (process disclosure), or a more general fact about him- or herself (personal disclosure).

Process Disclosure

This involves therapist self-disclosure of immediate here-and-now reactions, intentions, or limitations. These responses are used primarily to focus on the relationship between client and therapist, often to work through what is occurring in the relationship or to clarify misunderstandings. Process disclosures convey a sense of presence and immediacy. For example, the therapist may share his or her *internal responses* to the immediate here and now process between client and therapist when that is appropriate and facilitative, for example,

T: As I listen to what you're telling me, I'm feeling moved to tears.

Process disclosures can be used to let the client know about the therapist's *limits* or limitations, particularly when something is interfering or could interfere with the therapist's ability to focus therapeutic attention on the client:

T: I think I should let you know that I am not feeling that well today. I've got a bad cold, so if I seem a bit tired that's why!
T: I think I really misunderstood you there. Maybe you could tell me again so that I could try to get it clear.
T: I'm sorry, I don't feel comfortable meeting with you socially outside of therapy.

Personal Disclosures

The therapist may also occasionally disclose personal information involving his or her experiences outside the therapy session. These responses are fairly rare, as they risk distracting the client from his or her own experiencing. Thus, personal disclosure is only done when it is likely to be facilitative to the client, such as when it is needed in support of the Therapeutic Bond. One such situation occurs when the client requests personal information, for example,

C: Do you have kids?
T: Yes, I have a three-year-old.

In this instance, refusing to answer an appropriate question might communicate a lack of genuineness on the part of the therapist (Therapeutic Bond) and discourage client openness (Task Collaboration).

GENERALLY "OUT-OF-MODE" NONEXPERIENTIAL INTENTIONS

"Out-of-mode" or nonexperiential response intentions are generally to be avoided when the therapist is working experientially. These response intentions are out of mode because they violate the basic principles that guide the treatment, particularly Growth/Choice and Empathic Attunement.

Giving News

As noted earlier, therapist *interpretations* as typically defined in the literature (Brenner, 1976) are intended to give the client new information or expert evaluation about him- or herself. It is not that interpretations are "bad"; rather, they are simply not in line with the underlying principles, tasks, and processes of the Process-Experiential approach. Interpretations violate the Growth/Choice principle because they set the therapist up as an expert on the client's experiencing, creating the risk of disempowering the client. Interpretations, particularly theory-guided interpretations that link two different areas of the client's life, also violate the Empathic Attunement and Experiential Processing principles: they are outside the client's current frame of reference, may distract the client from further experiential processing, and can encourage the client to shift into purely conceptual processing (i.e., intellectualizing).

When therapists with previous psychodynamic training begin to use the process-experiential approach, they sometimes have trouble giving up interpretations. One of the authors (RE) was helped through this "weaning" process by the observation that however clever an interpretation might seem to him, it would almost certainly have turned out to be inferior to the client's own eventually arrived at idiosyncratic self-understanding.

Providing Solutions for the client by offering advisements about their problems is also "out of mode," in much the same way as Giving News through interpretations. Both responses set the therapist up as an expert and run the risk of disempowering the client; in addition, therapist advisements encourage behavioral problem-solving at the expense of experiential exploration. Although homework may be used, it is always discovery-oriented awareness homework. The aim of such homework is to help the client to become aware of experience, not to change behavior directly.

It is sometimes difficult for therapists with previous experience in behavioral or cognitive treatments to move away from a central focus on providing solutions through advisement. The aim in the process-experiential approach is not to provide clients with solutions but, rather, to help clients access primary adaptive emotions so that they can develop their own idiosyncratic, personal solutions. Again, general advisement or behavioral homework are avoided in this approach not because they are "bad" but because they are not consistent with the underlying principles of the approach.

Directing Content by telling the client what to talk about in the session is also "out of mode," and violates the Growth/Choice principle. As noted earlier, the therapist may and frequently does direct the process (*how* to explore), but he or she does not direct the content or topic (*what* to explore) in a deliberate manner.

Offering Expert Reassurance

Offering Reassurance is a response intention that is "partially out of mode." In other words, the therapist avoids responses which seek to reassure the client in a direct, "expert" manner. This includes praising or giving "pep talks" to the client, minimizing problems, predicting positive outcomes, or attributing positive characteristics to the client (e.g., "You are a bright person with a nice smile"). Such *content reassurance* responses might appear to support the Therapeutic Bond principle, but are "out of mode" because they set the therapist up as an expert "evaluator" and provider of environment support (violating the Growth/Choice principle) and usually interfere with client exploration (violating the Experiential Processing principle).

On the other hand, the therapist does offer the client support indirectly through the "process reassurance" provided by Empathic Understanding responses and a prizing, supportive Experiential Presence. In addition, he or she may occasionally use a personal, genuinely felt supportive process disclosure to offer personal support:

T: I feel really touched by what you explored today.
T: I feel glad for you and excited about this "new you."

However, it is important that such responses be shared as personal experiences of the therapist, not as expert evaluations.

Disagreeing/Confronting responses involve reacting negatively to the client in some way and include negating, differing, pointing out contradictions, blaming, and criticizing the client. It should be clear that such responses violate virtually all the treatment principles of this approach and should be avoided at all costs.

Being "Out of Mode" Experientially

Although the preceding responses are generally "out of mode" for this approach, conditions do arise in which it is advisable for the therapist to "go out of mode" for a brief time. These include such situations as when it is clinically necessary to do so (e.g., with acutely suicidal clients), or when a potential interpretation or advisement is interfering with the therapist's concentration. In such situations, the therapist may give the response as a process disclosure, that is, from his or her point of view, saying something like "I find myself wondering if this is linked to. . . ." the therapist says it briefly, without elaborating or repeating it, or attempting to give news or advice to the client. The therapist then returns to the primary task, which is to promote experiencing and exploration of what is salient for the client. Clearly, "out-of-mode" responses are avoided wherever possible, and they should be delivered in such a way as to minimize the disruption to the therapeutic process and be evaluated for their impact on the client.

SUMMARY

In this chapter, we have described the array of response intentions and associated types of therapist response found in the process-experiential approach, devoting most of our attention to the essential experiential intentions, consisting of Empathic Understanding, Empathic Exploration, Process Directing, and Experiential Presence. These response intentions express the dual nature of the therapy, as it balances the client–therapist relationship and the therapeutic work. On the one hand, Empathic Understanding and Experiential Presence primarily support the relationship. On the other hand, Process Directing primarily supports the therapeutic work. Finally, Empathic Exploration, perhaps the most characteristic response intention of the treatment, attempts to marry relationship and work within one response intention.

These essential therapist intentions provide the building blocks for the therapist operations to be described in the succeeding chapters on specific therapeutic tasks. They may be supplemented by an additional set of response intentions, which include Experiential Teaching, Process Observation, and Revealing Self. These have more limited roles and are often used for repairing difficulties in the therapeutic process or relationship. Finally, therapists are urged to avoid out-of-mode intentions and responses such as Giving News (interpretation), Providing Solutions (general advisement), Directing Content, Offering Expert Reassurance (content reassurance), and Disagreeing/Confronting.

THE
TREATMENT
TASKS

I N THE FOLLOWING CHAPTERS we present manuals on each of the six specific therapeutic tasks of the process-experiential approach to facilitating emotional change. The task markers, therapist operations, and client end-states of these are outlined in the table on page 138. Each task chapter is self-contained and includes a theoretical description of what needs to be changed, a description of the task-intervention strategy, of the process of client change in the task, and of the moment-by-moment therapist operations in the intervention strategy.

It is important to note that these tasks are generally not worked on until at least the third session and only when an initial alliance has been established. In addition, all of the tasks are engaged in only in the context of the empathic relating described in the previous chapters. The first few sessions, as well as the beginning of each session, can thus be viewed as involving a generic treatment task, that of Empathic Attunement and Exploration of Feelings. This general task is described briefly below.

EMPATHIC ATTUNEMENT AND EXPLORATION

The therapist begins treatment by entering the client's internal frame of reference and listening to the client. The therapist experiences empathic understanding and communicates this to the client. The therapist in this process continually attempts to understand and respond to the client's perception of inner and outer reality at that moment without imposing

Marker–Operation–End State Table

Chapter	Marker	Operation	End State
8	Problematic Reaction Point (Self-Understanding Problem)	Systematic Evocative Unfolding	New view of self in-the-world-functioning
9	Absent or Unclear Felt Sense	Experiential Focusing	Symbolization of Felt Sense; Productive Experiential Processing
10	Self-Evaluative Split (Self-Criticism, Tornness)	Two-Chair Dialogue	Self-Acceptance, Integration
11	Self-Interruption Split (Blocked Feelings, Resignation)	Two-Chair Enactment	Self-Expression, Empowerment
12	Unfinished Business (Lingering bad feeling re: specific other)	Empty-Chair Work	Forgive Other or hold other accountable, Affirm Self/Separate
13	Vulnerability (Painful emotion related to self)	Empathic Affirmation	Self-Affirmation (feels understood, hopeful and stronger)

some external view of reality. It is important to note that this is a continuing process of actively responding in an ongoing manner, as opposed to listening for long periods of time and then providing a single summary type of understanding. This manner of ongoing responding creates and conveys responsiveness and deeper involvement and provides moment-by-moment support of exploration.

The therapist, throughout, is neither agreeing nor disagreeing with the client's view but is simply trying to sense what it is. The therapist is attending to the intended message that the client is attempting to communicate, listening for what *is* said not for what *is not* said nor for some conclusion or picture that can be drawn about the client from what is being said. The therapist's intention is to communicate understanding, *not* to offer the client insight into something of which they are not aware. The therapist is thus engaged in an *active* effort to understand the client's experience and not a *passive* listening process. Empathic understanding is not simply a process of setting up good rapport or engaging in a friendly listening process. This is done in most therapeutic approaches and is often mislabeled as being empathic. Rather, in being empathic, the therapist actually tries to get a feeling of what the client is saying, to take it in, and "taste" what it is like to be the client in that moment. The therapist then communicates this understanding and has the client check this against his or her experience. The client then corrects and extends the therapist's perceptions, and then the cycle starts again with the therapist trying to get the feel of that. The level of therapist inference about what the client experience means is kept low, although the therapist's focus is of necessity selective, attending to that which is most live and poignant in the client's expression.

The skills of empathic responding have been written about extensively, and rather than repeat these here, we refer the reader to original sources (Rogers, 1951, 1961; Gendlin, 1968, 1974; Rice, 1974) and to available skill-training material (Martin, 1983). We however again wish to emphasize here the important distinction between the skills of empathic understanding and empathic exploration (Rice, 1983). Understanding responses emphasize the communication of understanding and serve to maintain safety and an atmosphere conducive to exploration. Exploratory responses, as well as communicating understanding, selectively leave the focus of attention on the aspect of the client's communication that is most fresh, live, and central to his or her current experience, thereby promoting exploration of that which is as yet unclear or is most novel. In this type of response one does not reflect back the client's feelings/meanings as a finished product but, rather, as an open-ended exploration of what the client may be feeling.

There are thus two different ways of empathically following the client, one which conveys that one has fully grasped the client's emotional meaning, the other, which pushes for further exploration. This is communicated not only in the content but also by vocal quality and manner of expression. Thus an Empathic Understanding response conveys a quality of "so that's what it is" or "I see what you mean." However, in an Empathic Exploration response there is often a tentative following quality conveying "I'm not sure, is this what it is?" This can even be thought of as, at times, engaging in empathic nonunderstanding in which one is attempting to understand what is not yet clear as opposed to conveying that one does understand.

The Empathic Understanding responses are the most important way for the therapist to create the empathic accepting climate. This communicates to clients that they are valued for who they are and this helps them to experience themselves as worthwhile. They accept their own feelings, trust their experience, and feel comfirmed in their own existence.

The Empathic Exploration responses facilitate engagement in productive differential exploration. Exploratory responses stimulate deeper experiencing and facilitate symbolizing of new aspects of experience not previously in focal awareness. These responses guide attentional allocation to focus on the as yet unclear edges of experience and help differentiate experience into greater particularity. They help to get at the differentiated idiosyncratic feel of experience as well as to integrate this into new levels of meanings. For instance with a therapist's response such as "So that left you with this angry feeling. Sort of a like a rising up in your stomach?" the client attends to the inner experience, symbolizes it as a "definite" anger, then differentiates it into a "steely, rightful" anger, then integrates this into "feeling wronged at being so misused," and translates this into an action tendency by vowing to "not allow this to happen again."

Once the empathic exploration process described above has been implemented, the crucial process of therapy has begun, and the client has entered into a process of attending to and symbolizing his or her own experience. This process is inherently therapeutic. In addition it is out of this internally focused process that markers of affective problems will arise and afford the therapist further opportunities for differential intervention. It is to a description of these markers and interventions that we now turn in the following chapters.

SYSTEMATIC EVOCATIVE UNFOLDING AT A MARKER OF A PROBLEMATIC REACTION POINT

A BASIC ASSUMPTION of a process-experiential approach is that each client needs to access and change self-in-the-world cognitive/affective schemes that are interfering with adaptive, satisfying, and growth-enhancing functioning. A further assumption is that identifying such schematic areas does not involve "diagnosis" in the usual sense but that the presence and the structure of such dysfunctional schemes can be identified by means of client process "markers." These markers not only indicate the potentially important involvement of tacit dysfunctional schemes, but even more importantly, they indicate the client's current readiness to focus on relevant puzzling issues in his or her life. Furthermore, the marker also indicates the mode of accessing and reprocessing of these relevant schemes that is likely to be most effective at this point.

People in therapy often recount an incident in which they found themselves reacting to some person or situation in a way that they felt to be unexpected, exaggerated, or unreasonable, recounting such incidents with a sense of puzzlement. These problematic reactions may not always seem to be of primary importance, and they may often be discounted by the therapist as simply the recounting of stories. Nevertheless, the Evocative Unfolding of such problematic reactions can lead to important self-discoveries. Their significance lies in the fact that the clients are aware of some discrepancy between their own actual reaction, and their view of an appropriate or self-consistent reaction, and are thus motivated to explore and understand it. Clients can become vividly and irrefutably aware of their own meaning construals concerning the impact or potential impact of the stimulus situation and the connection between their construal and their own problematic reaction. Furthermore, exploration can lead to awareness of their broader dysfunctional emotion schemes that underlie their own construals.

The marker for a problematic reaction point does not yet indicate the content of the relevant dysfunctional emotion schemes, but it does indicate the presence and operation of some dysfunctional scheme. When new situations are encountered, if they evoke a particular schematic structure through the similarity of its salient features, the whole structure is activated, thus determining the person's response. In the unfolding of problematic reaction points, the primary mode of client engagement that the therapist attempts to facilitate is experiential search (described in Chapter 2). This experiential search process in the unfolding of problematic reaction points involves a mode of engagement in which clients are able to get in touch with the edges of their own emotionally toned inner experience. This enables clients to reexperience and recognize important aspects of their experience that had not been fully processed previously. The therapist uses Systematic Evocative Unfolding to facilitate this process in the client.

WHAT NEEDS TO BE CHANGED?
THE UNDERLYING PROCESSING DIFFICULTY

The things that need to be changed in these events are the dysfunctional cognitive/affective self-in-the-world schemes by which the person's experience is filtered and which guide internal and external reactions to situations in their everyday lives. Many of one's self-in-the-world emotion schemes are consistent with, and integrated into, one's conscious experience of self, and thus they guide one's responses to situations in ways that feel self-consistent.

On the other hand, some emotion schemes that are influential in guiding one's reactions have never been really integrated into one's conscious experience of self, and yet they may be strongly activated by particular classes of stimulus situations. These situations contain some stimulus feature that is highly relevant to some emotion scheme that is not in awareness, and thus this particular feature activates this scheme. When one of these self-relevant tacit schemes is accessed, it becomes the trigger for some unexpected and puzzling internal or external reaction. Tacit emotion schemes are, of course, present for everyone and may trigger somewhat unexpected reactions for many people. For some people, however, there are a number of powerful tacit emotion schemes that influence experience and behavior in dysfunctional and puzzling ways. Some of these problematic reactions may not initially be viewed by the client as highly important, whereas others may be viewed as having serious consequences. In either case their evocation and exploration can lead to the accessing and reexamination of emotion schemes that have been centrally involved in important and troubling areas of one's own functioning.

Many of the dysfunctional tacit schemes were probably initially formed in early childhood, and strong emotional-motivational forces were involved in their construction. But an important theoretical assumption underlying our approach to change is that it is not the repressed memory of the early experiences, leading to unconscious motivation or defensive mechanisms, that is influencing the present functioning. Our assumption is that these schemes are maintained because potentially relevant new experiences are repeatedly processed through these dysfunctional tacit schemes that are automatically applied to the situation. Thus these new experiences are distorted and assimilated into the old structure, and change does not take place. The significant point is that it is these tacit self-in-the-world emotion-laden schemes that are influential in guiding perceptions and generating external and internal reactions in inappropriate, puzzling, and seemingly self-inconsistent directions. It is the recognition and reexperiencing of these puzzling reactions that can lead to accessing, reexamining, and ultimately to reorganization of the relevant tacit schemes, and thus to basic changes in one's conscious experience of self. We view the systematic evocative unfolding of problematic reaction points as a valuable strategy for enabling clients to access, reexamine, and restructure dysfunctional emotion schemes that are influencing their feelings and actions in directions that are interfering with their own relationships, satisfactions, and goals.

OPPORTUNITIES FOR INTERVENTION: THE MARKER FOR A PROBLEMATIC REACTION POINT

Clients often spontaneously describe particular incidents in which they found themselves reacting in a way that they felt to be unexpected, unreasonable, or otherwise problematic. These problematic reactions may involve either an external, behavioral reaction or an internal response such as a strong emotion. The marker that signifies client's readiness for engaging in the experiential search required in the unfolding of the problematic reaction should contain three elements as follows: (1) The client recounts a particular instance of a reaction in a particular situation. (2) The reaction that is felt as problematic is the client's own, not that of someone else. (3) There is some indication that the client views his or her reaction as problematic, not simply as an unfortunate consequence of someone else's behavior.

The clearest examples of such incidents are those in which the clients recount the incident with a real sense of surprise, as if they had somehow violated some expectation of themselves. For instance a client said "Suddenly I just got furious at my dad. I practically freaked out. It was weird." There can still be a useful marker, however, even if there is not strong surprise, provided that there is some sense of puzzlement, of the reaction not being fully understandable. For instance, another client said "When the professor was discussing that, I found myself getting a bit uneasy. I don't always agree with him, but the uneasy feeling seemed kind of odd." The reaction that was viewed as problematic may be recounted as behavioral rather than involving an internal reaction. For instance when a client said "I *knew* this wasn't a good time to talk with my dad, but I just went anyway; it was stupid," there seemed to be no explicit awareness of an inner reaction that led to this behavior. But as the reaction unfolded an important emotional reaction emerged and was explored.

It is important that the reaction should involve a particular incident rather than be stated in a general form. If a client states that he gets wholly panicked when he has to speak up in class, the therapist asks if the client can think of a particular recent incident. If he cannot at this point recall one that feels alive, the therapist may suggest that the next time this happens the client might remember it, not try to analyze it, but bring it up in the next session.

Sometimes Problematic Reaction Point (PRP) markers appear to be rather closely connected to issues with which the client is struggling in therapy, while at other times they may seem to be totally unconnected with presenting problems. In our experience either one may prove to lead to a valuable exploration. The former type may be more tempting because of its possible relevance to the client's presenting problems, but it may be more difficult, in this case, to keep clients from prematurely generalizing about some seemingly related issues before they have fully unfolded the PRP. On the other hand, the seemingly unrelated episode may at first seem irrelevant, but the exploratory path may eventually lead to some extremely relevant self-understanding. For instance a client, when he first came in, said "While I was coming here I saw a little puppy-dog that was obviously lost and hunting desperately for a way home. I can't get it out of my mind, and I keep wanting to cry." Although this seemed unrelated to any issues that had previously come up, the unfolding of this PRP led to an extremely poignant exploration of one of the client's deepest fears.

An essential characteristic of PRP markers is that the clients are *owning* their own reaction, seeing it as emanating from themselves rather than simply attributing it to the situation or to another person. In exploring problematic reactions, it is the recognition and owning of one's own puzzling reactions that is the entry point for a self-examination of some broader area of functioning that has not previously been owned or questioned.

HOW DOES CHANGE OCCUR?

The basic assumption in this approach is that having people focus on and explore a *particular* unexpected or dysfunctional reaction to a *particular* stimulus situation enables them to reexperience and explore a whole processing cycle that led to a reaction, external or internal, that does not fit with their own self-expectations. The kind of inner tracking involved in this exploration is very different from generalizing, or speculating, or attempting to analyze the experience. It is a process of experiential search, in which the unfolding process provides an opportunity to track a whole sequence of cognitive/affective processing, involving potentially important, but tacit, schemes that are relevant to unsatisfying, puzzling, or disturbing modes of functioning. In this process of experiential search clients can track a real-life processing sequence in a vividly reevoked, but slowed-down manner. They can be deliberately self-aware in this nondefensive climate. It is a real-life experience, and yet it can be reexamined at each step in order to recognize the perceptual trigger, the immediate construals made, the affective responses, and the self-relevant personal meaning implications of these construals and affective responses. This is an experiential search process, involving becoming aware of a complicated series of inner-process data that would otherwise have been inaccessible to awareness. It is as if the client is walking slowly through the experiencing process instead of running through it.

In this slowed-down reexperiencing and reexamination clients can recognize the stimulus ingredient that was salient for them at that moment and thus served as the trigger for the unexpected reaction. They can reexperience and become aware of their own meaning construals and the internal emotional reactions stimulated by these construals. Even more important, in further exploration, they can recognize that this kind of selective construal exercises a controlling effect on their emotional reactions and modes of functioning in a much broader range of experiences.

One vitally important feature in this exploration is that this experiential search is self-motivated. Clients are aware of some discrepancy between their view of an appropriate or self-consistent reaction and their own actual reaction and are thus motivated to explore and understand it. They are challenging themselves to understand the reaction, but it is not primarily an intellectual, conceptual analysis. They are reliving the experience but doing so with focal attention and maximum allocation of processing capacity. In some ways it is like any good inner self-exploration, but it has a special quality. The client is temporarily distanced and freed from the automatic assumptions and expectations that were generated by the old scheme. This enables the client to look freshly at the experience while a whole new set of questions guides the search. By engaging in this process of experiential search, the client can arrive at new meanings that are more accurate representations of his or her own in-the-world experience.

The effects of this evocative unfolding process have been studied by means of sequential analysis (Wiseman & Rice, 1989) and comparisons of the outcomes of those clients who resolved the PRP with those who did not reach resolution (Lowenstein, 1985; Rice & Saperia, 1984).

The Model of the Unfolding of Problematic Reaction Points: Necessary Client Steps to Resolution

The model of the evocative unfolding of problematic reaction points is shown in Figure 8-1. The steps of the model are described in detail below. In addition, a short form of a rater's Degree-of-Resolution Scale devised for research purposes is shown in Table 8-1. This indicates six degrees of resolution and can be used as a guide to estimate how far along in the resolution process one has progressed.

Stage I. Positioning for Exploration

The first stage begins when clients mention a situation in which they reacted in a way that somehow did not make sense to them. This reaction need not necessarily be related to any of the issues that have been the focus of the therapy, but there is a sense of puzzlement expressed. The reaction is felt by the client to be unexpected, inappropriate, maladaptive, or otherwise problematic. In response to the therapist's tentative and questioning reflections, the client identifies the aspect of his or her reaction that was felt to be problematic and confirms that it was indeed puzzling. Then the therapist suggests that this might be an interesting and important area to explore in detail. If the client agrees and seems motivated to engage in this exploration, the next stage begins.

STAGE I: Positioning for Exploration	1. The Marker: Problematic reaction stated
	2. Confirms what was felt as problematic and agrees to explore
STAGE II: Experience Reevoked	3. Vividly reenters scene and begins reexperiencing
	4. Searches for and recognizes the salient element in the stimulus situation
STAGE III: Tracking the idiosyncratic meaning of the stimulus as construed	Attends separately to affective reaction and/or subjective construal of stimulus situation

5. Attends to emotional reaction to perceived stimulus	6. Attends to nature of own subjective construal of stimulus as perceived

Meaning bridge: Partial resolution—recognizes causal link between reaction and construal of stimulus impact

STAGE IV: Recognition and reexamination of own mode of functioning (self-schemes)	7. Although still experientially involved, is able to stand back and examine own mode of functioning in the context of own needs, wants, fears, values, shoulds, and personal qualities
	8. Broadens the exploration and reexamines own mode of functioning in other situations

Resolution: New awareness and understanding of important aspects of own mode of functioning in a way that restructures the issue. There is a new awareness of what he/she wants to change, and a sense of having the power to make the changes

FIGURE 8-1. Unfolding problematic reaction points.

Stage II. Step 3. Client Vividly Reenters the Scene

After clients have already identified the reaction that felt problematic and have agreed to explore it in detail, they are facilitated in engaging in a vivid reexperiencing of the situation just before the reaction was triggered. They are encouraged to convey to the therapist an immediate feel for that particular situation and for their own inner experience at that point. If facilitated by the therapist in the ways to be described below, clients are usually able to recapture a very vivid description of the external scene and to reexperience their own internal state just as the reaction was triggered. It is this vivid reentry that sets the stage for a client's detailed, slowed-down reexperiencing of the incident, with an emotionally involved but exploratory stance.

TABLE 8-1. Degree-of-Resolution Scale: Unfolding Problematic Reaction Points

1. Client describes an unexpected, puzzling reaction of his/her own.

2. Client has "reentered" the scene and is recalling and reexperiencing the time when the reaction was triggered.

3. Client recalls salient aspects of the stimulus situation. Explores both own internal affective reaction to situation and own subjective construal of potential impact of the stimulus situation.

4. Reaches "meaning bridge." Has discovered the link between his/her problematic reaction and own construal of potential impact of stimulus situation.

5. Recognizes this as an example of a broader aspect of own mode of functioning that is interfering with own needs and wants.

6. Reaches "resolution." Gets a whole new view of important aspects of own mode of functioning and what self-changes he/she wants to make. Is beginning to feel empowered to make the change.

Stage II. Step 4. Searching for and Recognizing the Salient Aspects of the Stimulus Situation

Once the scene has begun to come alive in this experiential fashion, clients are encouraged to become aware of the aspect of the situation that felt salient for them and was associated with the reaction. This should not be a process of systematic analysis but a spontaneous recognition of the aspect that had an impact, the thing that stood out for the client. For some people it will be an instant recognition of "The tone of his voice" or "Everybody staring at me when I walked in." For others it will be a more internal sense of impact: "Walking in the door and seeing them all discussing things, I felt useless somehow." This recognition places the salient aspects in focal awareness, thus enabling clients to begin an intensive exploration of the idiosyncratic meaning that this situation had for them.

Stage III. Tracking the Personal Meaning of the Stimulus Situation as Construed: Attending to Stimulus and Reaction Sides

This stage of the exploration is a complex and sometimes lengthy one. Clients are reexperiencing these episodes in a live and vivid but slowed-down fashion, with an exploratory stance. At some points in the exploration they will be attending to their own perception of the situation and its construed meaning. At other times the focus will be on their own internal reactions, such as apprehension or sadness. It is important for clients to reexperience and explore both their internal "feeling" reactions to the stimulus situation and the nature of their own perceptual construal of the situation. Both of these aspects of their reaction may be important in leading to an awareness of the nature of their own idiosyncratic construal of the personal meaning of the situation.

This exploration is usually more effective if a client's focus is not on both sides at the same time. As will be illustrated in the next section, on the functions of the therapist, it is important for the therapist to reflect them in a way that leaves the focus on one side or the other. As the exploration continues, however, the stimulus side and the inner reaction side will begin to merge, yielding a new awareness of one's own experience at that point. This "tracking" stage of the exploration is completed when the client spontaneously recognizes that the reaction that seemed so problematic was a direct response to his or her own idiosyncratic meaning construal of some features of the stimulus situation and the emotions aroused by the nature of this construal. This spontaneous recognition provides the "meaning bridge" between the puzzling spontaneous reaction and the nature of the automatic construal of the self-relevant impact or potential impact of the stimulus situation.

First Change Point

Although the whole continuing process of experiential search is important, there are two points at which some decisive change occurs. At this first change point, the "meaning bridge," clients discover the link between the nature of their own construal of the personal meaning of the stimulus situation and the reaction that had seemed so inappropriate and puzzling. They discover that their puzzling reaction was actually quite consistent with their own meaning construal of the situation at that moment and with the feelings aroused by this construal. A tacit self-relevant emotion scheme had been cued by some aspect of the situation rather than the scheme that the client would have regarded as most appropriate to the situation.

The meaning bridge provides a vivid new understanding of the client's own idiosyncratic construal of the stimulus. This realization of the construed meaning of the stimulus brings a whole self-relevant schematic structure into focal awareness in a compelling way. For the self-relevant tacit emotion scheme has now been accessed and is potentially available for exploration. This spontaneous recognition and owning of one's own construal and the possible consequences following from this construal usually provide the stimulus for a broader self-exploration, which becomes the focus of Stage IV.

Stage IV. Recognition and Reexamination of Relevant Self-Schemes: Broadening, Deepening, and Owning

The awareness that their own puzzling reaction had been a direct response to their own construals of the stimulus situation and the feelings thus aroused usually provides clients with the stimulus for a broader exploration. There is usually a spontaneous recognition that the way they were functioning in this situation was an instance of a more pervasive mode of functioning, one that now feels inconsistent with their own self-expectations, satisfactions, and goals. This self-recognition usually provides the stimulus for a self-guided search process that is much more than an intellectual analysis. It is as if the wants, fears, values, and beliefs about self are being "tasted" in relation to each other.

This deliberate tasting process is a set of complex internal operations that is too nonlinear to describe systematically, but it is quite recognizable from the client's voice, experiential focus, and general manner. For instance, a client had recognized at the meaning bridge that if she were left alone at a party for even a minute or two, she felt ignored, and she construed it as rejection. As the process continued, she began to broaden the exploration, thinking about and exploring other situations when she had felt that sense of total rejection. The exploration also lead to a deeper awareness of how much she feared rejection, indeed, how rejection seemed to threaten her whole sense of self. But as the exploration continued, she began spontaneously to describe and explore areas in which she had developed a clear and positive sense of self, one that she clearly valued. Finally, she realized that, although she enjoyed attention, she no longer really *needed* this confirmation that she was a worthwhile person.

Second Change Point

Resolution is reached when clients achieve a new awareness of their own mode of functioning in a way that restructures the issue. Though still experientially involved, they now have a sense of what they want to change and a sense that they have already begun to change. This resolution point is usually accompanied by an upward mood shift. Following this resolution point, there is usually some further exploration and emotional tasting of one's own needs and wants, values and shoulds, fears and capabilities, but their relative emotional valences seem to have changed.

THERAPIST OPERATIONS

The Evocative Unfolding of a problematic reaction point is designed to bring the original stimulus situation vividly to life and to stimulate clients to reexperience and explore their own inner reactions and subjective construals of relevant aspects of the situation. Each of the five stages involves its own goal, and they are instigated in sequence (Figure 8-2). Each stage is made possible by the completion of the previous one. The primary focus until after the meaning bridge should be on one particular situation, rather than a generalization across situations and a broad identification of patterns. The reexperiencing and reprocessing take place within a basically client-centered relationship, in which the client is the expert of his or her own experience. Although the therapist will be quite process-directive at certain points, it is the client who will make the discoveries. The client mode of engagement in this event is Experiential Search, discussed in Chapter 2. An empathic and prizing relationship is maintained throughout the whole search process, but the emphasis is on helping clients to get in touch with and track the edges of their own affectively toned inner awareness in order to facilitate their discovery of crucial elements of their experience. Most of the therapist's interventions will be reflections, but many of these reflections will have an "open-edged" quality. They will indicate empathic understanding but will leave the focus on the client's inner experience that is just emerging. This is done in a tentative way, thus stimulating the client to check inside and correct it or carry it further.

STAGE I. POSITIONING FOR EXPLORATION
  1. Identifies relevant marker
  2. Verifies problematic aspect
  3. Suggests exploring the problematic reaction

STAGE II. EXPERIENCE REEVOKED
  4. Stimulates reexperiencing the scene
  5. Facilitates search for salience

STAGE III. TRACKING CONSTRUED PERSONAL MEANING OF STIMULUS SITUATION
  6. Maintains client's focus on emotional reactions to stimulus and/or
  7. Maintains client's focus on construal of demand characteristics of stimulus situation
  8. Acknowledges and focuses on client's spontaneous recognition of meaning bridge

STAGE IV. FACILITATES BROADER SELF-EXPLORATION
  9. Facilitates client's reexamination of self-schemes
  10. Facilitates broader reexamination of self-schemes in other life situations
  11. Acknowledges and focuses on client's new understanding of own scheme-guided dysfunctional styles and the new implications for self-change

STAGE V. POST-TASK
  12. Encourages client in brief discussion of what he/she has derived from the session

FIGURE 8-2. Therapist operations.

THE THERAPIST FUNCTIONS AT THE DIFFERENT STAGES OF THE MODEL

Stage I. Positioning for Exploration

This first stage begins when clients mention a reaction of their own in a particular situation that felt unexpected, peculiar, or inappropriate. The therapist needs to learn to listen selectively for such moments in therapy. It is easy to ignore these moments, viewing them as digressions from the major issues, but when they are reexperienced and explored, they can lead to important new self-understandings with broad implications. These incidents may provide a particularly useful entry point for clients who tend to stay in a recounting mode rather than turning inward. If the client's voice quality or the manner in which the incident is described conveys a sense of surprise, puzzlement, self-disappointment, or even self-disgust, exploring the incident may lead to further important self-explorations.

After the PRP has been stated, the first step is to confirm that it *is* felt as problematic and then to confirm just *what* aspect was felt as problematic. Sometimes a client may state a PRP as if it were viewed as problematic, but when he or she starts delving more deeply into it, it becomes apparent that it is viewed as an unfortunate but "natural" reaction to provocation. In that case an exploration is not likely to be productive. It is not always easy to tell in a sequence of responses which part is felt as problematic and which parts just follow from that. Both of these things can usually be checked, and an exploratory stance can be stimulated by responses such as the following: "So the part of your reaction that feels really exaggerated or peculiar to you is your extreme anger at that point...?" Another example would be: "And I guess you are saying that the part you don't understand is your getting so tense. You felt that you were really overreacting."

A client may initially point to one aspect of his or her reaction as problematic, but then, as the exploration begins, a problematic feeling prior to the feeling first identified comes into focus. If that happens, check that this prior one is the truly problematic part and, if confirmed, proceed with this new part.

If the PRP is stated as a general one, for example, "I always get scared in tutorials," one can ask for a recent example, or an example that stands out in the client's mind. Usually some relevant episode can be recalled in a live manner. If the client is not able to do this and continues to generalize, then the PRP is not workable at this point. In an ongoing therapy one can ask the client to notice the next time this happens, so that he or she can bring it in and explore it.

Sometimes, after clients state the PRP, they begin to react to their own reaction, starting to focus on how childish or self-defeating it was to react that way. Even though this "reaction to reaction" may be the liveliest part at this point, it is important not to get side-tracked by it, and to remember both that it is a secondary reaction, and that it is the exploration of the puzzling primary reaction that is likely to lead to new self-understanding. It is important not to let clients dismiss or invalidate their own primary reaction. One can maintain focus on the primary reaction with responses like the following reflection. "You feel that your response was self defeating, but there was *something* that made you extremely angry." The therapist here is not implying that the anger was "justified," but simply that something in the construal of the situation triggered the anger.

Although most clients do bring in some incidents in which they reacted in a puzzling, problematic manner, there are some clients who never seem to question their own reactions spontaneously, always viewing them as natural, though perhaps regrettable, responses to provocation. With these clients it may be productive to define and describe a PRP, mentioning that it is a kind of experience most of us have sometimes, and to suggest that they try to notice such times. Then if they do find themselves reacting in a way that feels somehow problematic, they should not to try to analyze it, but to bring it in to the next session. This should not be stated as a directive, but following the procedure does sometimes enable people to reexperience and explore areas that prove to be extremely important.

After the reaction that is felt as problematic has been identified, the therapist suggests that it might well be valuable to go back into this experience and explore it in detail. If the client agrees, then the next stage is begun. During this first stage of the unfolding process the therapist has three goals: (1) to establish and maintain the focus on the reaction that was actually felt to be puzzling; (2) to diffuse any strong secondary emotional reaction; and (3) to establish an empathic climate in which there is a mutual agreement to undertake a shared journey of exploration.

Stage II. Step 4. Stimulating Reentry into the Scene: Experience Reevoked

In this phase the goal is to have the client reenter and vividly reexperience the scene just before the problematic reaction was triggered. It is extremely important to have the client describe it as vividly as possible. This stimulates the reconstruction and reentry into the stimulus situation. This also enables the therapist to get a real experiential feel for the whole experience, which thereby enables him or her to make more empathic and meaningful reflections.

The therapist might start this explicitly by saying "I wonder if we could go back and visualize the scene so I could get the flavor of it." Or one might say "I'd like to get a feel for the situation. I guess you were sitting there—and he was standing over you . . . ?" In starting this way one uses the parts that the client has described, in order to get the experiential reentry started. Sometimes one tries out things to give the client something to check against, but it should be done in a very tentative manner. For instance one might say "I get an image of you driving along, and there are cars all around you, and maybe one jammed *right* behind you . . . ?" Usually one starts with the more external details and then moves to a more internal feeling. It is important, however, to remember that the client's feelings, attitudes, and thoughts at that point are also part of the situation just before the reaction was triggered and may therefore be part of the trigger.

Once the scene has truly come alive the therapist can reflect the scene just before the reaction was triggered and then just at the time when the client reacted, and thus one can get a feel for the moment when things actually changed. For instance if the client has described feeling uneasy or irritable right from the beginning of the experience, but it is still not clear just when these feelings became exaggerated, it is important to use a tentative sense of when things changed. One might say "So you were sitting there feeling comfortable and sort of quietly happy, I guess. . . . and then something changed."

When the therapist sees that the experience has come alive in a vivid fashion and been reexperienced, it is time to move to the next substage. It is important not to get so caught up in scene building that one ignores the fact that the client is really ready to move constructively to the next stage.

Stage II. Step 5. Searching for Salience in the Eliciting Stimulus

Once the scene has come alive, clients may spontaneously become aware of the aspect of the situation that was salient for them, and thus triggered the reaction. One can facilitate this process by searching tentatively for salience, but it is extremely important not to try to anticipate what this may be. What may seem obvious to the therapist may not have been the crucial element for the client. Some possible responses may be "There was just something about his face . . . or the way he said it . . . I don't know . . . ?" Or one might say "And there was just something about that that got *to* you . . . ?"

Sometimes clients mention spontaneously their own feeling reaction to something happening in the scene even though there is no explicit recognition of salience. For instance one client said "They were shovelling snow and having fun and laughing and all playing together, and I suddenly felt left out, even though I knew that I wasn't." The client's linking her discrepant feeling reaction to their happy playfulness clearly indicated the salient element in the scene. Whether it is recognized directly or indirectly, this sense of salience is the entry point for the client to start exploring his or her own subjective construal of the situation. This places the salient aspect in focal awareness, and it is the nucleus of the subjective construal.

If the search for salience starts to become primarily intellectual, the therapist returns the focus to the reevoked situation. It may be necessary to explore salience a number of different times before something clicks. Although this recognition of salience is a very useful entry point for undertaking the next stage, its nonemergence should not block for too long the entry into Stage III. For some clients salience may not emerge until entry into the stimulus-processing side in Stage III.

The following example is a shortened and condensed transcript of the first two stages of the model: Positioning for Exploration and Experience Reevoked.

Stage I. Positioning for Exploration

C1: So its been a rough week, getting an important essay done and trying to get ready for the exam that's coming up. I'm really tired. (*sigh*)

T1: I should think so. Just worn out.

C2: Yeah (*sigh*). In a way I feel good to have really concentrated on it. . . . to have done all that work (*pause*). But I found myself feeling kind of uncomfortable in a funny way.

T2: Feeling good about all you've done. But then . . . I'm not sure . . . uncomfortable . . . sort of uneasy? [Tentative reflection to stimulate further differentiation of feeling]

C3: Sort of . . . but maybe more resentful.

T3: Kind of resenting what you'd had to do? [Tentative identification of target of resentment]

C4: Resenting something. I'm not sure. I sat down to rest last night, and my dad asked me what I had accomplished. And then when I told him, he said "You've worked hard. I'm proud of you." I should have felt good, but I didn't.

T4: You would have expected to feel really pleased, but somehow you just *didn't*. [Leaving emphasis on puzzling aspect of reaction]

C5: No, I didn't feel good. It was strange. But maybe I was just feeling too tired. Maybe that was it.

T5: You were feeling worn out. But it seems as if you're still feeling a bit puzzled by it. [Maintaining focus on her sense of puzzlement]

C6: Yeah.

T6: I wonder if we could go back to that incident last night and explore it a bit—try and get a feel of what was happening for you. [Obtaining agreement to explore]

C7: O.K. It *was* kind of weird.

Stage II. Experience Reevoked

T8: So you had worked all week and all that day, I guess . . .

C9: Yeah.

T9: And you came into the living room where he was sitting and sat down. Feeling kind of tired but OK? [Building the scene just before reaction]

C10: Yeah, exhausted, but I was kind of pleased with myself.

T10: So you came in there, feeling good about all you had accomplished. And then your dad looked up . . . ? [Reflecting mood before reaction and then shifting focus to moment when reaction was triggered]

C11: No. He stood up and said "so what have you accomplished today?" . . . I guess I felt kind of uncomfortable right then.

T11: And that's when you started feeling uncomfortable? [Identifying beginning of reaction]

C12: Yeah, I think so. And then he said "I'm proud of you" and then I felt *really* uncomfortable.

T12: So there was just something about what he said . . . ? Or the way he said it . . . ? [Searching for salience]

C13: Yeah . . . sort of . . . like his tone of voice . . . like he was patting me on the hand and saying "You're a good little girl."

Stage III. Tracking the Idiosyncratic Meaning of the Stimulus Situation as Construed

This phase of the unfolding is a complex one, involving two different kinds of exploratory focus. Client and therapist will probably move back and forth between the two sides a number of times during exploration, but it is important that the "open edge" of the therapist's reflections and reflective questions should be on only one side at a time. It is important to enable clients to reexperience and explore both the nature of their own perceptual construal of the situation and their own internal feeling reaction to the stimulus situation.

Each of these aspects of their own reaction may yield a differentiated awareness of the nature and implications of their own idiosyncratic construal of the personal impact of the stimulus situation at that moment. Although both sides are important, the client is able to attain a more vivid experiential awareness, especially in the early part of the exploration if he or she is able to focus fully on one side at a time. Attending to both sides at once usually leads to "packaging" rather than to new explorations. Each side requires a separate and different kind of attentional focus. For instance if the client were exploring an incident involving an emotional reaction such as inner sense of disquiet, in response to her father at some particular point, the therapist might respond "When he looked at you in that way, you suddenly felt kind of uneasy . . . sort of apprehensive?" This clearly leaves the focus on an internal exploration of the particular flavor of the feelings aroused. On the other hand if the client's focus at that point seemed to be on exploring the nature of the father's expression, the therapist might respond "There was something about the look on his face that got to you—something in that tight . . . stern look . . . ?" This leaves the focus on the client's visual image of the father's expression.

As the exploration continues, the two sides will begin to merge. For instance the experience of feeling uneasy and apprehensive may become "I somehow felt undermined, as if he didn't think I was worth anything—that he didn't trust me." Or "that smug look on his face" that has been identified made her feel "weakened and diminished."

The therapist should not be over-constrained by the model. Reprocessing by means of experiential search works best when the client has time to check inside, perhaps sit with it for a moment, and then respond. Also, the therapist may need to slow down, to get a flavor of what the client is saying and experiencing. If the "meaning bridge," the first of the two major change points, is slow in coming, one should be willing to tolerate the blind alleys, but one should then take the client back to the situation and its salient aspects.

Step 6. Exploring the Differentiated Quality of the Client's Affective Reaction

When the client's problematic reaction is an affective one, and it is expressed in a live and present way, it would be wise to explore the feeling side first. One tries to facilitate the client in getting a more differentiated awareness of the idiosyncratic quality of the feeling. Most of the emotion language used in everyday life for more complex feelings is usually just shorthand. Helping clients to get a differentiated awareness of their feeling reactions will involve the therapist and client in trying out differentiated descriptions, and the client then checking them inside, and rejecting, modifying, or ideally, carrying the inner awareness a bit further. The feeling isn't just sitting there, waiting to be described, but it can be reexperienced by the client in a more differentiated fashion as the exploration continues.

It is helpful to use a vivid fragment of the scene to stimulate the feeling but to leave the emphasis and open edge on the feeling side. For instance, if the client has just mentioned feeling afraid, one might say "As you sat there, hearing his voice, the fear started oozing up." If the client hasn't mentioned a clear feeling, one might say "So there she was yelling at you, and you were feeling . . . I don't know . . . really strange . . . ?"

There are many different possible feeling qualities for any particular basic emotion. There can be flaming anger or corroding anger, or helpless anger. Also most feelings have "messages" in them. For instance fear may involve the appraisal that "Something awful is going to happen." Or it may involve an action tendency such as "a kind of shrinking." As the exploration of the affective reaction unfolds, it may become more differentiated in a number of ways. It may become a more idiosyncratic description, not just "anger," but a kind of "cold, knotted, wrenching anger." Or it may involve a different target for the anger: "I wasn't so much angry at them; I was angry at myself." Or the new facet of the feeling may emerge: "I was angry, but I was a bit afraid too." Or it may involve a shift: "I realize now I wasn't so much angry . . . It was the hurt that really mattered."

Bodily sensations can be important in getting a differentiated feeling, but the client's statement of them needs to be carried further. For instance, if the client said "My hands were clenched," one could push toward feeling awareness, by saying something tentatively: "Hands in fists, I guess . . . just ready to lash out?" Or if the client said "My throat felt tight," one might ask "I'm not sure . . . what was the feeling there?"

As one gets a more precise differentiated awareness of the feeling, it will probably take on a stimulus-related quality. Anger may turn into "I just wanted to put my fist into his smug face." Or fear may become "I felt just terrified by it, as if I might get overwhelmed by what they were doing." This may lead naturally into a shift to focus on the way in which the stimulus was construed. If the feeling doesn't continue to differentiate and seems to be getting less alive, then it is wise to move back to the stimulus situation as an entry point to a focus on the stimulus side.

Step 7. The Stimulus Side

On this side the therapist is trying to facilitate the client's focus on his or her own subjective construal of the situation, and to enable him or her to become more aware of the particular subjective flavor of the construal. (Sometimes this side will be accessed before the affective reaction side, but the approach to the stimulus side is fairly similar in either case.) The therapist tries to help the client to reenter the scene with a high level of vividness and arousal so that there will be some real reexperiencing. But it is also important for clients to keep a part of their attentional energy in a deliberately exploratory stance. One can use the awareness of salience that was reached in the previous stage as an entry to the client's exploration of his or her own subjective construal. There are a number of possible ways of doing this. For instance, if the client has identified "that smug look," one can say something about the smug look—"I'd like to get the flavor that smug look had for you." Or one could try out something that the salient feature implies. For example, when the client was exploring feeling pressured by traffic, the therapist might say "Almost like that car is right in your back seat." Although the therapist makes vivid reflections, it is important to make them in a tentative fashion and not in a way that imposes one's own expectations.

The therapist is trying to stay with the client's subjective construal as it unfolds, listening for any bit of newness and picking it up. As in any good experiential therapy, one will be reflecting the edges that seem to feel live and new for the client. It is also important to remember that there will probably be several blind alleys along the way. What seems to be a promising new track may peter out or become intellectualized. A number of times during the exploration one may have to go back to the scene, exploring for salience and unfolding new aspects of the stimulus construal.

If stage III of the exploration is successful, the clients come to a spontaneous awareness of the nature of their own subjective construal of the self-relevant impact, or potential impact of the stimulus situation and of the affect thus aroused. They recognize the causal link between the nature of their own construal of the stimulus situation and the nature of their own puzzling reaction and recognize self as agent in this construal. We call this the "meaning bridge" because the client has discovered and *owned* this important causal link. It is important for the therapist to acknowledge this recognition.

The following example is a shortened and condensed version of Stage III. This client had mentioned with a sense of puzzlement that he had been so bothered by cars driving behind him that he had turned up his rear-view mirror and left it up for a week. After the initial two stages he began to track the personal meaning of the stimulus situation by tracking the feeling side and the stimulus side.

C1: I just got so *bothered* by all those cars coming up from behind me.
T1: Yeah. I get a picture of you sitting in your car—all those cars behind

you. They're going too fast . . . or doing something . . . [Bringing scene alive, and a questioning entry into salience]

C2: Yeah, they're . . . They seem to come up behind me and put pressure on me . . . to *do* something.

T2: Oh . . . I see . . .

C3: The road wasn't even that busy. But because they're there, I have to speed up or something. I don't know whether he is satisfied to be back there . . . behind me.

T3: Mhmhm.

C4: Because he's there I feel like I have to do something.

T4: Oh. I see what you are saying. If he hadn't been there, you'd just be able to go driving along. [Focus on impact on client]

C5: So I either have to go faster, or pull over.

T5: And, I guess, then you'd feel more comfortable inside. [Focus on inner reaction]

C6: I . . . yeah. I'd feel more comfortable if nobody was behind me.

T6: Kind of a free feeling, I guess.

C7: Yeah, I can't relax when people are right behind me.

T7: I guess you are saying that when there is a car right behind, you have this real sense of responsibility. [Focus on construal of demand characteristics of stimulus situation]

C8: Yeah, that's right.

T8: There's something about having all those cars around that really gets to you. [Probing for particular impact of stimulus]

C9: I seem to be preoccupied with what's going on behind me all the time.

T9: It's always there.

C10: I don't know why. I just feel I have to . . .

T10: I'm not sure what it feels like inside, kind of angry feeling . . . or . . . ? [Tentative focus on emotional reaction to stimulus]

C11: I don't feel angry very often . . . So I guess it would be more the anxiety.

T11: Kind of an anxious, shaky feeling . . . [More differentiated emotional reaction]

C12: I don't feel angry at those people. The anger is more directed toward myself.

T12: I'm not sure . . . toward yourself?

C13: Well, if I'm so concerned about these people behind me . . . well . . . maybe I'm not thinking enough of myself.

T13: Yeah . . . thinking of what *you* need. [Recognition of beginning of meaning bridge]

C14: Should I be so concerned about satisfying these people, or maybe concerned about myself as I go along.

T14: Yeah . . . I see . . .

C15: And maybe it's at that time . . . when I turned up the mirror . . . maybe I decided that I was going to be concerned about myself.

Stage IV. Exploring Own Mode of Functioning: Broadening, Deepening, and Owning, Leading to Resolution

After the new understanding at the meaning bridge clients usually spontaneously begin to recognize that the way they were functioning in that situation was an instance of a more pervasive and general mode of functioning that is inconsistent with their own self-expectations. This recognition seems to motivate them to engage in a much broader experiential search process. This self-guided exploratory search process is facilitated by the therapist in ways very much like any good Client-Centered exploration, trying to avoid intellectual analysis and maintaining a focus on the client's own inner awareness as the search proceeds. The search usually broadens out, exploring other kinds of situations in which these construals are made, leading to similar kinds of internal or external responses. It is still clearly an experiential search process, but it seems to be guided by the client's own implicit questions. "What is this personal style? What is it for? How does it fit with the rest of my experience?" It is as if the needs and wants, values and basic beliefs are being "tasted" in relation to each other. In facilitating this self-guided experiential search process, the therapist's empathic responses should reflect the newly emerging edges of the client's self-exploration, but they should not anticipate the areas toward which the search should move, or try to direct it toward particular conclusions. This experiential search process is an idiosyncratic and very important one.

When this search process is successful, the client eventually arrives at a "resolution." Resolution is defined as a new awareness of important aspects of one's own modes of functioning in a way that restructures the issue. Though still experientially involved, one now has a sense of what one wants to change and an emerging sense of having the power to instigate the change.

The following example is a shortened and condensed version of Stage IV—Recognition and Reexamination of Own Mode of Functioning.

This client had described her own reaction when a close friend had asked her casually "How are things with David?" David was the man with whom she had a close, serious relationship. She had felt startled and affronted and had snarled angrily at the friend. The client felt that her own reaction had been unreasonable, unexpected, and weird.

When the therapist suggested that this reaction might be worth exploring in detail, the client, C, agreed, saying that "there is something inside here that is making me distrust people." As C explored her own reaction further, she realized that the question about "things with David" had evoked for her the entire relationship with David, and especially her own discovery of evidence that he must be engaging in a relationship with another woman. Even though she still cared about him, her own trust was diminishing. She realized that, even though the friend had simply been asking a casual, friendly question, her own hostile, defensive reaction had been triggered by her feeling of "being caught snooping." Even though she knew that she hadn't found it deliberately, she still felt guilty and defensive. After she had reached this meaning bridge, the exploration broadened and deepened. She began to explore her complex feelings of guilt and then began a broader exploration of her own values.

C1: It's like I'd feel guilty even though I know I'm really not.

T1: I'm not sure . . . guilty? [Encouraging further elaboration]

C2: I've done something wrong, whether I found out by accident or not, I would still be incriminated because I found out.

T2: So somehow, feeling that it's wrong to be seeing these things, even though you weren't intentionally looking for them. You should be looking the other way when you saw them . . . or . . . ? [Tentatively reflecting focus on values]

C3: Mhm. That's the way I felt. . . But also I guess . . . if I didn't know, it wouldn't bother me, and I wouldn't have to deal with it.

T3: Then you wouldn't have to get into it?

C4: It's not that I don't want to deal with it. But I know that if I tell him I know these things, he'll get very defensive. He'll go nuts!

T4: So, here is the kind of information that would be crucial for you. But you feel you can't go on with him this way.

C5: I can't trust him now because he's let me down before. I'm automatically thinking bad things.

T5: So there's something about . . . bringing up this evidence . . . something wrong about bringing it up . . . ? [Refocusing on values]

C6: The way I found it out doesn't feel right . . . He didn't tell me about it.

T6: Kind of . . . you don't have any right to know . . . ? [Further focus on values]

C7: But I *do* know now, and I think I'm owed an explanation. But he'll think I am a real snoop. He'll be furious with me.

T7: So . . . I'm not sure . . . You feel you need an explanation?

C8: I have to learn to deal with the fact that I *know* these things. Am I just going to harbor these bad thoughts?

T8: And there's just something about harboring these . . . I don't know . . . It scares you? [Focusing on emotional impact]

C9: Like I'm ready to burst! One more thing and I'm just going to burst.

T9: Kind of all these feelings that you are holding tight inside, sitting on them, not letting them out. [Reflecting the tension]

C10: Almost like *I'm lying* in a way, because I can't speak my mind . . . I can't be open enough. And I'm usually so open . . . it's crazy. Usually, with anybody I'll tell them right out . . . and they don't get angry with me. And I didn't get angry when somebody did that with me, because they were being honest with me.

T10: It's really important for you to be honest, to speak your mind out. [Reflecting crucial value]

C11: Truth and honesty are the number one, cardinal rules. If I can't be honest, and I can't . . . like forget it . . . I don't even want to be near you!

T11: So you feel that there's something very wrong about not speaking your mind out to David. [Application of crucial values to situation]

C12: Yeah. I'm just completely uncomfortable . . . I just felt awful within myself when Jane asked "How are things with David?" Like I'd done something wrong.

T12: So it's almost as if you were catching yourself for not being honest. [Referring back to meaning bridge]

C13: Yeah . . . I feel like a liar and I feel devious, and I'm very insecure with David because I feel like I haven't been true to my own cardinal rule. I can't be honest because of his reactions . . . but then I'll feel guilty . . . See, to me, when you do something wrong and you're honest about it, the person still has the right to be angry at you. But that can lead the way to . . . They can forgive you. You have been honest and their trust hasn't been betrayed.

T13: So there's something about betraying the trust . . . [Emphasis on exploring crucial values]

C14: I'm betraying my *own* trust. I feel like I'm lying and I'm betraying myself.

T14: There's just something crucial about being so . . . open and honest. [Returning to basic value of honesty]

C15: I can't keep untruths locked in. I hate it! I can't stand it! . . . Lying was just "no go" in our family. If you wanted to do something that they didn't agree with, you told them. And then if they didn't like it, they would discuss it with you, and you would arrive at some kind of compromise.

T15: So, you learned there was a way of sitting down with people, discussing things, and coming out with what's on your mind, and things kind of worked out from there. [Honest discussion as solution]

C16: That's the most important thing for me. Without that honesty. I can't remain in this relationship. It's no go!

Near the end of the session the therapist usually asks clients what they got from the session, whether it led to any new ideas. This may be valuable for clients who have reached resolution, enabling them to focus on the new awareness that was most important for them. It may also be valuable even if a clear resolution has not been reached, but some worthwhile exploration seems to have taken place. This enables clients to articulate for themselves a clearer awareness of some of the new aspects that have emerged from the exploration. It may also motivate them to become aware of relevant experiences in the coming week.

CHAPTER 9

EXPERIENTIAL
FOCUSING FOR
AN UNCLEAR
FELT SENSE

T HE CENTRAL ASSUMPTION in Experiential Focusing is that there is an experiential "felt sense" that exists independently of our attempts to symbolize it (Gendlin, 1974, 1981, 1984). In our terms this "felt sense" emerges from implicit emotion schemes that can be accessed by internal attending and experiential processing. The felt sense is an implicit higher-level meaning, the sense of something that includes thoughts, feelings, perceptions, internal actions, and context. In addition to attending inwardly to the felt sense, it is therapeutically useful for the client to develop some form of symbolic expression for the felt sense, in the form of a label, metaphor, or image. Thus, the central process in Focusing is the full articulation of emotion schemes, that is, cognitive/ affective structures that integrate a variety of levels of processing including bodily sensory experiencing and verbal propositional represen-tations.

Note, however, that we are taking a "dialectical constructivist" (cf. Pascual-Leone, 1991) view of the relationship between experiencing or felt sense and conceptual symbol. As we see it, the label is constructed as a description of the emotional processing, but it is not arbitrary (not just any symbol will "fit"). At the same time, the symbol also "constructs" the felt referent in the sense of giving it shape and influencing its nature. Thus, there is a circular interaction between the symbol and the felt sense, with emotional experiencing changing as it is symbolized (Gendlin, 1984, 1990).

At a more basic level, however, Focusing addresses two key client task skills that are of general importance in experiential processing, namely, the ability to develop an internal imaginal "working space" and the ability to attend to one's inner felt sense. In this context, Focusing can help the client develop a clearer understanding of the difference between experiential processing and purely conceptual processing; thus, it may be of value early in therapy.

Our formulation of Focusing as an intervention within the broader context of a process-experiential approach is adapted from Gendlin (1981) and relies in part on Leijssen's (1990) description of the "microprocesses" of Focusing. An important aspect of this view is that it describes Focusing as a "modular" task, consisting of a number of relatively self-contained "subtasks" or "microprocesses." As a result, Focusing can either be carried out as a complete task, or specific subtasks can be utilized as appropriate in particular therapy situations.

THE "FOCUSING ATTITUDE"

Focusing is usually presented (e.g., Gendlin, 1981) as a six-step process (plus a seventh, "carrying forward" step). However, Leijssen (1990) has proposed that the essence of this task is a more general "Focusing Attitude" adopted by both client and therapist. In this view, Focusing is not a technique or a skill but, rather, a natural process that emerges spontaneously in the right environment and with the right preparation. She describes this attitude as one of waiting patiently in the presence of "the not yet speakable, being receptive to the not formed" (p. 228). The client and therapist must temporarily set aside their verbal-conceptual activity and preconceptions, a process similar in some ways to Eastern meditation practices but directed toward a specific object, the inner, felt sense.

WHAT NEEDS TO BE CHANGED?
THE UNDERLYING PROCESSING DIFFICULTY

In Chapter 4 emotion schemes were described as complex structures that always contain both nonverbal-experiential (bodily-somesthetic, expressive-motor) components and symbolic or verbal-conceptual components. In addition, we argued that experiencing is more accessible to conscious attention and choice when it is linked to verbal-conceptual elements.

It follows from this that an important dysfunctional process is the absence of either verbal-symbolic or experiential elements in a person's processing of his or her emotional experience. Often, the experiential element is missing; that is, the client is unable to "focus" his or her attention internally on a particular experience. Instead, the client operates in a purely conceptual mode, either thinking and speaking abstractly or intellectually without the experiential referent, or else attending externally, describing situational details (often in circular fashion). In either case, there is no actual immediate awareness of the associated inner experience. In a sense, then, one could say that the processing difficulty is one of an "absent" felt sense.

Alternatively, the client may be able to attend to some particular internal experience without being able to portray it adequately in words or images. In other words, the felt sense is present but "unclear." Because the verbal-conceptual element is missing, the client is left with a vague sense, usually of something being wrong or left unsettled.

As we discuss in the section that follows, these two difficulties give rise to variants of the basic Focusing marker, which in turn suggests how Focusing can be varied to help different clients develop functional emotion schemes.

OPPORTUNITIES FOR INTERVENTION: UNCLEAR FELT SENSE

The primary marker for Focusing is an Unclear Felt Sense. In addition, there are two variant markers, which define a general "process task" of helping the client to develop an internal working space and initial Attending mode of engagement. The variant markers signal opportunities for work that will lead up the primary Unclear Felt Sense marker.

Unclear Felt Sense

In Gendlin's writings, the prototypical marker for Focusing is an Unclear Felt Sense, that is, a vague sense of something not right, often a crankiness or a generalized sense of foreboding or anxiety, that things are "out of kilter" or slightly "off" in some way that one cannot put one's finger on. This marker has three identifying features: first, the client makes reference to a particular internal experience (versus an abstract, general, or external experience). Second, he or she describes difficulty in articulating or symbolizing this experience. Third, he or she expresses some distress or disturbance in connection with the experience. For example,

C: I don't quite know what I'm feeling about the break-up. I just sort of feel like something's not right, but I'm not sure what's going on.

C: I'm feeling kind of upset right now, but I'm having trouble putting it into words.

C: I know there's something going on inside me about my new job. I wish I could put my finger on it.

Variant Markers

With the Unclear Felt Sense marker, the client presents a clear task to work on. He or she has already contacted an internal felt sense and wants help in clarifying it. Often, however, the client has not yet arrived at the point of experiencing an internal felt sense. Thus, common variant markers for Focusing occur when the client speaks extensively without reference to his or her experience, and the therapist's empathic and exploratory reflections do not help the client develop an internal focus. This is the case when the client is either externalized ("circling") or stuck.

For example, the client may be speaking in a distanced, externalizing manner, often talking in circles around a topic without getting to what is important to him or her. Often, the client continues to talk on the surface or in an abstract manner, skipping over personal details of his or her actual experience, in spite of the therapist's use of empathic and exploratory reflections. We will refer to this variant marker as "*Externalized*."

There are four identifying features of Externalizing: First, either client or therapist has the experience of going in circles and not getting to what is emotionally involving or important to the client. Second, the experience of circling is immediate and current. Third, the therapist's efforts to deepen the process using empathic or exploratory reflections have not been successful. Fourth, the client either directly expresses or confirms a sense of being on the surface or circling.

It is very important for the therapist who senses that the client is in an external or abstract, circling mode to check this out rather than assuming that he or she is correct. It often happens that the client has a purpose or task that he or she has not yet made clear, or it may be that the therapist is being impatient and needs to wait for the client to "spiral in" to what is important to him or her. A general experiential inquiry often accomplishes this:

C: . . . (absently): And I don't know what he's going to do with all those other people in my department after the first of the year. You know, this new generation of managers are only interested in profits, not like when I was starting out, you know?

T: I'm wondering what you're experiencing right now as we're talking?

C: I was just feeling like I was going on and on, and not saying anything.

On the other hand, the client may express feelings of being

overwhelmed, scattered, tangled, confused, disorganized, or generally anxious; or blank, stuck, or empty. Clients may feel torn "in four different directions." (Being torn in only *two* ways is a marker for Two-Chair Dialogue; see Chapter 10.) Basically, they may have so much going on or may be so anxious or depressed that they feel paralyzed and unable to proceed in the therapy session. Sometimes, their speech and manner may appear either agitated or depressed. This variant will be referred as *Stuck*, and is illustrated by the following:

C: I don't know what to talk about. I've got five million things running through my mind, and I can't seem to concentrate on anything!

C: My mind is a complete blank right now. I know that I was thinking about some things to talk about on the way over here, but right now I can't think of any of them.

THE PROCESS OF RESOLUTION

The Client's Change Process in Focusing

Experiential Focusing consists of a series of six or seven subtasks, referred to as "steps" by Gendlin (1981) and as "microprocesses" by Leijssen (1990). The first of these steps is an option "Prefocusing" step, as indicated in Figure 9-1, whereas the last step provides a bridge to other activities. The figure depicts the current performance model for Focusing, an idealized model of the complete set of steps through which a client moves in resolving an Absent or Unclear Felt Sense. We will describe each step first from the point of view of client performances and then from the point of view of potentially facilitative therapist operations. In addition a short form of a rater's Degree-of-Resolution Scale devised for research purposes is shown in Table 9-1. This indicates six degrees of resolution and can be used as a guide to estimate how far along in the resolution process one has progressed.

Preliminary Step: Clearing a Space

The complete performance model for Focusing assumes that the client begins in an externalized or stuck state, as indicated by the presence of one of the variant markers. The first subtask or step is thus for the client to develop an adequate internal "working space" for experiential processing. The client can accomplish this by a series of internal actions, including becoming comfortable and relaxed, imagining an inner place where impressions and feelings form, finding a productive "working

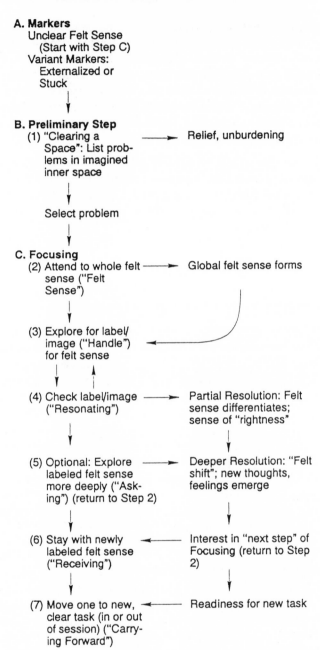

A. Markers
Unclear Felt Sense
(Start with Step C)
Variant Markers:
Externalized or
Stuck

B. Preliminary Step
(1) "Clearing a ⎯⎯⎯⎯➤ Relief, unburdening
Space": List prob-
lems in imagined
inner space

Select problem

C. Focusing
(2) Attend to whole felt ⎯⎯➤ Global felt sense forms
sense ("Felt
Sense")

(3) Explore for label/
image ("Handle")
for felt sense

(4) Check label/image ⎯⎯➤ Partial Resolution: Felt
("Resonating")   sense differentiates;
                              sense of "rightness"

(5) Optional: Explore ⎯⎯➤ Deeper Resolution: "Felt
labeled felt sense   shift"; new thoughts,
more deeply ("Ask-   feelings emerge
ing") (return to Step 2)

(6) Stay with newly ◄⎯⎯ Interest in "next step" of
labeled felt sense   Focusing (return to Step
("Receiving")   2)

(7) Move one to new, ◄⎯⎯ Readiness for new task
clear task (in or out
of session) ("Carry-
ing Forward")

FIGURE 9-1. Revised performance model for Experiential Focusing. Adapted from Gendlin (1981) and Leijssen (1990).

TABLE 9-1. Degrees of Resolution for Focusing Task

1. Nonengagement: Client presents or confirms Unclear Felt Sense (or feeling Externalized or Stuck) but does not engage in Focusing.

2. Clearing a Space: Client imagines an inner space, lists, selects problem or experience to focus on.

3. Felt Sense: Client attends to whole felt sense; attains global felt sense.

4. Finding a Handle: Client explores, tests (resonates) appropriate labels or images for felt sense, until the right one is found.

5. Felt Shift: Client explores labeled felt sense more deeply, until bodily sense of discomfort eases and experienced lack of clarity dissipates.

6. Carrying Forward from felt shift: After staying with new, changed feeling ("Receiving"), client explores implications for change outside of therapy.

---

distance" between self and problems, listing and setting aside immediate problems, and selecting one problem to work on. This "Prefocusing" step is referred to as "clearing a space" and is essential for everything else that follows. It is accomplished when the client arrives at a sense of a friendly, accepting internal space in which he or she feels separate from but in contact with his or her own problems. This usually results in an experience of relief and a readiness to select one problem in order to move on to the next step. Clients who present the primary marker, Unclear Felt Sense, have generally either completed this step already or can accomplish it without delay.

Felt Sense

The Felt Sense step has three prerequisites: First, the client is now able to form an internal "working space" (i.e., is not externalized or stuck). Second, the primary marker for Focusing is present; that is, the client is experiencing an unclear internal "felt sense." Third, the client feels safe in allowing him- or herself to experience painful or ambiguous experiences in the presence of the therapist. Having reached this point, however, the client may still not be attending to an internal felt sense of a selected experience or problem and may not yet be using the internal working space productively.

Therefore, the next subtask is for the client to place his or her inward-turned attention onto some specific unclear "object" of experience, in order to allow a holistic felt sense to form. This turning of attention to a specific unclear or difficult internal object occurs in the initial step of Focusing proper, referred to as the "Felt Sense" step. Experiential objects typically include an unclear, painful internal aspect or difficulty in oneself, but they might also include the client's internal experience of or reaction to another person or external situation. In this step, the client attempts to experience the unclear experiential object in a divergent (vs. convergent) manner, trying to let him- or herself sense as many different aspects as possible. This step has been successfully completed when the client adopts the Focusing attitude of inward-turned receptivity and allows a complex, rich felt sense to form.

Finding a Label or "Handle"

The client is ready for the next step of Focusing when he or she is both attending to a complex inner felt sense and feels ready to go deeper. However, a global sense of "what the problem is all about," is not enough for optimal emotional processing, since the verbal symbolization is still missing. Therefore, the next step is for the client to develop an initial verbal label or pictorial symbol for the nonverbal felt sense, by means of a kind of "dialogue" with it. The client does this by asking him- or herself for a descriptive label for the felt sense, searching inwardly, then waiting for an answer to emerge spontaneously. These symbols often take the form of qualities or adjectives, such as "twisted" or "cold as Lake Superior."

The dialogue initiated in this step is continued in the next step, where the emergent labels are checked or "resonated." In these two steps, the client is in the Experiential Search mode of engagement (Chapter 2), seeking a label that "hits the nail on the head." The Labeling step is accomplished when a potential label or "handle" emerges, although the client may return to it later.

Checking or "Resonating" a Label

Once the client arrives at a potential label for the felt sense, he or she is ready for the next step of Focusing, referred to as checking or "Resonating" (Gendlin, 1981). Having a potential label is often not enough to bring an uncomfortable or unclear feeling to resolution; to begin with, the label may not "fit" the client's felt sense. Therefore, potential labels must be checked against the felt sense and adjusted until a sense of "rightness" occurs, a process analogous to tuning a musical instrument. The Checking step of Focusing often involves an extensive back-and-forth search between a series of labels and an evolving felt sense. When the client finds the right label, this is usually marked nonverbally by a more definite manner and more open, friendly contact with the therapist (Iberg, 1990). The completion of the Checking stage, finding the "right" label, successfully resolves the "process task" of facilitating productive experiential processing through integrating verbal-conceptual and nonverbal-experiential elements. The client-checking step is also a useful microprocess for other times in therapy, such as when the client is engaging in overly-abstract or intellectual self-speculations.

Asking: An Optional Step When Reaching Resolution Is More Difficult

In the full Focusing model, the client might continue with an optional next step, referred to as "Asking," in which he or she continues the dialogue with the now-labeled felt sense, exploring and differentiating it more deeply by means of various self-directed probes in order to reach a fuller resolution, or "felt shift" (Gendlin, 1981). This continued exploration often leads to new thoughts and feelings. Furthermore, if the client began with the task of not only clarifying but transforming a troublesome experience, then symbolizing may not be sufficient. Although finding the right label is often enough to precipitate fuller resolution, a common consequence is a clearer formulation of a problem that needs further work in order to resolve.

The client's task in the Asking step is thus to take a successfully symbolized felt sense that is still experienced as troubling or in need of a full resolution, and to explore it in different ways, until a "felt shift" occurs. The client does this by continuing in the Experiential Search mode. He or she again uses the method of inner dialogue with the felt sense, taking an open, exploratory attitude while addressing questions inwardly and waiting to see what arises spontaneously. In doing so, the client "loops" back through the preceding three steps (Felt Sense, Labeling, Checking).

Full resolution usually carries with it clear verbal and nonverbal indicators, including absence of hesitancy; open, happy facial expression; and experiences of physical relief, freedom, or satisfaction (Iberg, 1990; Leijssen, 1990). In instances of partial resolution, these are either absent, or present to a much lesser degree.

Receiving

Once the client has arrived at resolution, either through finding an appropriate label or through a deeper felt shift in something that had been troubling, the client is ready to "receive" the new label, understanding or changed feeling. The underlying process in this Receiving step of Focusing is self-reflection on the impact of Perceptual Change (as described in Chapter 2); this helps to consolidate change and overcome the internal processes which typically undermine emergent change. It is important for the client to review, "savor," "taste," appreciate, or dwell on what is new or different. This helps the client to plant the change firmly in memory and to enjoy the self-esteem-enhancing sense of accomplishment that accompanies a felt shift. Without this step, the new clarity and understanding might be forgotten or lost track of.

However, the emerging experience labeled in Focusing is often experienced as "primitive" or childish. It is thus likely to activate internal conflict, especially Self-Evaluative Splits. In particular, some clients tend to discredit any steps forward they might have made by criticizing or attacking themselves (Leijssen, 1990). For this reason it is important for the client to take a moment to review and enjoy any changes before attempting to test these in the "real world" (see Carrying Forward, below). Having delayed criticism and practical application in order to review progress, the client is free to reflect on and to "savor" change, until he or she experiences a spontaneous readiness to go on and an openness to whatever comes next.

Carrying Forward

The felt shift naturally excites the client's interest in pursuing its implications, either for further self-understanding or for action outside of therapy. After consolidating the achieved change, the client often feels "ready for more." This self-motivated "Carrying Forward" process often takes the client back into further exploration in the form of continued self-exploration in the introspective Attending and Experiential Search modes (looping back to the Felt Sense step, see Figure 9-1); often the client moves ahead to develop additional tentative new understandings of the wider connections and issues implied by the resolution of the Focusing. On the other hand, the client may spontaneously express interest in pursuing the extra-therapy implications of resolution by deciding or preparing to take some new action, such as confronting or being more open with another person. In other words, the client may show in-session evidence of Problem Change impacts (see Chapter 2).

THERAPIST ATTITUDE AND OPERATIONS USED IN FOCUSING

Having described the steps through which the client may pass in resolving an Unclear Felt Sense, we now turn to the therapist attitude and interventions used to facilitate the client's process.

Focusing Attitude

As noted earlier, the Focusing Attitude is required of both client and therapist. The therapist must wait patiently for what is not yet clear or verbalized in the client (Leijssen, 1990). This attitude fosters a therapeutic environment in which clients feel safe enough to tolerate ambiguity and to give up control by their purely conceptual, nonexperiential processes. If Focusing is attempted in a situation in which the client does not feel safe, he or she will experience it as threatening.

How does the therapist enact this Focusing Attitude? In essence, the therapist follows the three relationship principles spelled out in Chapter 6, as reflected in the three recommendations made by Gendlin (1984), Leijssen (1990), and Mathieu-Coughlan and Klein (1984): First, the therapist should listen empathically to "every bit of communication." Second, the therapist should be continuously genuine or present to the client as an experiencing person. Third, he or she should introduce the client to the Focusing process a little bit at a time, during sessions.

The therapist operations in Focusing, given in Table 9-2, will now be described. In addition, we provide two running examples (adapted from Clark, 1990), each of which illustrates different aspects of the client processes and therapist operations involved.

Preliminary Steps: Helping the Client Prepare for Focusing

Ideally, the client accomplishes this preliminary step quickly and spontaneously and moves on to the steps of Focusing proper. If, however, the client is having difficulty spontaneously clearing a space (that is, if the variant Externalized or Stuck markers are present), then the therapist can facilitate this step by drawing on any of a number of different interventions that appear to be needed and are likely to facilitate matters (see also Table 9-2). Thus, it is usually a good idea to confirm the marker and elicit the client's agreement to try the intervention. If the client is tense, the therapist might suggest taking a deep breath or two and relaxing; if the client is confused, some process information may be given (e.g., on the use of a "focal point").

The therapist then asks the client to imagine an internal space, usually an imagined room or a clearing in the forest, then suggests that the client allow successive problems to emerge (e.g., suggesting that the client ask "What is keeping me from feeling good about myself?") and then suggests the client imagine setting the successive problems aside (e.g., in a box, niche, jar). Throughout, the therapist speaks slowly and meditatively in order to model the focusing attitude and to allow the client time to carry out the suggested internal actions.

TABLE 9-2. Therapist Operations for Focusing

A. Preliminary Operations
  1. Help client prepare for Focusing
    a. Confirm marker and obtain client's agreement to try intervention.
    b. Help client get comfortable.
    c. Suggest client imagine internal space.
    d. Suggest that the client allow successive problems to emerge, then imagine setting each aside.
    e. Ask client to select one problem to focus on.

B. Opening Operations: Beginning of Focusing
  2. Facilitate development of an internal felt sense.
    a. Suggest that client direct attention inside to problem.
    b. Encourage client to encompass the whole felt sense

C. Exploration Operations: Later Steps of Focusing
  3. Facilitate client finding label or "handle" step
    a. Listen for and reflect potential labels.
    b. As needed, encourage client with focusing prompts.
    c. Facilitate emergence of potential labels.
  4. Checking or "Resonating" a Label
    a. Direct client to check labels against felt sense, as needed until fit occurs.
  5. Help client explore labeled sense more deeply ("Asking" step)
    a. As needed, use General, Crux, and Felt Shift Direction questions.

D. Closure Operations
  6. Help client "receive" new or emerging experience
    a. As needed, suggest client "stay with" the new experience, or temporarily set self-criticism aside.
    b. Offer empathic exploration and genuine prizing of progress and sense of progress.
  7. Carrying Forward:
    a. Listen for, reflect new connections or possible actions in the world.

Most of these interventions are illustrated in the following example of a female client who had been having repeated difficulties in the session with feeling blocked; the example starts with the Stuck variant of the Unclear Felt Sense marker.

Example 9-1

C1: (*pause*) I don't know what to talk about. I'm stuck. (*pause*) [Potential client marker]

T1: What's that like, that stuckness? [Exploratory question to confirm marker]

C2: I don't know, it's just all these things, and they're driving me crazy. I feel kind of all tangled up inside. [Clear form of client marker]

T2: (*speaking slowly*) OK, there's something we can try here, to try to untangle things. You want to give it a try? [Obtain client agreement to carry out task]

C3: OK.

T3: OK, Here we go. (*pause*) You can close your eyes or you can look at a point someplace. [Instructions for task]

C4: (*nods*)

T4.1: Either way, whatever you're comfortable with. But you probably won't want to look at me because that might distract you. Can you get yourself comfortable, take a deep breath?

C,T: (*simultaneous deep breaths, then pause*) [T models nonverbal aspect of Focusing, slows self down for guiding Focusing]

T4.2: Maybe let some of the tension out. Just take a minute for yourself. (*pause*) OK? Ready to go on? (*pause*) [Relaxation instructions]

C5: (*nods*)

T5: Now I'm going to ask you to imagine a space inside yourself, a place where you feel things. I picture it as a clearing in a forest, or a room (*pause*), and I'm going to ask you to ask yourself (*pause*) "What's bothering me now?" Ask yourself, "Why don't I feel great right now?" (*pause*) and see what comes. As it comes, say it to me. (*pause*) Just take them one at a time, OK? [Suggest imaging internal space and allow successive problems emerge]

C6: Mhm.

T6: "What's bothering me right now?" (*pause*)

C7: I'm thinkin' about my dad.

T7: OK, there's the business with your dad. (*pause*) OK, take that business with your dad, and put it aside. Can you do that? [Process Suggestion for setting problem aside]

C8: Mhm.

T8: Now, ask yourself "What else is bothering me right now?"

C9: The thing with Ed.

T9: OK, The thing with Ed. Now take the thing with Ed and put it aside, push it to the edge of the space. OK? (*pause*) Got that?

C10: Mhm.

T10: OK. Repeat the process. "What else is bothering me? What else?" (*long pause*)

C11: My cousin.

T11: OK. The stuff with your cousin. OK, take that and put that aside to the edge. Ask yourself again, "What else is there that's bothering me?" (*pause*)

C12: My daughter.

T12: Your daughter. OK, there's some trouble with her. OK, take that and put that aside. What else is bothering you? (*pause*)

C13: My job.

T13: Your job. OK, take your job, put it aside. "What else is there?" (*long pause*)

C14: My mother.

T14: Your mother. OK? There's the trouble with your mother. Put that aside also. (*pause*) Ask yourself, "What else is bothering me?" I'll keep asking you till you run out of things, OK?

C15: (*laughing nervously*) All the men I ever knew.

T15: OK, so there's all of the men you ever knew, sitting there in a group, right? A crowd of them.

C16: Mhm.

T16: OK. This whole *business* with men, in general. Take that and put that aside, too. (*pause*) *What* else? Is there anything else, that's bothering you?

C17: No.

T17: OK, So you've got a space, a *clear* space. Can you imagine that clear space? [Suggestion to attend to internal clear space]

C18: Mhm.

T18: OK? How's that feel? [Checks for resolution of clearing space step]

C19: (*chuckles*) Feels good.

After successfully generating and clearing the imagined internal working space, the client prepares for the next step of Focusing by selecting one problem to attend to. If needed, the therapist can coach the client in the process of letting one problem "select itself."

Example 9-1, cont.

T19: Can you go back into your space (*pause*) and pick one of those things to focus on. Let it come. Don't pick it intellectually. Just see which one feels most important to you right now. (*T closes eyes, softens voice*) The *one* thing that feels *most* important to you right now. (*pause*) Say to yourself, "Of all those things, which one's bothering me the most right now. Which one needs my attention right now?" (*pause*) Just let it come. [Task instructions]

C20: (*pause*) I guess the thing with Ed.

At this point the client is in a "ready-to-work" state. She has entered the Attending mode of engagement, imagining an internal working space, creating a good working distance between herself and her problems, and selecting a particular problem or experiential object to focus on.

Facilitate Development of an Internal Felt Sense

Although clients sometimes move spontaneously into it, the Felt Sense Step is the most difficult one for many clients (Leijssen, 1990).

Therefore, it is often useful for the therapist to suggest that the client direct or redirect his or her attention inside to whatever is unclear or troubling. In doing this, the therapist encourages the Focusing Attitude of receptive waiting in the Attending Mode of engagement; the therapist allows the client to take his or her time. It may also be useful for the therapist to encourage the client to adopt a divergent attitude of trying to encompass the entire scope of the felt sense, "all of what that is about"; this may be valuable for helping the client to bypass any tendencies toward premature closure or narrowing of attention. Finally, it is important for the therapist to attend to and explore any signs that the client does not feel safe with this process (Leijssen, 1990). (These operations are summarized in Table 9-2.)

The following excerpt continues our previous example.

Example 9-1, cont.

C20: The thing with Ed. [i.e., is what is bothering me the most right now]

T20: OK, so that's the most troubling thing right now. (*pause*) Can you put that into the middle of that space inside? Not too close or too far away from you? [Preparing the client to attend to problem]

C21: Mhm. (*pause*) Well, he hasn't caused the pain that the others have.

T21: Can you pull it as close as you can, imagine it right there? [Directing client to attend to problem]

C22: Mhm.

T22: All the stuff with Ed, what that's all about. Not too fast, don't put words on it yet. All of it, the whole thing, can you feel it? [Directing client to attend to whole sense]

C23: (*nods*)

Note that the Felt Sense Step occurs largely in silence; as soon as clients begin to try to put the experience into words, they are in the next step. Thus, as illustrated in T22, the therapist may suggest that the client not try to symbolize the experience quite yet, in order to prevent premature closure and to allow the felt sense to emerge fully before attempting to put it into words.

Facilitate Client Finding a Label or "Handle"

Clients typically progress to this step spontaneously, without any direction or prompting from the therapist. Thus, the most important thing for the therapist to do at this stage is to listen empathically and to reflect on what the client is saying; a common and useful response here is for the therapist to listen for and repeat key descriptive words (potential handles; Leijssen, 1990). At times, when the client is having trouble putting an experience into words, the therapist may encourage the client with prompts such as:

T: What word or image comes to you now as you let yourself feel this whole sense of _____?

T: What is the most important quality in this feeling?

In addition, the therapist can also allow potential labels or images to emerge in him- or herself; however, it is very important that these not be imposed on the client and that they not distract or throw the client off-track.

This step is nicely illustrated by the following example, which comes from a male client who is Focusing on his feelings about his abusive older sister:

Example 9-2

T1: OK, What's the feeling like right now? [Attend to Felt Sense]

C1: It's hot.

T2: It's hot. (*pause*) OK. Can you describe the quality of that heat? Either a picture or a phrase? (*pause*) What's the heat like? (*pause*) [Labeling prompt]

C2: It's like a (*pause*) gas stove, the one particular section of it. Like you're boiling coffee. [T: Mhm] And there's a fire underneath that.

T3: Uh-huh. (*pause*) So there's fire in it, and it's boiling something on top of it.

C3: Yeah. (*pause*)

T4: But only one part of it. What's the rest of it? (*pause*) [Elaboration prompt]

C4: It doesn't feel that intense.

Note that T4 involves an attempt at helping the client to differentiate and elaborate his meaning in C2.

Help Client Check or "Resonate" Labels

The therapist's most important job in this step of Focusing is helping the client to maintain the contact between felt sense and potential labels until the sense of rightness or "fit" emerges. Thus, as needed, the client is directed to check the label against the felt sense; if hesitant, the client is encouraged to continue going back and forth between felt sense and symbols until he or she does achieve a "fit."

As noted earlier, therapist interventions to foster the client Checking process from Focusing may be useful at other times in therapy.

Thus, it is useful for the therapist to listen for the occurrence of Checking "micromarkers." These most often appear in the form of intellectualized self-speculations, for example,

C: (*glibly*) Maybe I'm trying to pay him back for all the times he let me down.

In addition, clients sometimes make negative assertions of experiencing (i.e., say they are *not* feeling something); or therapists may offer a word for the client's felt sense. In these various instances, it can be useful to suggest that clients check the potential label against their experience.

Our first Focusing example contains an explicit Checking step and therefore is worth returning to here:

Example 9-1, cont.

T23: (*slowly*) Now that you have a sense of all that bothers you with Ed, try to find a word or picture that captures it. Just let it come. (*pause*) [Labeling prompt]

C24: (*tentatively*) The word that comes to mind is "control."

T24: (*slowly*) OK, check that against what it feels like. (*pause*) [Checking prompt]

C25: Unsure. (*pause*)

T25: "Unsure." (*pause*) That fits better. (*pause*) Now check "unsure." [Checking prompt]

C26: (*sighs*) (*more firmly:*) Anger.

T26: That, too, that fits?

C27: (*nods*)

Here is another instance of the Checking step, taken from our second example of Focusing; the client is exploring his anger toward his sister when a Checking sequence spontaneously emerges. Note that in this second example the client ends up with a complex image for a complex feeling.

Example 9-2, cont.

T8: So, ignoring your sister would keep you from building on the (*pause*) bank of anger. [Offers metaphoric reflection]

C8: On the reservoir. Right. [Corrects metaphor]

T9: Uh-huh. (*pause*) The reservoir. So it's like a vat.

C9: (*laughs*) A lake.

T10: Oh! A *lake*, of boiling oil huh? Is that it?

C10: No, just a lake. [Checks and corrects therapist version]

T11: Just a lake. (*pause*)

C11: Lake Superior, something like that. Hudson Bay.

T12: Uh-huh. (*pause*) It's a pretty big lake.

C12: Yeah. (*pause*)

T13: Do you have a sense of that lake in you now? (*pause*) [Felt Sense prompt]

C13: Yeah, my perception of it is, it's cold.

T14: (*whispered*) Cold.

C14: (*firmly:*) And that's the way I see my sister sometimes. (*pause*) She's either cold or (*pause*) a banshee. If I had two words to describe her those would be the two.

Help Client Explore Labeled Sense More Deeply (Optional Step)

Gendlin (1981) and others (Clark, 1990; Hinterkopf, 1984) have described a series of three types of questions therapists can offer to clients to help them to resolve experiences that continue to be troubling after they are labeled successfully. These are General questions, Crux questions, and Felt Shift Direction questions. These questions are variants on the initial question of the Felt Sense Step ("What is this all about?"), and they help the client to loop back to that step in order to process the troubling experience more deeply.

General questions are used first, to encourage the client to engage in further differentiation of the label, usually taking the form,

T: What is so (*Label*) about this (*problem*)?

as in:

T: What is it that's so "twisted" about this feeling you have when your wife asks you to do things?

If needed, the therapist can next try a "*Crux*" question, often in the form of

T: What is the crux (*most important part, worst part, bottom line, heart*) of this (*label*) feeling?

as in:

T: Ask yourself, "What is the heart of this 'twisted' feeling in me?"

Finally, *Felt Shift Direction* questions are used when the other methods have been tried and the client is still "stuck." As Gendlin (1981) notes, these questions are analogous to "looking at the back of the book" for the answer to the math problem so that one can figure out the intervening steps. The therapist asks the client to imagine what it would be like if the problem were resolved, for example,

T: Now what I want you to do is direct this question toward that burning feeling. (*pause*) "What would it take (*pause*) for this to change?"

Such questions, used sparingly and at the right time, may help the client to access the crucial "sticking point" which prevents resolution.

Help Client Receive New or Emerging Experience

The therapist can facilitate the client step of Receiving by doing several things (Leijssen, 1990). First, as in the other tasks, it is important for the therapist to be able to recognize resolution when it occurs. He or she watches for the two Receiving step micromarkers, described earlier: a felt shift or sense of resolution; or self-criticism of emergent new experience or emotion schemes.

In Example 9-1 (the female client with the problem with her male friend), after the client labeled her discomfort with Ed as anger caused by his "treating me like a game," she began to blame herself and moved onto another task (a Self-Evaluation Split). Thus, the "process task" of helping her to get unstuck and find a therapeutic task were resolved, and she became more energetic and Task-Focused; however, the "content task" of resolving her conflicts about how to deal with Ed still remained and was not directly addressed by Focusing.

In the second example, 9-2, resolution actually occurred when the client identified the double image for his experience of his sister in turn C14; therapist and client explored this for several more minutes, then moved more clearly into the Receiving step.

As the client reviews and explores the change and its meaning, the therapist carries out empathic exploration and genuine prizing of both the progress and the client's sense of self-appreciation. In example 9-2, the therapist helps the client to identify with his good qualities and to separate himself from his abusive older sister:

Example 9-2, cont.

C21: My sister can't express love, even to her grandchildren.
T21: What does that evoke in you?
C22: Maybe I feel a little bit of pity for her. (*pause*)
T22: How about you, where are you right this minute?
C23: I know I'm doing better than she is on that score. It just seems natural to me to express love.
T23: It feels like you've got something on her. What's that like?

C24: I like that. It feels real good. And I don't think she'll ever feel that.

T24: Tell me more about that. What's the quality of that?

C25: It's warm.

T25: It's like, you can give yourself a little hug about that. (C, T *laugh together*)

Finally, if self-criticism is present, the therapist gently suggests that the client try at least temporarily to set it aside. If needed, the therapist suggests that the client "stay with" the new experience. Here is an example of a therapist response that does this:

C: Wow, that anger sure has gotten me into a lot of trouble; I wish it would go away.

T: So part of you feels that these rebellious feelings get you in trouble sometimes, but I guess they really are there for you. Can you just let yourself feel them some more for a little while?

Carrying Forward

The therapist's job in this last stage is straightforward: to listen for and empathically reflect the new connections or ways of acting as these begin to emerge, tentatively, in the client. In addition, Leijssen (1990) suggests that the therapist might also offer prompts to encourage this process of translation, such as,

T: What have you discovered now? Where does this leave you?

Often the Carrying Forward step is an impact of in-session Focusing that is accomplished outside the session. For example, on his postsession questionnaire, the client in Example 9-2 described how he was carrying forward the work illustrated above: "Perhaps I could empathize with my sister in the future and decide if there could be any possibility of a real relationship, or just forget her and purge the anger I feel toward her." If it had come up in the session, the therapist could have reflected and helped the client to explore this new direction.

DEAD-ENDS AND COMMON MISTAKES IN FOCUSING

Where do therapists most commonly err in carrying out Experiential Focusing? Leijssen (1990) has outlined a number of frequent mistakes that therapists need to guard against, including impatience, rigidity in following the model, ignoring the therapeutic relationship, and inappropriate use of "bibliotherapy."

Therapist impatience reflects a difficulty in maintaining the "Focusing attitude," which involves waiting in a state of openness for whatever emerges in the client's experience (Leijssen, 1990). Given the existence of an explicit set of six steps that lay out the process to resolution, the therapist may be tempted to "push the model," for example, by trying to get the client to focus on a felt sense before a good working distance has been achieved, or by pushing the client to symbolize the felt sense before it has been allowed to fully form, or by encouraging action before resolution has occurred.

Therapists also err when they follow the Focusing instructions too closely, often by forcing clients to go back through steps they have already passed. Clients differ widely in which steps of Focusing they traverse easily as opposed to with difficulty, requiring great sensitivity and flexibility on the part of the therapist. It is common for particular steps to be bypassed or even, at times, done in reverse order! It is for this reason that the full Focusing process described here is not typically carried out in therapy. Instead, the therapist uses whichever steps are called for by virtue of the nature and pattern of markers. When full Focusing is done, it is usually only carried out once, early in treatment.

Therapists can also create problems when they do not adapt Focusing language to specific clients (Leijssen, 1990). For example, some religious clients may be uncomfortable with locating a felt sense in their body because they regard it as untrustworthy and "sinful"; whereas others are simply not used to thinking in terms of an internal working space and find suggestions to attend inward puzzling and embarrassing. Other clients are put off by the "California-speak" of terms such as "felt sense" or "handle." Leijssen (1990) also points out the related problem of therapist and client using the technique to avoid real contact with each other, or as an excuse to ignore the client's experience of the therapeutic relationship.

CONCLUSION

As we have noted Focusing is a modular task made up of different microprocesses, each with its own micromarkers (Leijssen, 1990). Focusing can lend itself to use a complete task, or substasks can be used to help clients to work more effectively in sessions. In addition, it is important to emphasize that Focusing should not be taught systematically in therapy. It should instead be implemented in a flexible manner and adapted to the client's immediate needs (Gendlin, 1984, 1991; Leijssen, 1990; McGuire, 1991).

TWO-CHAIR
DIALOGUE AND
SPLITS

AS WE HAVE STATED, dysfunctional states occur because of underlying schematic processing difficulties. These difficulties arise from the content, structure, and organization of the emotion schemes through which one processes information about the self and the world. Specific types of processing difficulties can be related to specific types of interference with, or blocking off of, more adaptive emotional processing.

WHAT NEEDS TO BE CHANGED? THE
UNDERLYING PROCESSING DIFFICULTY

One of the major ways in which organisms interfere with their adaptive functioning is by the incorporation of societal standards, attitudes, and ways of thinking and acting that are to differing degrees at odds with their more basic needs, goals, or concerns (Perls et al., 1951). For a variety of different reasons, cultural and family influences often overwhelm individual preferences or requirements. These influences often reinforce the overriding of one's personal needs and preferences for the sake of complying with perceived social norms or the approval of others. Therefore, people often lose their ability to discriminate from among the various environmental resources those that will best meet their needs and are personally acceptable and unacceptable. In addition, the processes of discriminating one's own needs and the defining of oneself in relation to the environment are often difficult because they require some capacity to tolerate conflict and difference with others. People often incorporate values, standards, and judgments about how they ought to be and do not subject these to discriminative processing, selecting what fits for them and rejecting what doesn't. Then, the "shoulds," "oughts," evaluations, and expectations of other people come to exert an undue influence on their subsequent experience and behavior. It is important to note that the incorporation of external standards and evaluations often does not occur by conscious decision. Rather, these standards and evaluations are tacitly acquired and are incorporated into schemes. There they operate automatically and exert influence that people are not fully aware of.

When these automatic standards and evaluations operate so as to prohibit or suppress organismic feelings and needs, people experience a sense of confusion and struggle and find themselves unable to decide on clear courses of action. Or, having decided, they find themselves failing to execute their plans. The important issue here is that in this type of conflict, both the self-evaluative process and the organismic feelings and needs are often evoked automatically, largely out of the person's awareness. What is in awareness is the resultant sense of struggle and confusion or the inability to decide or act. At times, the global conflict itself may be in awareness but the specific self-evaluative and organismic processes underlying the conflict are not in focal awareness.

The general schematic processing difficulty that needs to be changed in this task is the simultaneous evocation of two opposing schematic structures involving incompatible behaviors, thoughts, feelings, and desires, either or both of which may be out of awareness. Of special significance in this form of disturbed functioning are the two sets of conflicting schemes. One is based on emotion schemes representing biologically adaptive emotions and needs, and the other set involves negative evaluations and introjected standards based on social learnings that oppose the feelings and desires. These schemes are evoked simultaneously by some internal or external cue, or they are evoked sequentially in response to each other. This leads to the experience of conflict. It is the conflict between schemes containing societal shoulds and those containing organismic feelings and needs that must be brought to awareness and changed.

Failure to recognize needs and wants leaves the person unclear and confused, whereas failure to meet the standards and values produces negative self-evaluation and loss of self-worth. In addition, the dominance of the negative evaluative scheme in these conflicts often leaves the person immobilized and can lead to anxiety, depression, loss of self-esteem, and other symptoms. For example Greenberg et al. (1991) noted that it is the combination of the negative cognitions of the critic, plus the intensity of the hostility or disgust of the critic toward the self that is important in producing some forms of depression. It is the intense hostility of the critic that overides the self's ability to respond actively and activates the weak/bad modular self-organization so characteristic of depression (i.e., depressive scheme).

Certain verbal and paralinguistic markers of these conflicts emerge in therapy. The markers of two aspects of self in opposition we have labeled "splits". A number of different split markers have been identified, each with its own characteristic verbal features and representing different types of conflictual processes (Greenberg, 1979). The first split, the one dealt with in this chapter, is the "conflict split."

OPPORTUNITIES FOR INTERVENTION: CONFLICT-SPLIT MARKERS

The marker of this type of split is a verbal statement by the client that two aspects of the self are in opposition. This is accompanied by some verbal or paralinguistic indicator that the person currently experiences a sense of struggle or coercion between the parts. The two parts in opposition are often clearly identified as two different "I" states. There is often a linguistic juxtaposition indicator such as "but" or "on the other hand" that sets the two "I's" in opposition. A prototypic split is: "On the one hand I do want to settle down and get married, but on the other hand I just can't decide if this is the right time and the right guy. I get so confused." The two "I's" represent two aspects of the self in opposition, and the statement "I just can't decide . . . I get so confused" indicates the sense of struggle, both verbally and vocally.

We have found that in instances of stated conflict of this type, the client generally is experiencing a conflict between standards and values on the one hand, and organismic emotional reactions and needs or wants on the other (Greenberg, 1984). We have come to focus on these splits as highly significant opportunities for change and have found that many conflict splits develop into dialogues involving *self-evaluations or self-coercion*. Thus, a conflict such as, "part of me wants this, but another part wants that," generally develops into some form of conflict between "shoulds" and "wants." For example, in our study of decisional conflicts (Greenberg & Webster, 1982), a conflict between wanting to stay or leave the city rapidly became a conflict between "you should stay" versus "I want to leave." More direct markers of self-evaluation or injunction often appear. Thus "I should do this, but I can't" or "I shouldn't do this, but I can't stop" is a frequent type of marker indicating the operation of some form of injunction. The statement "I want to do this, but I'm not competent" or "I'm too shy" indicates the operation of some form of self-evaluative processing. *Self-evaluative* and *self-coercive* splits are the most prolific and important types of conflict splits.

A prototypic marker from an actual session follows: "I should be able to do more. I'm just so damned lazy, I should get up and get going. I have to mow the lawn, do all the things that need to be done, instead I just laze around and do nothing. I just can't seem to get motivated." When an explicit verbal statement of a conflict split like this emerges, it indicates an experienced conflict between two parts of the self. In this case, we assume that the client is involved in a particular type of schematic processing difficulty in which opposing sets of schemes are being activated. The conflict is characteristically between societal "shoulds" and/or self-critical evaluations on one side and organismic feelings and associated needs and wants on the other. Although each scheme or set of schemes contains feelings, needs, and beliefs, we have repeatedly observed that one set, the internal critic, initially involves more conceptual processing. We refer to this as the "internal critic," and it is heavily weighted toward "shoulds" and negative evaluations. The other set, which we refer to as the experiencing self, involves predominantly more experiential processing and is more heavily laden with affective reactions, needs and wants.

Implicit Markers

Often markers of conflict splits occur with one aspect of the self implicit. Examples of these occur in the form of negative self-evaluations such as "I'm worthless," "I'm a failure," "I'm bad," or in the form of self-coercive statements such as "I should work harder," "I shouldn't be angry" in which one aspect of the self, the speaker, is evaluating, condemning, or coercing a second aspect of self-experience or behavior, which is not explicitly referred to. In addition, certain other statements about emotional states can be construed as indicating implicit splits but need to be explored to check if this is the case. Thus statements such as "I feel guilty, depressed, or hopeless" can be seen as involving one part of the self negatively evaluating another part of self, and statements such as "I feel afraid, unsure, or anxious" can be seen as one part of the self frightening the other part by catastrophizing about the future or constructing a threatening view of the past or the future.

Markers of Attribution of Conflict

On occasion, an individual may experience the critical aspect of a conflict split as though it were originating in someone else, for example, a 21-year-old man who wants to travel abroad is in conflict because as he says "my father thinks it would be wise for me to finish college first." Statements of this kind, putting self-desires against another's impeding evaluations or injunctions, represent markers of possible attributional splits in which the self-evaluation or coercion is attributed to another. Rather than the marker acting as a diagnostic indicator that the person is attributing, it is used as an opportunity to explore if there is an internal conflict.

The assumption put forth here is that the individual, having been exposed to the negative evaluations or expectations of parents, teachers, and others, learns both to be self-critical or self-pressuring and to expect this from others. This expectation leads the individual to become attuned to and sensitive to minor indications of criticism or expectations in others. In other words, the individual constructs schematic representations including both negative evaluations or expectations of self and anticipations of negative evaluations or expectations from others. These schemes are the filters through which experience is automatically processed. Unaware of this processing bias, new experience, which may disconfirm these expectations, is not easily available. In an example such as the one above, we assume that the client may be failing to some extent to recognize his own doubts about leaving college, and he may be attributing them to others or focusing on the opposing or critical comments of others rather than on his own internal doubts. In the above example, it is likely that the father does in fact disapprove of the plan. But if the client himself were clear about what he wanted to do, he would not be as sensitive to his father's views. Instead, he would experience the problem in a different fashion, perhaps focusing on practical issues such as the feasibility of traveling without his father's support.

As long as individuals attribute externally and experience others as being critical, they may not only be unable to resolve their internal conflicts, but they may also experience themselves as being victimized and controlled by others' views. Individuals who have discriminated, and either assimilated or rejected what they have introjected from others, are more readily able to distinguish personal values and standards from the evaluations and expectations of others. They generally are not immobilized by the criticism, opposition, or expectations of others.

In the attribution of evaluation or opposition, clients may report that they want to do something but cannot because someone else disapproves or disagrees. As we have said, the assumption is that an individual's difficulties in shrugging off the criticisms or opposition of another and making his or her own decisions is not primarily a result of the controlling actions or negative opinions of the other. The impediments to decision and actions are a person's own internal conflicts between what that individual believes he or she should do versus what the person wants to do.

A further form of experience that can be viewed as an indicator of an attribution split is that of shame and embarrassment. Here the shame indicates that one views oneself as an object of scorn, disgust, or contempt in the eyes of the other and as inferior, smaller, and weaker. Shame or embarrassment are thus implicit markers of attributional splits. The interesting issue is that generally people feel ashamed without the other being critical or contemptuous. This is because people have developed internal splits of self disgust/contempt that lead to shame. The ashamed state can be seen as the attribution of disgust/contempt to others or as imagining being contemptible/disgusting in the eyes of the other. There is, then, a complex internalized process of shaming the self. The experience of shame is therefore a good implicit marker of an attributional split, and Two-Chair Dialogue is an excellent means of explicating this process of internalized shame.

HOW DOES CHANGE OCCUR?

The basic assumption in this intervention is that having the person engage in a dialogue between opposing sides of the self will help bring these sides into creative contact with each other to develop an integrative solution. This is not a process of talking about a conflict or exploring why the conflict is experienced, rather, it is a living-through of the conflict in the present in order to forge new solutions. In terms of the modes of engagement described in Chapter 2, it involves the *active expression* of each side of the conflict to each other, *attending* to elements of experience in each side, as well as an *experiential search* process to access the tacit schemes involved in generating the experience of each side. The dialogue offers an opportunity for two aspects of experience to be brought into awareness at the same time and to be given the opportunity to fully express themselves to each other in an explicit and slowed-down fashion. Thus, covert internal dialogue is made overt with the opportunity afforded to each side to more fully articulate and explore its position. This makes the construction of a new synthesis more possible by virtue of the dialectical process of the contact of opposites.

In the process, change involves a form of self-acceptance in which people are able to accept their needs and wants, which may themselves evolve in the process of being acknowledged. The fundamental issue is how to bring the "shoulds" and needs into harmony, how to transform negative evaluation of one's wants into self-acceptance, and how to satisfy needs in a manner acceptable to one's values and standards. This involves reevaluating "shoulds" and standards to discriminate which aspects of these are truly held self-values and acknowledging previously disowned feelings and needs. Once one has clarified one's internal values and one's needs and wants, resolution occurs by facilitating development of a new organization to incorporate both in a harmonious fashion. This we call integrative self-acceptance, in that the two sides become more integrated and mutually affirming. No longer is there a disaffiliative relationship between the sides. They now accept each other and are integrated into a more self-accepting, nonconflictual response to evoking situations.

Change in this task involves predominantly active expression and experiential search processes. In the expressive process, each side is experienced more clearly and is engaged in dialectical contact with the other side by actually expressing out loud its point of view. This process of active expression vividly brings experience into awareness and brings opposing aspects of experiencing into direct contact thereby creating the possibility for the construction of a new organization. In the experiential search process, the experience of a particular side is developed by attending inward to the internal experience of that side in order to symbolize what is experienced. This process occurs predominantly in the experiencing chair although it appears at times in the other chair, especially when this chair softens its critical stance.

We have studied the process of resolution of conflict splits in a variety of different client populations and have developed a model of the steps to resolution (Greenberg, 1984). Intensive analysis of the in-session performances of clients who resolved conflicts in the context of Two-Chair Dialogue were compared with the performance of non-resolvers. This has resulted in the empirical identification of measurable components of successful resolution

Model of the Resolution Process

The model of resolution is shown in Figure 10-1. The path to resolution involves a number of stages and steps. The dialogue can be broken into three main stages: Opposition, Identification and Contact, and Integration. These are described in detail below. In addition, a short form of a rater's, Degree-of-Resolution Scale devised for research purposes is shown in Table 10-1. This indicates six degrees of resolution and can be used as a guide to estimate how far along in the resolution process one has progressed.

Opposition

In this first stage of the dialogue, after initially *roleplaying* the two sides, the client becomes more involved, leading to an activation of the schemes governing this conflict. The *harsh criticisms*, the "shoulds," the

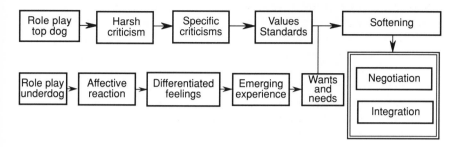

FIGURE 10-1. Refined performance model of conflict resolution.

expectations, and the self-evaluations then emerge in one chair, which we refer to as the critic. Meanwhile, the *affective reactions* to these criticisms emerge in another chair, which we refer to as the experiencing chair. The initial emotional reactions in the experiencing chair are predominantly reactive affects, either feelings of helplessness and submission or more rebellious anger and defiance. As the dialogue unfolds, the critic become more *specific*, referring to concrete episodes in the person's life. The criticisms become more detailed and are expressed with appropriate manner and feeling. Now the client's lips curl as they express condemnation, their fingers point and wag as they chastise, and the voice and posture match the content. These expressive motor and affective signs signal that the schemes are beginning to be activated. These signs are

TABLE 10-1. Degree-of-Resolution Scale (Short Form)—Splits

1. Description of a split in which one aspect of self is unaccepting of, or coercive toward, another aspect.

2. Criticisms, expectations, or "shoulds" are clearly expressed to the self in a concrete and specific manner.

3. The client's primary underlying feelings in response to the criticisms emerge.

4. Needs and wants associated with a newly experienced feeling are clearly expressed.

5. The client genuinely accepts his or her feelings and needs. Compassion, concern, and respect for the self may be shown.

6. There is a clear understanding of how various feelings, needs, and wishes may be accommodated and how previously antagonistic sides of the self may be reconciled in a working relationship.

then brought clearly into focal awareness and are further elaborated. This helps further activate aspects of the schematic associative network.

Identification and Contact

In the experiencing chair, the initial affective reaction is differentiated into a more complex set of feelings until, eventually, some more core primary feeling is acknowledged, perhaps a feeling of sadness or loneliness. When this feeling is fully heard, both by the person him- or herself and by the therapist, *a new feeling* somewhat different from the earlier feeling often emerges. Perhaps this is the angry feeling of not being heard. This feeling is then elaborated into the *want or need* leading to, for example, an assertive statement of the need to be validated.

In the resolution process, the critical chair now makes a shift from an essentially blaming, outer-focused position to a more self-focused, self-exploratory, and self-expressive stance. Rather than "You have failed," the critic now says "I have always wanted to be more than just a somebody." The change in focus is noticeable in the voice, which becomes more internally focused and exploratory, and in expressive stance, which becomes internal and self-expressive rather than external and blaming. Now the person in the critic chair begins to discriminate his or her own *values and standards*, formulating and stating personal hopes and ideals. At this point, the person is poised at a stage in the dialogue in which there is a dialectical confrontation between internal values and standards and organismic needs and wants. The fact that the opposing tendencies are now fully acknowledged in awareness and fully owned provides the soil for a new synthesis—the construction of an integrated resolution.

Integration

The formerly critical chair now *softens* and adopts a more affiliative stance toward the organismic concerns of the experiencing chair. The organismic concerns also become more open to *integration* by acknowledging the concerns of the other chair when necessary. Depending on the nature and content of the conflict, resolution occurs in different ways with different degrees of predominance of the original sides in the resolved state. Thus, at one end of the continuum there is a total predominance of organismic need integrated into the self, which has essentially rejected the "should" as not containing anything of value. At the middle of the continuum is a type of a *negotiated*, compromise resolution, recognizing and incorporating aspects of both sides. At the other end of the continuum is a less frequently observed type of resolution, involving the letting go of a need in favor of an ideal. It is important to note here that acceptance of organismic need does not refer to the encouragement of the expression of impulse. Impulsive behavior, rather than being an expression of a need, occurs more out of lack of recognition of the true needs of the self. The needs being accepted in this process are those that enhance the survival and growth of the organism.

An important observation we have made from our study of resolution is that the critic appears to soften in two noticeably different manners. One is the *softening into compassion* in which one part feels a type of understanding support for the vulnerability of the self. Another is a *softening into fear* in which the previously harsh critic expresses anxiety about ceasing to exist or being overwhelmed by an assertive need or want. In softening into compassion, resolution occurs by self-acceptance. In softening into fear, resolution occurs by the newly assertive part of the self acknowledging the fear of loss of control, or the fear of destruction of the controlling aspect, and by its providing some type of reassurance. Finally, two general forms of resolution appear to occur. One is an explicit negotiation between the two sides and the other is a more spontaneous integration in which the two sides cease to be disaffiliative and simply feel more integrated.

In summary, the two crucial resolution processes appear to be: (1) the expression of feelings, wants and needs from the more experiential self-organization; (2) the softening of the previously harsh critic in the more cognitive self-organization. The change process seems to be one of reaching some form of self-acceptance that involves an integration of different aspects of the self. In order for the person to experience self-acceptance and integration, the individual needs to discriminate both his or her own personal values and standards and his or her own feelings and needs. This occurs by the client identifying which of his or her standards and evaluations are external and by reevaluating or rejecting those that are incompatible with the self's true needs. Clients also need to be able to identify and acknowledge what it is they truly and primarily feel and want, as opposed to their more secondary reactive feelings and wants. This process involves both becoming aware of the automatic evaluations and standards and acknowledging and claiming one's primary feelings, action tendencies, and the needs associated with these feelings.

Therapeutic Intervention

Therapeutic intervention involves helping the client engage in a dialogue between the opposing aspects of the self until a core conflict emerges between an experiencing aspect of the self and a self-evaluative/coercive aspect. The therapist facilitates the client in identifying with each aspect and helps bring them into psychological contact with each other by directly expressing thoughts and feelings to each other. The process goal is to help the person listen to these expressions and respond to them until resolution is experienced. In life, these opposing aspects of self are often kept separated from each other in order to avoid direct conflict. Therefore, they never have the opportunity to engage in the dialectical process of the confrontation of opposites necessary to create a new synthesis. In this intervention, the opposing aspects are brought into contact with each other to allow the conflict to be faced and to run its course.

Therapeutic work involves an ongoing process of clearly separating the client's experience into two sharply differentiated aspects: self-evaluations and injunctions on the one hand;, self-experience on the other. The therapist's task is to develop the client's experience along these two separate tracks. At times he or she directs the process to facilitate separation and contact between the parts, always following emerging shifts in the client's experience and carefully tracking the emergence of the "critic" and the emergence of the "experiencer." At other times, the therapist directs the client to actively express by suggesting the client make statements to the other chair, or to attend to and exaggerate verbal and nonverbal behavior. At yet still other times, the therapist facilitates experiential search by reflecting feelings and validating and supporting the client's emerging experience. The therapist aims to help the client move from a vague sense of two opposing deadlocked aspects to two aspects listening to each other. The therapist's task then is to facilitate a dialogue between the two hostile sides and to help the two sides differentiate. This is done in order to help create an experience in which the client is willing to relinquish the struggle for self-control and the process of self-condemnation and put energy into listening and hearing the self.

In this intervention, the therapist is not a definer of the client's reality and does not determine which "shoulds" are societal and what feelings and needs are primary and organismic. Rather, the therapist facilitates the client's exploration and discovery from the client's own experience of what is alien and introjected, and what is organismically congruent. The therapist style is experimental and exploratory stimulating clients to try things out in order to see what they experience and to take on only what fits their experience. Throughout, the therapist adopts an empathic and caring stance, not an authoritarian distant one. For this reason, when reading the transcripts below, it is important to read in the vocal, facial, and postural cues conveying concern and involvement and to remember that the manner and tone of the therapist's engagement is egalitarian and warm rather than controlling or more knowing (see Greenberg, 1990).

THERAPIST OPERATIONS

This intervention process will be described in terms of pre- and postdialogue stages, and the three stages of the dialogue, Opposition, Identification and Contact, and Integration. Each stage involves a number of specific types of therapist operations that are shown in Table 10-2 and are discussed below.

Pre-Dialogue Stage

In this stage, the goal is to engage the client in the task. This is done in two major ways.

Establishing Collaboration

Once a client marker has been identified, the therapist establishes agreement with the client to work on the split as the focus for the therapy session. The therapist suggests the focus (as described below under identifying the two aspects of self), provides a rationale, and enlists the client's agreement to work on the split. This establishes a process goal.

TABLE 10-2. Therapist Operations

Predialogue Stage
  1. Establish task collaboration
  2. Structure the experiment

Opposition Stage
  3. Identify the two aspects of self
  4. Separate and create contact between the two sides
  5. Promote taking responsibility for each side's position

Contact Stage
  6. Promote client's awareness of automatic self-criticisms and injunctions
  7. Increase the specificity of the client's self- criticisms and injunctions
  8. Identify core self-evaluations and injunctions
  9. Access and express underlying feelings in the experiencer
  10. Encourage recognition of and affirm wants and needs of experiencer
  11. Increase awareness of values and standards

Integration Stage
  12. Focus critic on inner experience when softening appears and promote expression
  13. Facilitate negotiation or integration

Postdialogue Stage
  14. Create meaning perspective

Structuring the Experiment

The therapist then structures the experiment by introducing the idea of a dialogue between opposing sides by preparing the physical space, for example pulling over an extra chair, or indicating what it will be used for. The therapist also reassures the client that it may seem strange at first to dialogue with an empty chair and conveys to the client the experimental attitude of "let's try this and see what happens." Once goal and task agreement have been established, the therapist proceeds with the following sequential steps:

Opposition Stage

In this stage the goal is to separate out the opposing sides and to bring them into contact.

Identifiying the Two Aspects of Self

At the beginning of the experiment, the therapist listens to the client's report of the conflict and helps to identify the two opposing aspects as clearly as possible, often by reflecting the split: "So it sounds like part of you wants to do this but another part is really afraid." After establishing agreement to work, using Two-Chair Dialogue, the therapist then helps the client to fully develop each side of the conflict. This is done by directing the client to begin by speaking from the side of the conflict that seems more "alive" at the moment. For example, "Which side are you more in touch with right now?" Then, the client may either speak from within that side, "Can you speak from that side? What do you feel or want?" or express something from that side to the other side, "Tell the other side what you feel or want." Usually, the client will be able to discern which side is more alive quite easily. If not, the therapist suggests where the client might begin, based on his or her observations of the liveliness of the client's verbal and nonverbal communication. Often, the initial liveliness is located in the aspect of self that expresses itself in a harsh, self-critical, blaming manner.

This aspect of self, one that Perls described as the "Topdog" (1969) seems to lecture and attack the other aspect of self, as though it were addressing a true other, not the self. To increase the client's experience of separating out two conflicting aspects of self, the therapist directs the client to change chairs before speaking from the opposing aspect. The therapist may summarize and restate the harshest or most critical point made by the critic and then inquire "And what do you say in response to that?" Often the response is a self-defending, self-excusing one, characteristic of what Perls describes as the "Underdog." The therapist must ensure that the client not get stuck in the accusations and counteraccusations that are characteristic of these postures. It is as though each side has its own prepared, well-rehearsed, often-delivered speech to which the other side does not listen.

The therapist avoids this dead-end by refining each aspect of the conflict and having the experiencer attend inward to its felt reactions to the accusations. The therapist helps the dialogue unfold by listening carefully to both the content and style of each aspect as expressed by the client. In addition, as will be described below, the therapist makes explicit both the "what" and the "how" of the self-criticisms. The goal is to distill out the core criticisms and to help the client become aware of, identify with, and express the way in which the criticisms are delivered. This helps capture the affect and the intensity of the critic. Thus, in working with a client who begins a dialogue with a global evaluation such as "You're useless," the therapist promotes elaboration and differentiation by asking the client to "Be more specific and tell yourself what's useless." This is done until the client arrives at a core criticisms such as "You're so cowardly." After this the therapist might also bring to awareness *how* the person is relating to the experiencer by asking "Are you aware of how you're talking to yourself, of the tone in your voice?" If the client becomes aware of a scolding quality or a contemptuous quality, the therapist then asks the client to proceed by scolding or being contemptuous and to exaggerate this quality.

The therapist also concentrates on helping clients in the experiencing chair to attend to their current primary emotional experience in response to the criticisms. It is by this inner attending that the clients get past their initial reactive affect and move toward differentiating their more primary feelings. By helping the client refine each aspect and access underlying feeling, the therapist creates a forum where contact and negotiation can take place.

The Dynamic Process of Identifying the Two Aspects

It is important to recognize that this stage involves an ongoing, dynamic process of identifying and refining opposing aspects of the personality, rather than the identifying a single split. If the true opposition in the personality is not identified, the dialogue will not be an emotional, change-producing, experience. Rather, it will be a more conceptual, role-playing, experience. As the dialogue proceeds, the split must be continuously refined by separating out the developing opposing aspect of self. Thus, a person may start with a split, "I should do this but I can't." The aspect saying "I can't" may then differentiate into two sides, "I want to, but I'm afraid." This then becomes a new split in which "I'm afraid" splits into one side expressing the fear-producing experience, "If you do this, you'll make a fool of yourself" and the other side the effects of this such as "I feel hopeless or frightened."

An example of correctly identifying the opposed forces is given below. A client talks initially about her difficulty in separating from a relationship. She first presents a split of, "I should leave him but I can't." This develops in the chairs into, "You should leave him" versus "I want to stay." As "I want to stay" is explored, by actively expressing this aspect of experience, it differentiates into a new split, "I'm afraid to be without him." The experience of fear is then explored in the two chairs in terms of what creates the sense of fear. The therapist asks her to explore how she creates the fear by saying "Come over here. How do you make her afraid? Can you experiment with this? Try to make her afraid right now." She first discovers that she produces fear both by reminding herself of past loneliness and by anticipating future pain. The therapist encourages her to explore even more deeply by asking her to continue to enact how she makes herself feel insecure. She begins to enact some of the core insecurity producing internal appraisals, and she expresses the subtle yet powerful self-processes that produce her feelings. This may involve appraising herself as worthless, as without substance, or as despicable. In addition to appraising herself, she also begins to enact the more action-related aspects of her internal insecurity-producing procedures.

The goal here is to get at both what people say and what they do to themselves. Thus, certain internal fear-producing procedures, such as intruding in on oneself and making oneself disappear or destroying oneself, are enacted and experimented with until they create a current experience of the fundamental insecurity that is central to the experience. The enactment of these procedures accesses the automatic action sequences that were discussed in Chapter 3. They are controlled by schematic procedural processing, as opposed to the declarative processing that accounts only for the content of what is said rather than for what is done. Once the fundamental opposition, that of fear producer and basic insecurity have been clarified, the dialogue proceeds through its further stages in which the client's basic insecurity is then deepened and explored. Eventually, her internal resources and organismic potentials and confidence are contacted. These then challenge the fear producer, which softens its stance, and the two sides negotiate a relationship of greater support.

A conflict dialogue often begins with the Topdog occupying a "coaching" position saying "Do this, do that," "Be more confident, speak up," apparently designed to be helpful. This coaching has the opposite effect, making the person feel insecure and unsure. The paradox of coaching, or telling someone or oneself what or how to do things, is that it contains the implicit assumption that the person doesn't know how to do it, or isn't good enough. This coaching dialogue needs to evolve into one side, the self-evaluative side, evaluating the experiencer. This helps clarify that the self comes to feel unsure by this process of self-criticism and that the true opposition is between a critic and an experiencer.

Another type of dialogue in which it is important to identify the true opposing aspects is one related to depression and anxiety. In depression and anxiety, coaching can often act to worsen the symptoms. This occurs by the critic "shoulding" the person not to be depressed or anxious. The critic's behavior only exacerbates the depression or anxiety and needs to be transcended in order to relieve the disorder. Thus, dialogues of "You should get moving; don't be so depressed or anxious" and the response from the experiencing self "You're right," need to be differentiated into a more fundamental opposition or the core conflict. This is the conflict between the critical stance creating the depression such as "You're worthless" and the depressee's initial response of "I feel bad." Or the conflict between the catastrophizer's anxiety-creating "You'll fail" and the organisms resulting insecurity "I feel unsure." Once these true opposing aspects of the dialogue have been identified, the dialogue will proceed more fruitfully.

Facilitating the true opposition in the person's experience or identifying the core conflict is crucial, because if this is not done the dialogue will not develop and will become a confused intellectual exercise. Thus, the therapist works sensitively to refine the split until the true opposition occurring in the personality at the moment has been identified. The opposing sides are then put in contact with each other.

Separate and Create Contact

In order to maintain separation and contact, the therapist asks the client to speak from the experience of one aspect of self (that which is more lively for the client at the moment) and to direct statements to the other aspect. The experience of separation is enhanced by having the client change chairs when he or she shifts to speaking from the experience of the opposed aspect. Contact is created by having the client express feelings and wants to the other chair. When this occurs, the dialogue tends to take on a life of its own, as each side comes alive and is richly expressed.

Promote Taking Responsibility for Each Side's Position

Throughout this stage, the therapist continuously suggests that the client speak from the experience represented in each chair. This is helped by encouraging the making of "I" statements when speaking from the experiencer to capture feelings and by making "You" statements when speaking from the other chair to capture the blaming quality of this side. Each side needs to own and express itself, rather than talk about its experience or talk about the other part's experience. The goal is to express the experience of the side that one is occupying at that moment.

Example of the Opposition Stage

An example of an early stage of a dialogue is given below:

C: It's the feeling I have when I do certain things. It's, I would like to do them and not feel guilty but I can't. I just feel bad. [Conflict split]

T: Uh-huh.

C: I'd like to do them and feel any human being has the right to do them so I have a right to do them, but I don't feel that. Instead I make myself feel guilty.

T: Can you come over here and lets experiment with this, how you make yourself feel guilty? Can you try? Making her feel guilty and not feel that she has the right. That's seems to be what you're struggling with. [Structures experiment]

C: A human being has so many hours on this earth and you shouldn't waste any of them on frivolous, pointless, unproductive activity (tapping her foot).

T: Are you aware of your right foot. [Identifying aspect of self]

C: Yeah School Teacher!

T: Right. Right. Be a school teacher, go with that foot. [Promote responsibility for that side]

C: You should value what you have been given. (points her finger and taps her foot. Laughs) Get good use out of it.

T: And not fritter away . . .

C: And not fritter away your time, your life, in useless activities.

T: Will you tell her what you expect from her. [Promote awareness of injunctions and criticisms]

C: I expect you to be useful. (*pause*) I expect you to be adult (*yeah*) grown up. Play is for kids who don't know any better. Play is for kids who haven't learned any better. Play is for kids whose minds are undeveloped. When you're adult you should take pleasure in different sorts of things.

T: Will you change. What do you say? [Separate and contact]

C: [Experiencer] I get tired of using my mind all the time.

T: Uh-huh. You sound tired. Tell her. Tell her what it's like for you. [Identifying and promoting responsibility]

C: She doesn't care. (*snickers*)
T: Uh-huh. Leaves you feeling uncared for. [Empathic Exploration]
C: Yeah!
T: Tell her about it. [Promote responsibility]
C: I feel demanded on. I feel uncared for. (*pause*)
T: So what are you experiencing. [Experiential question to access feelings]
C: Stuck. (*sighs*) I'm . . .
T: Tell her this. [Process Suggestion to promote responsibility]
C: I feel stuck especially since I know!
T: Know what?
C: I know that when I use my mind all the time I use it poorly. I use a tired mind all the time, and I never have the chance to rejuvenate it.
T: Tell her this. [Process Suggestion to promote responsibility and contact]
C: (*sighs*) I never get a chance to recharge the batteries. I never get a chance to pause, that spot where you're really raring to go, where you have lots of energy, where you have a clear and narrow viewpoint of things.
T: Uh-huh so what are you really saying to her? What do you want? [Experiential question to encourage recognition of need]
C: I want . . . I want to do things that don't involve my head. I want to rest. Basically I want to rest.

In this dialogue the therapist identifies and separates out two aspects of self and has the client take each position. In addition the client begins to identify criticisms and feelings entering Stage 2 of the dialogue.

Additional First Stage: Identifying with the Attribution

When a dialogue begins with an attribution split, as it often does, the first stage prior to the opposition stage involves identifying the internal aspects of the attribution. Therapeutic work then begins with helping clients to discover that, if there are attributions, that an important source of evaluation or opposition is within themselves. This is accomplished by having the client enact the other's criticism or opposition in order to discover its internal source. This then adds a stage to therapeutic work at the beginning of the dialogue, before the opposition stage, which can be thought of as involving identifying with the attribution.

In this stage, the therapist directs the client to express the content and the manner of the other's evaluations or opposition. The therapist pays close attention to both the content, expression, and nonverbal behavior of the client in the role of the other and helps the client to become very specific in this role. As this unfolds, it usually becomes clear to clients that it is their own criticisms and doubts, or their own "shoulds" that are being voiced and not those of the other. This becomes clear from the degree of detail and concreteness of the criticisms or injunctions, to which an "other" could not have access. Thus, clients begin to recognize that the position attributed to the "other" represents a facet of their own view, one that has been unclear to them or of which they have been predominently unaware until now. The therapist then encourages clients to "identify with" this aspect of their experience, to recognize their own self-evaluations or coercion rather than continue to experience the evaluation or opposition as originating outside themselves. The dialogue then proceeds as a self–self dialogue between two opposing parts of self as described above. If the client does not identify the conflict as internal, it is then explored in its own terms as an interpersonal conflict.

Contact Stage

In this stage the therapist directs the client to change chairs frequently, attempting to facilitate access to and contact between the critic and the experiencer, using each to stimulate the other. The therapist works on refining the conflicting aspects to enable clients to formulate and identify with their deeper feelings and the associated wants and needs on one side and their own values and standards on the other.

Throughout, the therapist's main task is to help the client maintain the distinction between, and facilitate greater differentiation within and between, the two aspects of self. The therapist ensures that whatever is implicit in the client's verbal and nonverbal communication is explicated. In addition to listening to the content of the dialogue, this involves careful attending to the client's body, face, voice, gestures, noting any changes in these, and bringing these to the client's awareness. The client can then discover the meaning of these aspects of his or her communication and add them to the dialogue.

The following interventions are used in this stage.

Promote Client's Awareness of Self-Criticism and Injunctions

The therapist follows the self-evaluative track first listening for self-critical and self-coercive statements. This is followed by unfolding the dialogue and helping the client to specify the self statements. This is done by directing the client to articulate his or her set of expectations or the list of "shoulds," and to express them to the other aspect of self.

Increase Specificity of the Self-Evaluations and Injunctions

The focus here is on becoming more concrete and specific. Thus, the therapist intervenes at a statement by the critic of "You should work harder," with a question and process directive such as, "Can you be more specific? What should he do." This facilitates in the client's next statement, "Last night you shouldn't have given up at 10:30. You should have stuck with it at least another hour." The differentiation of the global "should" into more specific statements begins to reveal much more of the idiosyncratic content and quality of the person's criticisms. In addition to greater specification of the content, the therapist brings the client's attention to the manner and style of the self-evaluations, helping the client to become aware not only of what is being said, but also of how this is occurring. This is explicated as fully as possible by enacting the manner, such as being harsh or guilt-producing. The manner of relating to the self is often highly indicative of the person's character structure. Thus someone who is haughty and superior in their self-criticisms saying such things as "That's not good enough . . ." has this quality as a part of his or her personality and is quite different from someone who has a more cajoling and guilt producing style of criticism like "How can you do this . . .?" The process of haughtiness or guilt induction is then turned into content in the dialogue by asking the client to be haughty or cajoling. Clients then become aware not only of *what* their criticisms are but also *how* they themselves criticize, that is, their manner of self-relating. As the client engages in the specification and explication of self-criticism, he or she comes to realize experientially that the locus of criticism is within and is operating constantly with real affective intensity.

Identify Core Negative Self Statements

Identification of core negative self statements is achieved by heightening the key aspects of the negative self statements. Direct the client to repeat and exaggerate phrases or nonverbal expressions associated with self-disapproval. For example, if the client says "you're worthless" or sneers while criticizing, direct the client to "do this again . . ."; "do this some more . . ."; "put some words to this. . . ." This operation will intensify the client's affective arousal and help access core criticisms.

Access and Express Underlying Feelings in the Experiencer

Once the self-evaluative/coercive side has been developed fully, the therapist concentrates on the "experiencing" track. Here the therapist aims initially at accessing the client's feelings in response to the specific and heightened self-evaluations. The therapist may summarize, restate, or heighten the core evaluations or "shoulds" in order to elicit an affective response. The therapist then helps the client access primary feelings by guiding and, if necessary, teaching him or her, to focus inward and attend to emotion. The therapist might inquire: "What do you experience as that part says you're no good?" The client's response "I feel defeated" is then responded to with a reflection of the client's primary feelings. This reflection is followed by a directive, suggesting that the client express this feeling to the other chair in order to keep the focus on the dialogue between the parts. The therapist tracks the feelings as they change, focuses on emerging new experience, and encourages the exploration and expression of the emerging experience.

The client's productive engagement in this aspect of the task can be recognized in the client's manner of experience and expression. Rather than speaking glibly, expressing self-defense or making excuses (as the experiencing aspect does in the first phase of the dialogue), the client now searches experientially for words to match the feelings newly aroused in him- or herself. If the client has difficulty accessing underlying feeling, the therapist can help to further stimulate an affective response by getting the client to return to the self-evaluative track for a while. By repeating and intensifying the self-evaluations, the self's experience is finally evoked. In this intervention the criticisms in the other chair can thus be used as an aid to help arouse the client's feelings.

In addition to focusing the person internally on immediate experience in order to identify feelings, the therapist also promotes active expression of feelings. This process helps access feelings by enactment, as well as promotes contact between different aspects of experience. The therapist might say, "Tell her what you feel," suggesting the expression of the feeling to the other chair; or "What do you want to say to that side?"; or "Tell her about this." This process leads to a clarification and sharpening of the feeling and also builds the client's sense of identification with the feeling and his or her agency in its production.

The Emotional Change Process in this Stage

An issue of crucial importance in this stage of the dialogue is how one works with the painful feelings in the experiencing chair. Clients will experience and express intense feelings of sadness, despair, insecurity, exhaustion, and inadequacy, among others. How does one respond, and how does one facilitate change in these feelings? When someone enters a painful state saying "I feel weak" or "I feel sad," the therapist helps the client stay with the feeling rather than move away from it. He or she asks the client to immerse him- or herself fully in the feeling by suggesting "Stay with your sadness," or "Let it come, speak from it," or "Can you put some words to your feeling?" Essentially this facilitates the allocation of maximal attentional capacity to the experience in order to identify with it, to own it as fully as possible, and to symbolize it as accurately as possible. Once claimed as one's own and symbolized, the painful feelings are further differentiated and developed in phrases such as "I'm afraid life is passing me by," "I feel all alone and soft," or "In my softness I'm vulnerable." This attentional focus to and symbolization of evoked experience entails the creation of new meaning by a dialectical construction that involves both discovery and creation. Experience is symbolized and new possibilities are created. The continual operation of the growth tendency in the client and the therapist's empathic attunement to this growth tendency leads to the forward movement.

A key therapist intervention, following the identification and symbolizing of feelings, is the asking of Exploratory Questions that inquire into clients' experience, particularly their needs and wants. This facilitates elaboration and differentiation. It is useful to note that the question "What's it like inside?" asked in an exploratory tone is far more effective in facilitating symbolization than "What are you feeling." The former question promotes differentiated bottom-up description, the latter often engenders conceptual, top-down labeling.

This process of differentiation of feeling leads to the emergence of new experience and ultimately to the expression of needs associated with emergent feelings. One of the principles of affective processing has been stated as "one thing leads to another" (Polster & Polster, 1973; Greenberg & Safran, 1987). This is a type of "law" of process. In essence, processing affective information by attending to it, symbolizing *new features*, and differentiating and integrating these new symbols leads to the creation of new meaning and to the emergence of new experience. Thus, the experience "I'm afraid" or "I feel vulnerable" may evolve into "I feel delicate, and I like this feeling" when new features of the experience are attended to. Furthermore, the feeling "I feel unworthy," having been differentiated into "I did my best, you expected too much of me," may transform into "I feel angry" and finally into the assertion to the other chair, "You expect too much of me." Given that emotions are action tendencies based on appraisals in relation to needs, once the emerging emotion has been identified, it is crucial to identify the action tendency and need associated with it. "I feel exhausted" generally contains within it a tendency to pull back or cease effort and a need to relax. "I feel angry" generally contains a thrusting forward and a need to defend or break free of. However, it is important to note that all human experiences are ultimately idiosyncratic. There are different types of exhaustion and anger for different people and different types for the same person at different times. Thus, each feeling needs to be explored for its current unique action tendency and need.

When a client's pain or basic insecurity has been contacted in the experiencer, any tendency to move away from this discomfort is overcome by the support from the therapist and the collaborative alliance to work on this painful place by accepting it, staying with it, and allowing it to develop. The person might experience feeling shaky and unsafe, feeling existentially vulnerable—afraid of falling apart, or of collapsing, disappearing, or becoming chaotic. This is not an out-of-control, panic state. It is an allowing, experiencing process in which the person is in some way facing his or her pain, fear, or fundamental insecurity. This is done in the safety of the presence of another, who provides the acceptance and the security that helps the person to feel contained. Having allowed the pain or insecurity and experienced it in this safety, a transformational process occurs in which the person contacts his or her own inner resources, organismic capacities, and confidence. Paradoxically, this often occurs by owning and confidently asserting "I feel unsure" or "I feel like I don't know what to do." From this congruent and self-accepting base of feeling "what is," be that insecurity, or vulnerability, or pain, the person begins to feel more able to cope. It has been the struggle against this feeling and/or the desire to protect this aspect of the self that has utilized so much of the person's internal resources and attentional capacity and that has kept the person weak and split. The acceptance of the feeling by allowing it, and discovering that one survives the feeling, frees up internal resources that can be used to enhance coping with the *world* rather than coping with the *self*. It is this type of acknowledgment and expression of the organism's primary feelings that makes it possible for the critic to shift out of the self-blame.

Affirm Wants and Needs of the Experiencing Self

This affirmation of the wants and needs of the experiencing self is done by the therapist offering validation and support for emerging new feelings and the associated wants and needs as they emerge. The previously unacknowledged needs are affirmed and supported. At this point, the therapist may respond empathically to the client. However, such responses are to be followed by a direction to "tell this to the other part" in order to have the client actively express the feelings and needs to the other part. Once a client accesses and expresses underlying feelings, the person can eventually begin to make some more assertive feeling statements. For example, he or she may say: "I don't ever get a chance to be myself," which implies a need to be myself, or "I'm not perfect, you expect too much," or "I feel exhausted." When some feeling is expressed that implies a need or want, the therapist asks, "What do you want?" or "Tell her what you need." It is these needs or action tendencies that accompany feelings that provide the directional tendency of experience, and it is these that must be brought to awareness.

This expression of need in conjunction with the identification of standards described below then promotes the necessary contact between the expression of needs and wants and the values and standards. It is this contact that offers an opportunity for the creation of newness and synthesis.

Increase Awareness of Own Values, Standards, and Expectations

While the client is speaking from the "self critical" chair, the therapist helps him or her to focus on what is hoped for and to express these ideals. This is not an instructional intervention in which the therapist teaches the client to identify his or her values. It is an exploratory process designed to help the person symbolize the currently experienced core standards and values upon which the criticisms are based, as they emerge.

Example of the Identification and Contact Stage

This excerpt is taken from an ongoing dialogue in which the client, in the experiencing chair, is talking to both parents in the other chair. The integrated sense of her parents is being enacted to access the "shoulds" and expectations. In this case the parents can be viewed as internalized representations that carry the person's introjected conditions of worth or "shoulds."

C: (*experiencer*) But I know that if I was how you wanted me to be I'd be good. But I'm *not good*. I'm just me.

T: Yeah . . . OK Come over here. Tell her "You should be good. You should be . . ." How did they try to mold you? [Awareness of critic]

C: (*Moans, sighs. Voice lower, calmer*) Mom was always saying this facetious cute thing: "Whatever happened to that darling little child with the dimple?" (*sniff*)

T: Uh-huh. Say that. [Promote responsibility]

C: Whatever happened to that darling little child with a dimple in her cheek we used to have around here *that was so good?*

T: Yeah. Be these expectations, tell her how she should be . . . What are the core messages about how she should or shouldn't be . . . ? [Identify core evaluations]

C: She shouldn't make any waves. She shouldn't try to disrupt the family.

T: You shouldn't . . . [Responsibility]

C: You shouldn't disrupt anything here.

T: Can you make this some specific situation? What shouldn't she disrupt in the family? Tell her. [Increase specificity]

C: It's just a big catalogue. I'm thinking about being told "Why don't you fit into the family?" Don't be so noisy, you're too "other," be like us. (*Increased tempo*) Be loving, be giving, Do good deeds, go into the world, give of yourself, take care of people. (*slows down*). Be open, give to the world.

T: Yeah, say this again. [Identify core injunction]

C: But this is what I say to myself now.

T: Uh-huh. So tell her. What I'm hearing you say, somehow—you should be open and give to the world. [Identify core injunction]

C: You should be . . . soft . . . and nice (*sighs*) and brave (*voice breaks*) and smart . . . and . . . open and loving.

T: Yeah. You should be loving. [Core injunction]

C: You should be loving (*sniffs*) and you should be brave (*deep breath*).

T: Right . . . These are the two important things—loving and brave. Say it again. [Core injunction]

C: You should be loving and you should be brave. (*deep breath*)

T: Uh-huh. And what do you say? (*Indicates to change chairs*) [Separate and contact and access underlying feelings is experiencer]

C: Yeah. And I *can't*. (*sobs*)

T: Uh-huh. Stay with this feeling. [Support and access underlying feeling in experiencer]

C: I just can't. (*sobs*) I don't want to.

T: Say this again. [Affirm wants and needs]

C: I don't *wanna*.

T: Yeah. Again.

C: (*More deeply, slowly, emphatically*) I don't want to.

T: Tell her what you do want. [Recognition of wants]

C: I just want to be myself. I want to follow my path, do what I do, and do it well.

T: Uh-huh. I want to be allowed to be me and to develop my talents. [Affirm wants]

C: Yeah.

T: Change what does she say. [Separate and contact]

C: Well. It's not good to be selfish. It's not that you shouldn't be you, it's just that it's also important to contribute to others. Don't be only for you, give of yourself.

T: Change. [Separate and contact]
C: I don't want to sacrifice myself. I want to give, but I won't give myself up.

In this the therapist promotes identification of the introjected criticisms and works on making them more specific and on identifying the core criticisms. The client's underlying feelings and wants are identified in the experiencer, and a standard and value emerge in the other chair.

Integration

Focus Critic on Inner Experience and Promote Expression

Once the previously unexpressed organismic needs have been expressed, the blaming has stopped, and the standards and values have begun to be articulated, the therapist directs the client to change back to the self-evaluative track. Here the therapist checks for signs of whether or not the critic is softening, observing if there is any indication of the critic beginning to reexamine its position relative to the experiencer. If there is a shift of state, the therapist helps the client focus inward by asking the critic "What are you feeling right now toward the experiencing self?" The newly accessed feelings contrast noticeably with the harsh criticism and blaming feelings initially expressed and may include concern, understanding, and respect for the self. These are expressed to the experiencer.

Facilitate Negotiation or Integration

Negotiation or integration should be facilitated between the two aspects of self by shuttling back and forth between the two aspects and having each express their own perspectives and want. Sometimes explicit negotiation is facilitated; at other times, the spontaneous emergence of a new integration is consolidated.

When the critic's underlying feelings have been accessed and expressed, the therapist explores the client's response to this shift. In the experiencing chair, the client now expresses a new, more assertive perspective. The therapist will recognize this in the client's more confident tone and manner of expression. As the therapist directs the client to shift between these two positions, the client often will begin to experience a coming together of the two aspects, as though the differences between them have melted into a single more unified perspective. An example of the Integration stage is given below. The dialogue begins with the client moving to the critical chair.

C: [experiencer] I need space just give me some space.

T: Uh-huh. Change.

C: [Critic] Hmm . . . Well I'm not disappearing. I must warn you that right now. [T: Uh-huh] There's no way you're getting rid of me.

T: What do you . . .

C: I'm lurking around.

T: What happens, what happens when she says give me space? [Focus critic on inner experience]

C: Well . . . I'm kind of fearful. (*Voice becomes more internally focused*) I, I experience myself kind of backing up in a way, but I'm watching.

T: Tell her what you fear for. [Express inner experience]

C: Um . . . yeah . . . I'm really scared for you . . . I'm really scared that a . . . you're going to get hurt [T: Yeah] and a . . . that a . . . I'm scared of the future sense, not so much in the present [T: Uh-huh] I don't think. That's interesting. Yeah I suddenly have this feeling like . . . like . . . like what happens ten years from now. (T: Uh-huh) . . . A . . . a . . .

T: What do you feel towards her? [Express inner experience]

C: Oh . . . very protective [T: Uh-huh] . . . I . . . just realized I feel a lot of love for her too [T: Uh-huh] Uh-huh . . . But I just don't want her to get hurt.

T: Yeah, tell her.

C: And a . . . I don't want you to get hurt. And what I'm doing is watching out for you. What I'm doing . . . is using my . . . my talents or . . . abilities, or whatever it is . . . my awareness . . . um . . . and watching out for the part of you . . . that . . . in watching out for you . . . yeah. Um . . . and trying to . . . make sure you don't get hurt. Trying to make sure that you make wise decisions and . . . um . . . don't run off with . . . stars in your eyes.

T: Uh-huh . . . So over here.

C: [Experiencer] (*chuckles*) Well, you see, but I want to run off with stars in my eyes. (*laughs*) That's the whole point. (*laughs*) Um . . . I think you've missed the whole thing . . . um . . . I don't mind you watching, and I don't mind you making . . . you know, comments and, I don't mind you a . . . bringing up things . . . but you can be such a wet blanket . . .

T: Uh-huh (*laughs*) . . .

C: And I really don't want you around. Well I want you—No that's not altogether true. I want you to be there . . . for me to call on if I need you . . . but stop being such a wet blanket.

T: So what do you want from her? [Facilitate negotiation]

C: When you see I'm about to make . . . some disastrous decision, then you could step in. But for the rest of the time, let me . . . let me breathe [T: Uh-huh] Give me room. Don't stifle me.

T: Hm . . . So . . . can you change? What . . . [Separate and contact]

C: *(sigh)* Yes, but you should be very thankful I'm here . . . Yeah I'm, I'm . . . I may be stifling and I may be . . . [T: Uh-huh] . . . a . . . distracting, and I may put the brakes on a lot of stuff, but . . . you know, you still need me . . . because I keep you out of a lot of trouble . . . a lot of jams . . . yeah . . .

T: What do you experience? [Attend inward]

C: I've stopped breathing [T: Uh-huh] I'm just holding everything absolutely still . . . ummh . . . I cut things off. [T: Yeah, yeah] Yeah . . . I kind of . . . I hang on umm . . . I don't, I don't . . . you know, go with things . . . I put on brakes.

T: So what do you need from her? [Recognition of need]

C: Hmm, what do I need of her? What do I need from her?

T: 'Cause it sounds like you kind of get frightened. [Conjecture]

C: Well . . . I get frightened in a way, yeah . . . um . . . I want her to listen to me . . . um . . .

T: Right now, what do you want her to listen to? [Facilitate negotiation]

C: . . . Oh, I feel really . . . like a . . . I feel like I should be—well, over there.

T: OK. Change.

C: Um . . . hmm . . . right now I think I've heard you . . . And a . . . I heard you, you know, I heard your warning. I heard what you said.

T: Tell her what you heard. [Facilitate negotiation]

C: Well, I heard you say you know oh oh . . . a he's [the new man in her life] not dependable . . . you know, if you get involved with him, you're . . . you know, it's purely a . . . a short term thing . . . and . . . I don't put any stock in him, you know, I mean . . . I don't invest in it too much. [T: Uh-huh] I've heard all that . . . all those things you said . . .

T: And . . .

C: And I know, [T: Uh-huh] you know, that what you're saying about a lot of things . . . is perfectly true . . .

T: And I want . . . [Facilitate negotiation]

C: I want to risk it . . .

T: And what do you want from this part . . . [Facilitate negotiation]

C: Hmm—from that part of me.

T: Uh-huh.

C: I want you to trust me.

T: Change. What do you say. [Separate and contact]

C: I will trust you, and I also want you to pay heed to me.

In this transcript we see when the therapist hears a change in the critic she focuses the critic on her inner experience, and the critic softens into both fear and compassion. The therapist then facilitates a negotiation between the two sides.

Postdialogue Stage

Creating Meaning Perspective

In this phase, when appropriate, the therapist and the client talk about the client's in-session experience. This is done to help the client symbolize what has occurred and to extract personal meaning from the experiment. The new experience of self gained in the experiment is assimilated and integrated. When a resolution has not been reached, the therapist may summarize what has occurred and set awareness homework related to discoveries in the dialogue. Homework, is often used, such as becoming aware of the self-evaluations, becoming aware of the feelings and needs, or becoming aware of the manner the person adopts in delivering or opposing internal criticisms. In addition to becoming aware, the client may also be instructed to deliberately engage in any of the above processes during the week. This is done to bring them into awareness and under control by turning automatic processing into controlled processing (Greenberg & Safran, 1981, 1987).

Example of the Postdialogue Stage of the Task

T: Can you describe that to me, if you can. What do you feel like?

C: [Experiencer] Well I guess actually I'm sort of feeling a little bit more . . . um . . . don't know how to put it into words . . . um . . . just a bit more outlined. . .

T: Yeah, yeah . . . I understand that . . . you can feel that you're outlined.

C: Yeah you know, whereas that person always just seemed like—that person had a lot more to say . . .

T: But now you're feeling—are you aware of how you're sitting?

C: (*pause*) Like I always am. (*laughs*)

T: (*laughs*) You're holding you're head a little higher . . . [process observation]

C: Oh, really?

T: What's that like, . . . so what do you say to her?

C: Well . . . uh, that's something I needed to hear, actually. (*laughs*) Um . . . you know I need any support that you can give me, and as a matter of fact—or, if you can't give me support, then get the hell out of here . . . pack your bags . . .

T: Right.

C: . . . and go!

T: Right.

C: (*laughs*)

T: Right. So it's if you can't give me support, at least don't shoot at me.

C: Just don't be there, you know . . .

T: Right.

C: . . . just, just either have a void or something—oh mind you, that's not good either but . . . um . . . but I appreciate the support, and I think . . . *I need any support*, certainly from within myself, and I realize I need to fight to get the support I need and fight her off when she's putting me down.

T: Mhm.

C: . . . I mean, the only person who could take care of my life is me! And um . . .

T: Mhm. Can you say this again?

C: I said the only *person* who can take charge of my life is *me*.

T: Uh-huh.

C: And a . . .

T: What do you experience when you say this?

C: I feel . . . stronger.

T: Uh-huh, uh-huh.

C: I do . . .

In this excerpt the therapist alternates between facilitating the creation of meaning and finalizing some aspects of the integration stage of the dialogue.

CONCLUSION

It is important to emphasize that although stages and steps of a resolution process have been identified and specified, they need to arise spontaneously from the client in order for resolution to occur. They are in no way to be imposed on the client. The therapist's stance is one of facilitation, not modification nor instruction. The dialogue needs to engage the client in experiential, not conceptual, processing. The model and stages act as a map to help therapists recognize where they are and what processes to attempt to facilitate to keep the client on the path, or not veer too far astray. In addition, the model can be helpful in guiding therapists to not get in the way of the client's naturally attained steps to resolution.

TWO-CHAIR
ENACTMENT FOR
SELF-INTERRUPTIVE
SPLITS

T HOUGH EMOTIONS can be viewed as affective responses to situations, they also have social aspects. The experience and expression of emotion can have a social impact, and in this way humans have evolved processes of affective regulation. Affect regulation is both healthy and functional, however problems of under-control and over-control of emotional experience and expression sometimes arise. This chapter focuses on problems of over-control, involving the interruption or over-regulation of adaptive emotional experience and expression. Once one cuts off primary adaptive emotions, one loses contact with one's sense of self and one's needs. This can result in feelings of hopelessness and helplessness, cynicism, emptiness or alienation, and has been associated with a variety of psychosomatic symptoms.

In this chapter we focus on a second type of split, one involved in the interruption of emotional experience and expression (Perls et al., 1951). Both the marker and resolution processes of this split are slightly different from those of the conflict split. This split in which one part of the self interrupts a second part of the self was referred to initially as a subject/object split (Greenberg, 1979). It is now referred to as a self-interruptive split. This emphasizes the essential difference between this split, which involves interruption of expression, and conflict splits, which involve self-evaluation or self-coercion. Both types of split involve a conflict between two aspects of the self. However, the processes involved in self-interruptive splits emphasize interruptive *activity* against the self, as opposed to *evaluation* or use of coercive *power* against the self.

WHAT NEEDS TO BE CHANGED? THE UNDERLYING PROCESSING DIFFICULTY

Organisms function optimally when they are able to experience their primary emotional reactions and the needs associated with them, and they are able to integrate these with awareness of what the environment can offer to satisfy their needs. In order to attain satisfaction of the need, a person must act on the environment appropriately. However, awareness of needs does not ensure need satisfaction, nor does it specify the means whereby the needs will best be met. It does however provide the end goal, the attainment of which will result in greater organismic satisfaction and balance. How the need is to be met satisfactorily is a complex psychological process. It involves utilization of existing resources, past learnings, and where necessary, the development of new skills. People generally benefit from being able to obtain from the environment actively and assertively that which is required to function effectively. However, when biologically adaptive action tendencies oriented toward need satisfaction are interrupted or interferred with, the organism becomes frustrated and unable to meet its needs.

The self-interruption event to be discussed in this chapter focuses on dysfunctional instances of overregulation. This is defined as the interruption of organismically natural expression and the associated needs. It should be differentiated from healthy self-regulation, which involves a conscious choice to hold back emotion when socially appropriate or personally beneficial. An example would be the choice to hold back anger during a public meeting. Unhealthy overregulation involves the consistent, automatic, unconscious interruption of emotional reactions and expressive tendencies, and it leaves the person disempowered and without a response.

People can learn to hold back organismic expression and assertive action. This happens when adaptive attempts at satisfying needs have been constantly thwarted, ignored, or punished. Thus, attempts to express the need or act on the environment to satisfy it are prevented. Not having one's needs recognized, validated, and responded to, is painful. It can lead to the decision not to allow oneself to be so disappointed or humiliated again, which in turn leads to the development of a set of interrupters or self-control processes to ensure that one is never again so vulnerable. This is tantamount to the decision "I'll never let myself feel or need again."

Alternately, in overwhelmingly painful or in crisis situations, the painful experience is adaptively staved off to protect oneself and allow one to cope. Not only are the adaptive action tendencies held back or interrupted, but the individual's emotional experience, which is associated with the action tendency, is also automatically prevented. In any current process of interruption, the individual operates as a divided self and is both the "doer" (the interrupter) and the "done" to (the interrupted). Any effort to make contact with the environment and the object of need is lost as the person becomes involved in automatic internal activity against self-experience and expression.

In the interrupting of expression, one aspect of the self automatically becomes organized to engage in some expressive-motor activity to control the expressive action of another part of the self. The activities that counteract emotional action tendencies are varied. They can range from muscular tension, to holding one's breath, or the holding back of the urge to cry or yell. These activities can also involve internal cognitive/affective operations, which also act to prevent or interrupt experience and expression. Internal operations, such as telling oneself to remain silent, mentally whipping or torturing oneself, silently verbally restraining oneself, or squashing one's feelings, all act to interrupt expression. When these interruptive actions against the self become chronic, people are unable to express themselves. When these self-interruptions become automatic, people feel empty, helpless, defeated, confused, and are unable to act to get what they need.

In schematic-processing terms, the particular emotion schemes involving emotional experience and expressive-motor outputs are being automatically prevented from entering consciousness and from governing processing. The interruptive process probably occurs as a function of a second set of schemes, which were developed to inhibit the expressive-motor and cognitive/affective responses of the self. These schemes guide the person in the interruption and avoidance of the experience. It is often threatening or painful feelings that are too overwhelming to the self that are controlled. Essentially this is done in order to prevent pain.

In the self-interruptive split, there is restriction of self-expression predominantly by internal procedural *action*. This differs from the process in conflict splits, which involves a more declarative process of making *evaluations* or *injunctions*. Rather than the evaluation "you're bad" or the injunction "you shouldn't," we have muscular squeezing or internal mental operations of restraining, suppressing, and demobilizing. The process of self-control and the interruption of expression characterizes this split. In reality, conflict and self-interruptive splits are not always distinct or easy to differentiate. There is overlapping class membership. But we have found it helpful to distinguish prototypes of these two different internal processes. One is based on evaluation/coercion, the other on procedural interruptive activity. Each marker has different implications for intervention and resolution.

In self-interruptive splitting, the emotion scheme may be activated in any given situation. But then, automatic processing leads to lack of awareness of the emotional experience and the expression of the associated action tendency is interrupted. That which is being interrupted is generally not in awareness. What *is* often available in awareness is the end result of the interruptive process or some awareness of the interruptive process. Thus, a person may be aware of physical pain, tension, or discomfort from the squeezing of muscles. Or there may be a loss of a sense of personal agency, or a passive, defeated sense of self often accompanied by a cynical view of the world. These are the effects of persistent automatic self-interruptions. Alternatively, a person may be aware of the interruptive process itself, squeezing down of tears or anger, or a rigid focusing of attention to stay away from inner experience. It is the interruptive activity that first needs to be brought into awareness. Only later will the expressive-action tendency that is being interrupted and controlled become available in awareness.

The goal in this intervention is ultimately to bring the interruptive tendency under deliberate control such that expression can be allowed into awareness and be executed in an appropriate adaptive manner. The expressive tendency that has been inhibited is not in and of itself as dangerous or painful to the self as is so often feared by the client. In some cases it is the automatic interruption or suppression of a tendency (such as anger, or a need for affection) that has led to it remaining primitive and undifferentiated. The continual frustration of the emotion can then lead to its disproportionate intensification. The tendency needs to be allowed and expressed openly in the safety of the therapeutic hour. Once people have stopped interrupting themselves and have re-owned their experience, they are free to begin to differentiate and develop their responses into appropriate expressions oriented toward need satisfaction. Thus, inhibited anger may be transformed from frustrated rage and hostility, into an assertion of needs and rights. Or, a feeling of desperate neediness and a desire to cling may transform into an ability to ask for what is needed.

OPPORTUNITIES FOR INTERVENTION— THE MARKER

Certain verbal and nonverbal markers of these self-interruptive splits emerge in sessions. The explicit marker for this type of split is a report or action conveying that one part of the self is engaged in a self-controlling action against self-expression. Clients often report feeling helpless or passive and experience themselves as "objects or victims" of some aspect of their own reflexive activity. They may say they are "squashing or "wiping themselves out," or feel squashed or wiped out. They may report engaging in some action against themselves, often self-punitive, such as "kicking myself" or "punishing myself." The basic linguistic structure is one of "I do something to myself," with "I" as the subject and agent and "myself" as the object and victim of the action. In addition, a current feeling of hopelessness, powerlessness, or resignation indicates that the split is being currently activated automatically, and that rather than just being talked about, the interruption is being experienced. It is more amenable to intervention by virtue of the fact that the interruptive process and the interrupted expression can more easily be brought to awareness because they are currently operating. It is important to note that in the self-interruptive split, the emphasis is not on the self-evaluation or even on the injunction, although some of both may be present. The emphasis in the statement "I kick myself" is on doing something to the self, that is, kicking. An example from a session follows.

> I just stop myself from feeling anything. Somehow, after cutting off my sexual feelings, I cut off all my feelings. I can't feel. I often don't know that I am feeling 'til a couple of days afterwards. I've just cut off my feelings about him now.

In addition to explicit verbal markers of interruptions, signs of physical and muscular squeezing can indicate the presence of interruptive action. So too can nonverbal activities, such as pinching oneself, hitting oneself on the forehead, or using one's hands self-recriminatingly to apply pressure to any part of the body. The interventive issue here is not one of interpreting these actions as self-interruptions but, rather, to bring them to awareness to facilitate exploration of the experience. It is important to accept that sometimes a scratch simply is to relieve an itch and is not a tearing at oneself. However, a report of physical tension can indicate an interruption or blocking of expression. For example, while talking about a painful experience, a client may report a band of tension around the head or chest. And when the band is experienced and explored, the client might discover that it is he or she who is doing something to create the band of tension. And, with facilitation, he or she might gain control over the previously automatic process. This could be done by the person actually identifying with the squeezing activity, by actually enacting the squeezing of the self, perhaps on a pillow. An example of this is a client saying

I feel all this pressure in here (*massaging and rubbing her throat and chest*). It's so hard to like . . . it's just one big vice. It's like a yoke here. I try to release it all the time. But I'm always in a vice, you know. Absolutely no release.

Other implicit markers are signs such as hopeless sighs, statements of resignation, and verbal or nonverbal expressions of hopelessness without explicit verbal markers of the split itself. These signs need to be explored for the possible presence of a self-interruptive process by asking clients what is happening and seeing if they articulate a self-interruptive split.

As we have said, the distinguishing characteristic of this type of split is the *interruption or suppression of self-expression*, as opposed to the negative evaluation of an aspect of the self as in conflict splits. The prototypic state is thus one in which an angry or assertive response to an environmental impingement is restricted and literally "held back" by muscular squeezing, clenching of the jaw, or tensing of the body. One part of the self can be construed as engaged *in an activity* against another part of the self. Thus, a report of feeling powerless, coupled with an indicator of an active–passive relationship between two aspects of the self, is a prototypic marker of a self-interruption split. Actual examples are statements such as "I feel suffocated, like I'm strangling myself" or "I'm just kicking myself," or an implicit marker "I've just given up trying to get what I need."

ATTRIBUTION OF INTERRUPTION

In the attributed form of self-interruptive conflict, clients may report that they feel powerless in relation to another. Or they feel as if someone "makes them feel" some feeling, be it depressed, powerless, hopeless, or embarrassed, humiliated, or clumsy. The assumption here is that the feeling of disempowerment and the difficulty in feeling entitled and in asserting oneself come ultimately from one's own psychological means of handling others. This is in contrast with having those feelings generated directly from the actions and statements of others. Although it is true that in political, economic, administrative, and bureaucratic ways people certainly are disempowered by others, in other types of situations, people who feel unentitled interrupt themselves. It is these psychologically based interruptive processes that need attention. Thus, a shared perspective that this is an internal process that is troubling the client needs to be established before that client may engage in a re-owning of the interruption. Otherwise, a therapist might mistakenly invalidate a person when it is actually the environment that is the oppressor or disempowering medium.

HOW DOES CHANGE OCCUR?

In this intervention, the client actively enacts the self- controlling or self-interrupting process, mobilizing the unexpressed and reclaiming the disclaimed action tendency. It is the actual engagement in the activity and the engendering of the passive state or its intensification that are so crucial to this process. And it is paramount that this happen *in the session.* Often the person is not aware of what is suppressed, but there is always some sign of the interruptive process. This is brought to awareness, exaggerated, and owned. The process involves flushing out a set of condensed and covert processes that occur almost instantly and converting them into an explicit extended process in real time.

In this process of differentiation, the client brings to awareness a variety of automatic processes involved in the interruptive process. Once the interruptive processes are owned, what is being interrupted becomes more available to awareness. The undoing of self-interruption involves the mobilization and expression of the suppressed tendencies. Also important in this event is a process of increasing physical activation in order to increase general level of arousal. The activity engaged in, such as squeezing a pillow, often involves hostility against the self. The increase in physical and emotional arousal then spreads to help increase the arousal of previously unexpressed hostile feelings (see Berkowitz, 1990). This process works by increasing the persons general level of arousal, thereby amplifying emotional experience. It also evokes or primes other anger or emotion schemes that have been suppressed.

The therapeutic task in this event is first to have clients become aware that it is *they themselves* who are the agents of the interruption or the blocking of self-expression. They then mobilize the interrupted expression. The expression of the interrupted emotion *empowers* the client and enables him or her to engage more actively with the world and more freely contact the environment. Thus, a person who feels hopeless after a setback can mobilize anger to assert his or her own boundaries and rights. Or, a person who feels isolated can mobilize sadness and distress to attempt to break through the isolation and make contact by asking or reaching out.

Self-interruption occurs by blocking the action tendency associated with an automatically activated emotion scheme. This blocking or interruption of expression is driven by the automatic activation of a set of schematically cued inhibitory expressive-motor and ideational responses. These responses may have been originally instituted consciously. They may have been seen as the best way to cope with the situation by controlling the self, and only later did they become automatic. Thus, healthy assertive expressions (such as anger at violation, or requests for contact when needy) are interrupted and prevented, leaving a passive and helpless sense of self. The key is to provide the person with a greater sense of control of his or her experience. This includes helping a person become aware that "It is I who am interrupting myself" rather than a view that interruption "just happens," or that "others are doing it to me." This is coupled with an awareness of the blocked emotion and action tendency. The previously automatic processing involved in the interruption is slowly transformed into controlled processing by enactment procedures (Greenberg & Safran, 1981). People are then able to bring the interruptive processing under greater control. They can then become aware of the interrupted feeling, can connect it to the relevant situation, and begin to learn how to express it in a constructive fashion. They are encouraged to use the impetus of this action tendency to act more assertively in the world.

Model of the Resolution Process

An intensive analysis of the process of the resolution of self-interruptive splits has led to the model of resolution shown in Figure 11-1. This model is a preliminary one open to further refinement. The resolution process consists of three stages: Enactment, Recognition of Agency, and Contact. These are described in detail below. In addition, a short form of a rater's Degree-of-Resolution Scale devised for research purposes is shown in Table 11-1. This indicates six degrees of resolution and can be used as a guide to estimate how far along in the resolution process one has progressed.

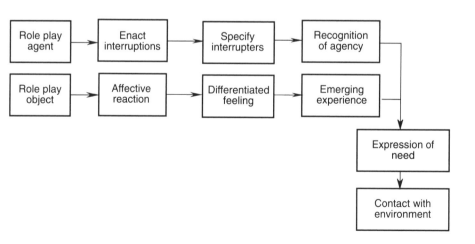

FIGURE 11-1. Resolution of Self-Interruption.

TABLE 11-1. Degree-of-Resolution Scale (short form)

Self-Interruptive Splits

1. The client is acting on the self to interrupt expression or describes how one part interrupts another part.

2. The client actively engages in a concrete and specific manner as the interrupter in the self interruptive process.

3. The client's feelings of passivity and resignation are contacted and differentiated.

4. The person clearly expresses the interrupted emotion.

5. The need associated with the emotion is clearly expressed.

6. The person, feeling empowered, envisages or plans new actions in the world to get the need met.

Enactment

The first step in this enactment is a highly deliberate *role play* of the interruption, in which the client takes the role of the doer and the done to, the active and the passive roles of the enactment. After role-playing the sides, the client becomes more involved, and this leads to the activation of the scheme's governing the self-interruptive process. The client begins to *enact* verbally and nonverbally the process of interruption, be it a squeezing or squashing action or a verbal and nonverbal rendition of wiping out oneself. After initial deliberate experimentation, a more fluid and spontaneous enactment begins to flow. As the client identifies with the interruption, the interruptive process becomes more *specific* and detailed. This is a sign that the scheme is activated and running. This involves the recognition by clients that it is *they* who are punishing, restraining, or stopping *themselves*. And it is *they* who are interfering with the experience and expression of their suppressed feelings and needs.

The ultimate key change process appears to be one of feeling sufficiently empowered to be able to actively contact the environment to satisfy one's need. In order to do this, clients need to become aware of the ways in which they interrupt their emerging experience. They need to become aware of their feelings and needs and to feel entitled to them. Even when there is no awareness or expression of the organismic feelings and needs, there is always some small sign of an interruptive process. This is where the work begins, as people become more aware of: (1) the fact that they are interrupting themselves; (2) how they idiosyncratically interrupt themselves. As people become aware that they interrupt themselves and how they do this, what is being interrupted slowly becomes more available to awareness.

In the self chair, people begin to experience in a more vivid manner their emotional reactions to being interrupted. They sigh in resignation, feel passive or hopeless, or in a knot. By focusing attention on and identifying with this feeling, rather than deflecting away from it, the bad feeling begins to differentiate from a global reaction to more specific aspects. As the enactment proceeds and the persons differentiate their reactions and how they are interrupting themselves, the experience and the expression that are being interrupted become more clear.

Recognition of Agency

As clients become aware of how they interrupt, and of their idiosyncratic means of interrupting, they begin to recognize that they are really the *agent* of this, not only the victim. As the feelings become more differentiated, a *new feeling emerges* and is expressed. This may be anger that was interrupted, a feeling of unsureness, or pain and defeat that was disallowed. The feeling, like anger, may be contact-oriented. Or like fear, it may be withdrawal-oriented. What is important is that now an emotion is felt, rather than the experiencing of blankness, numbness, or emptiness of interrupted emotional responses.

Contact

With the emergence of these new feelings and the recognition by clients that they have been interrupting, clients become again empowered to *express their needs*. And these needs are then associated with the newly emerging experience and action tendency. The need, be it a desire to push someone away or to reach out and bring someone closer, is then experimented with to find an appropriate expression. Once the suppressed feelings and needs are experienced, they are translated into expressive action, brought into *contact with the environment*, and differentiated. Thus an unmet need for love, or an overwhelmed need for autonomy or separation, are owned and asserted. Once the interrupted expression is re-owned, different ways of appropriately meeting the needs are explored, discussed, and experimented with. This helps to develop ways of being able to get what is wanted and needed. Often through lack of experience and/or anxiety, clients are not skilled in acting in the world to meet their needs and are helped by practice to refine their behavior.

The two crucial aspects of the resolution process, shown in Figure

11-1 are: (1) the recognition of one's own agency in the interruptive process and (2) the empowered expression of need.

Therapeutic Intervention to Bring About Change

The major therapeutic steps in this intervention are promoting the client's recognition of agency and the client's taking of responsibility for the self-interruption. The therapist facilitates the client's sense of control by helping the client to: (1) recognize that it is he or she who is the agent of the interruption, rather than feeling that it just happens or that someone else is doing it; (2) become aware of the blocked emotion and action tendency. As each emotion has a directional component, each feeling has its implication for action. Therapeutic intervention must facilitate explication of the want, desire, and action tendency implied by the recovered feeling (Greenberg & Safran, 1987).

When therapeutic work focuses on physical tension, the therapist helps the client locate the tension, discover how he or she creates his or her tension, and experiments with doing this deliberately, in awareness. This allows the client to slow down his or her automatic processing. As clients gain awareness of the motor activity involved in the creation of the tension, they begin to recover a sense of agency for these actions. As we have said, rather than feel that the tension or aches "just happen," the client begins to discover that "I am doing this to myself." As clients identify themselves as the active agent of their experience, they recover a sense of personal power. Once clients have identified with and re-owned the self-interruptive activity, they are helped to gain awareness of the interrupted feelings. With facilitation by the therapist, the client learns to express these constructively.

When the therapeutic work focuses on verbal or nonverbal expressions of powerlessness, the client needs to become aware of the active aspect of the self involved in creating the powerless experience. In this type of split, the active aspect is generally not in awareness. The therapist works with the client's report of his or her experience of passivity to help the client become aware of his or her own agency in its creation. If the client reports feeling suffocated, the therapist directs the client to "experiment figuratively with suffocating yourself. What could you do to produce this experience." First, the therapist helps the client to experience engaging actively in the self-interruptive activity, deliberately and in awareness. Then the therapist helps the client to intensify and differentiate the self-interrupting activity, until the client is able to recognize fully how he interrupts himself and what actions he engages in to do so. The therapist may have to help tease out the various levels of self-interruptive activity, helping raise the client's awareness of each aspect. This may include cognitive, affective, or motor aspects, and combinations thereof. The client may discover that he or she is constricting throat muscles to hold back expressions of anger or may discover that he or she is engaging in extremely harsh self-talk that is accompanied by chest tightness and feelings of being wiped out. The deliberate and conscious "doing" of the self-interruptive activity will bring the client to the experiential realization that "I am doing this to myself." This recognition, the owning of the disowned self-interruptive activity, is crucial for resolution of this split.

The therapist then helps strengthen and empower the organismically felt "need" aspect of self, in either or both of two ways: (1) by directing the client to intensify the self-interruptive activity in order to elicit a self-preservative organismic reaction; (2) if the organismic aspect is particularly passive, defeated, and resigned, by directing the client to heighten his or her experience of resignation, until organismic agency or reactance is mobilized.

Therapeutic work with self-interruptive processes involves acceptance and empathy for the client's experience including avoiding any stance of victim-blaming. At the same time, the therapist provides clients with the opportunity to experience themselves as agents in the construction of their own experience. In addition, the therapist needs to recognize and facilitate clients' experience of personal power.

THERAPIST OPERATIONS

The following stages of therapeutic work are covered below: the pre- and postdialogue stages; Enactment; owning of attribution agency; and contact stages. Each stage involves a number of specific types of therapist operations, which are shown in Table 11-2 and discussed below.

Predialogue Stage

Establishing Collaboration

The therapist obtains the client's agreement to work on the self-interruptive process by suggesting the self-interruption as a focus for work.

Structuring the Experiment

The therapist introduces and sets up the experiment, much as in Two-Chair work, but suggests here that one part of the self seems to be doing something to the self. It is often best at this marker to ask the client

TABLE 11-2. Therapist Operations

Predialogue stage
  1. Establishing collaboration
  2. Structuring the experiment

Enactment stage
  3. Separate and create contact
  4. Promote the client's owning of experience
  5. Increase client's bodily awareness
  6. Promote awareness of self-interruptive activity

Recognition of agency stage
  7. Intensifying the client's arousal as agent
  8. Differentiate self-interruptive aspect
  9. Promote client's awareness of agency in self-interruptive activity
  10. Increase client's awareness of the passive organismic aspect of experience
  11. Identify the interrupted expression
  12. Stimulate assertiveness in felt-need aspect

Contact stage
  13. Support emerging assertiveness of felt-need aspect
  14. Experiment with interpersonal expression of need
  15. Empower the client

Postdialogue stage
  16. Create a meaning perspective

directly, without much discussion, to "do this to yourself." This is done in order to get into the process rapidly and not miss the current experience of what the client is doing to him or herself.

Enactment Stage

Separate and create contact between the two aspects of self. This is similar to the process of working on conflict splits. Instruct the client to speak from within the experience of that aspect of self that is more lively for the client at that moment, and direct statements to the other aspect. Generally, one starts with the active part, the interrupter, in order to get the dialogue underway. The experience of separation is enhanced by having the client change chairs when he or she shifts to speaking from the other aspect.

Work generally begins with the therapist directing the client to enact the active aspect of self to make explicit both the "what" and the "how" of the client's self-interruptive activity. This may take one of several forms. It may involve guiding the client to enact the muscular squeezing that prevents tears, or to deliberately set one's jaw to keep from expressing anger. Or, it may involve the enactment of squashing or throttling oneself. If the client's experience is of physical, muscular holding back, the therapist works to increase the client's sensory awareness of the muscular process. If the client's experience is a combination of affective/cognitive/motor processes, the therapist helps the client to become aware of, articulate, and turn these into actions against self-expression.

Promote the client's owning of experience. Suggest that the client make "I" statements when speaking from within the experience of each aspect. The active aspect is asked what it does and is asked to do it to the passive aspect, which is asked what it feels.

The emphasis at all times is on having clients *do* things to themselves, rather than talk about them. In this process the therapist often inquires "how do you stop yourself from expressing that" in response to clients' statements that they are stopping themselves. This intervention seeks initially for a more conceptual awareness from the client. The client really has to think about how he or she does this. The therapist might help by conjecturing or offering possibilities. A coexploratory set is created to help identify how the interruptive process operates. This is then turned into an active expression by the suggestion that the person now does this to the self.

Increase client's bodily awareness. Direct the client to attend to the physical sensations associated with the active and passive aspects of the interruptive process. Offer the client observations concerning posture and other nonverbal expressions related to self-interruption, such as squeezing oneself, covering over one's mouth, or hitting oneself. Direct the client to locate sites of physical tension, tightness, pain, and anxiety in order to begin to discriminate the effects of the interruptive process.

Promote awareness of self-interruptive activity. Attend to client's verbal and nonverbal expression, and bring to the client's awareness any activity on the self such as a self-squeezing, self-chastising, or self-choking activity.

Once some initial idea has been formed about the self-interruptive process, the therapist then asks the person to experiment with how he interrupts or stops himself from expressing. Now the emphasis is on "doing" in order to discover how the self-interruption is achieved and then to identify the agent of the activity. Thus, clients experiment with doing things to themselves, such as smothering or silencing themselves deliberately and in awareness. Clients may be asked to do these things to a pillow or even, at times, to the therapist. The latter often highlights for clients how cruel the things are that they do to themselves, as the clients shrink from doing to another what they regularly do to themselves. The enactment helps people gain perspective on their self-interruptive activity and to experience themselves as active, in relation to the self.

Identifying with Attribution Stage

When the client presents an attribution of agency marker, the dialogue begins with an identifying process. Therapeutic work on attribution of agency begins with the client enacting the "other" doing things to disempower the self. The therapist directs the client to do whatever it is the other is experienced as doing. As these actions against the self become more detailed and specific, it generally becomes clear to clients that it is really *they, themselves* who are restraining, inhibiting, or disempowering themselves. The therapist then encourages clients to own or identify with what it is that they are doing to themselves. This constitutes the first step in working on a self-interruptive split and the self–self dialogue is then continued as described above in the enactment stage.

Recognition of Agency Stage

The goal in this stage is to help clients recognize that they are agents in the creation of their experience and to help them identify with the active aspects of self in the experience.

Intensify the client's arousal as the agent. Intensify the self-interruptive activity by instructing the client to repeat, or more vigorously exaggerate, an activity. Then instruct the client to add a voice to the central interruptive process. The therapist helps the client identify the idiosyncratic manner in which he or she interrupts the self. As this becomes more differentiated, clients become more and more aware that they are actually engaged in repeated, self-reflexive activity. The aim is to bring this activity under deliberate control, which in turn provides the opportunity for ceasing the activity against the self.

Differentiate the self-interruptive aspect. Help the client attend to and explicate the what and how of the self-interruptive activity. Ask the client "what are you doing to him or her?" (indicating the other aspect of self in the other chair), and help the client discover the unique style and manner (the how) of this activity.

An often-observed phenomenon is a person enacting the preventive function of squeezing or holding back of tears. As the clients do deliberately what is being done automatically to prevent the weeping, they become differentiatedly aware of what muscles are being squeezed and of how they are holding their breath. When they actually do these intentionally, the automaticity is overridden, and expression begins to flow.

Promote client's awareness of agency in self-interruptive activity. Instruct the client to experiment with doing the self-interruptive activity deliberately, in awareness, until the client truly experiences and realizes that it is he or she that is responsible for producing the anxiety or tension, or self-squeezing, or self-defeat, or depression. Homework is also given to continue the enactment outside of therapy to assist clients to become aware of how and also to deliberately interrupt themselves.

Expression

Increase client's awareness of the passive organismic aspect of experience. Have the client shift, physically, to the "experiencing" chair. Focus the client inward in response to the self-interruptive activity. Instruct the client to attend to the inner experience of passivity, resignation, or whatever is there. Initially, the client is totally identified with the passive aspect of self. In this enactment, the therapist guides the client in shifting back and forth between the enactment of the interruptive activity and the passive aspect until the experience of being interrupted is accessed.

Identify and express the interrupted expression. The therapist helps the client work through the passive, resigned, helpless position by focusing on the feeling until the newly differentiated organismic expression emerges into awareness. The client is directed to attend to any newly emerging experience or expression that was previously suppressed or to give voice to that which is known to be interrupted. The client is then encouraged to express both the feeling and the associated action tendency and, ultimately, the unmet need. When the expression is activated, the interruptive process has dissolved (at least for the moment), and the person is facilitated in expressing the feeling in whatever way seems most helpful.

Stimulate assertion of the felt need. This is done directly by asking what the person needs, but it may also be accomplished by two distinctly different means:

1. Direct the client to shift to the self-interruptive aspect and to intensify the doing of the self-interruptive activity. By increasing the organismic level of arousal by engaging in action and/or by provoking a reaction by the escalation of the interruptive activity, the core self is often evoked.

2. Heighten and differentiate the client's experience of passivity, hopelessness, resignation, and so forth. Help the client "stay with" and speak from these feelings. The therapist conveys to the client that one can only be where one is and that without acceptance of this, change is not possible. This leads to the emergence of the felt need and a response from the self.

Contact Stage

Support Emerging Assertiveness of Felt-Need Aspect

Help the client to specify the felt need. Offer support, validation, and encouragement for genuine expression of feelings and needs. Help the client become aware of the action tendency and the need implicit in the previously interrupted emotion.

Further therapeutic work involves having the client express the specific feeling and need in a more generalized fashion to others. It also serves to help the person make authentic contact with the environment in order to complete expression and meet needs. This stage involves helping the person both to generalize the ability to express and to translate the expression into appropriate expressive action.

Experiment with Interpersonal Expression of Need

Have the client identify an "other" to whom he or she might express the identified need; then structure a miniexperiment in which the client is given the opportunity to express this need to an "imagined other" in the empty chair, or directly to the therapist.

The person expresses the feeling to the interrupter, or, more often, to the imagined other to whom the response was originally directed but interrupted. The person might express the interrupted anger to the imagined police officer in the other chair for having given the client a ticket, to a boss for criticism, or to a friend because of hurt or rejection.

Empowering

Ask the client what he or she can do in the real world to get his or her need met. Then help the client to plan the next step toward action. This empowers the client to be proactive on his or her own behalf.

The therapist, supports the client in attempting this behavior outside the therapeutic setting. This stage involves differentiating the previously unexpressed and undifferentiated feelings and needs to allow their development into appropriate means of expression and need gratification. Thus, a newly accessed need for contact may need to be developed from an indiscriminate desire to be hugged or to disclose one's feelings to a more differentiated selection of appropriate time, place, and degree and manner of expression of the need. The therapist does not generally train clients in social skills but, rather, helps them experiment with new behaviors and learn what worked for them.

Postdialogue Stage

Create a Meaning Perspective

Discuss the therapeutic experience with the client. Help him or her evaluate and create meaning out of his or her experience of expressing and acting upon need. Homework can be given to assist the client to become aware of the interruptive process in the client's ongoing experience outside of the session. An example follows.

Example of a Two-Chair Enactment

The following event comes from the middle of a 16-session treatment of a woman who experienced depression, anxiety, and interpersonal difficulties. In reading the transcript, it is important to hear the therapist as empathic and concerned and as closely following the client. Directives are offered in a gentle and collaborative manner. There is a real sense of the client and therapist working together to combat her difficulties.

Predialogue Stage

C: Yes. I don't . . . I don't even . . . I don't want to think, I don't want to feel. I, I want to shut off all emotions. I want to, I want to stop, I, I, I'm trying to block everything so that I have no feeling. [Self-interruptive split]

T: It's like just too painful to feel.

C: I . . . yeah. I don't want to feel any more.

T: Yeah . . . I just don't want to feel. What happened? [Responding to client's facial gesture]

C: Well, I do have an image that comes up. [T: mhm] When I was very young, but I don't know whether that's the [same] rejecting or not.

T: Mhm. What, what's the image?

C: Well. I mean, I remember, I don't actually remember the occasion, I just remember the story. [T: right] I was told that when I was about five or something. Four. I was staying with my aunt. One of those times, I don't know why, but we were shunted around (mhm). And I got measles. And I was put in the basement for 2 weeks, or whatever. A maid would come down twice a day to bring me my meals . . . and . . . so (laughs) that was the image [T: yeah] I was feeling.

T: Feeling . . .

C: I was feeling maybe that's . . . maybe there was a real place.

T: Mhm, mhm. And what's the feeling? . . . being in the basement.

C: Well. Abandoned. I was completely abandoned. [T: mhm, mhm] I'm feeling, I'm just here forever. [T: yeah] And nobody is ever going to come and nobody is ever going to care, and . . . nobody is ever going to take me away from here. [T: right, right] (*client huddles over and puts her arms around herself*)

T: What's happening? What's this? (*points to her arms squeezing herself*)

C: (*laughs*) What's this? [T: mhm] It's a . . . I guess I do this when I sort of give up.

T: What's it feel like?

C: When I squeeze myself like this, so I . . . here we are again.

T: Be this hand. What do you do? This arm. [Promotes owning of interruptive aspect]

C: Well I'm holding in pain. [T: mhm] If, you know, I have this feeling in my stomach or in my throat, and I'm just holding it all in. [T: mhm, mhm] Yeah, I sort of feel like here we go again and I'm just settling in for the long run.

T: So it's a kind of a holding, holding in?

C: Yeah. And I just. That's just the only response I have. I . . . there's no point screaming, nobody will hear. [T: mhm. mhm]

Enactment Stage

T: So all you can do is hold, and hold it in. [C: yeah] Be these arms, and hold, hold in the pain. [Promotes owning of the active interruptive part]

C: That's what I am doing.

T: Yeah. Be the arms. Actually give them a voice. Speak to the pain. Tell her what you are doing and actually do it. Holding you in, or I'm containing you, I'm stopping you from screaming . . .

C: Well, the arms don't feel bad. They're quite protective.

T: right, right. So tell her this.

C: I'm protecting you. [T: Yeah, yeah] I'm protecting you, except there's nothing to protect you from except the pain you're feeling inside, and there's nothing I can do about that. [T: mhm] Except maybe if I hold you very tight [T: yes] it'll be smaller. I'll make the pain smaller. [T: right]

T: So actually you are trying to protect her, or . . .

C: Make her smaller. Reduce the pain.

T: Mhm. Change. Now can you be the pain? Be the pain. What is the pain like. This is important pain. [Promote owning of passive part]

C: The pain is simple. Very scary. [T: mhm] Cause it feels like it could completely overwhelm me. (*crying*) The pain, I think, is uhm, more threatening than what is happening outside because it's quite dark, but it seems more alive. [T: mhm]

T: I'd like you, if you can, to go into that pain, attend to it, and I want you to know that I am here and that you can come out. [Own experience and offer relational support]

C: (*cries*) What? I am not sure I can do this anymore. It's too painful. (*cries*)

T: So what happens?

C: What happens? [T: mhm] Well, I don't know. I feel like on the one hand I'm in here and on the other hand I'm here (*points to other chair*) [T: mhm]

T: Change. It's the "Don't feel it anymore," right? Stop her from feeling the pain. [Promote owning of interruption]

C: Stop her from feeling pain? Well, that will be easy. [T: mhm]

T: Make her not feel it anymore. How do you do this? [Promotes awareness of self-interruptive activity]

C: OK, she can feel pain allright. I'm just not going to notice anymore [T: mhm, mhm] You see, I can't stop her from feeling it.

T: I see, but I'm just not . . .

C: I just gotta get away, I gotta get out of here so I don't feel it.

T: Tell her. This is too . . . much I don't want to feel you.

C: Well, when I am here, and I keep the pain out, everything is going really well over here, my mind is back to normal. I feel like I've conquered all my demons, and then [T: yeah] quite accidently, I keep opening the door, and seeing that, [T: yeah] and feeling. In my stomach, and I just . . . it's always a terrible shock.

T: Mhm. Tell her, you're always such a shock.

C: Well, you're always . . . I hope . . . totally by accident I opened this door and there you are.

T: And then what do you do?

C: I close the door.

Recognition of Agency

T: Yeah. Be a door closer. How do you close the door? [Promote awareness of interruptive activity]

C: How do I close the door?

T: Yeah, Yeah.

C: I look the other way. [T: right, right]

T: Can you actually do that? With . . . do it physically. Look the other way. [Intensify arousal of agent]

C: (*laughing*) Look the other way. [T: yeah, yeah]

T: Tell her what you are doing. I'm . . . [Differentiate self-interruptive activity]

C: I'm turning around, and I'm going to stay until you're gone. [T: mhm, mhm]

T: Stay with it. I don't want to see you. I don't want to look at you. Whatever . . .

C: I'm going to do whatever I can do to forget that I noticed you. [T: mhm]

T: Change. What happens here now? [Awareness of passive experience]

C: What happens here? [T: mhm] I'm just here. [T: mhm, tell her] Well, you may ignore me, but . . . I'm always going to be here.

T: What are you?

C: What am I? [T: yeah] A little person huddled against the pain. [T: mhm]

T: What is the pain like? [Increase bodily awareness]

C: What is the pain? [T: yeah, what is your . . .] It's not . . . it's not terror [T: no] It's just . . . (sighs) . . . the inevitable emptiness.

T: Can you go into that and describe yourself as this painful emptiness . . . I'm . . . [Increase awareness of passive organismic experience]

C: Well, I'm not empty when I'm painful. [T: mhm] I'm full of suffocating, erasing, uh, pain. It's . . . it feels like it's gonna take over.

T: Can you actually be the pain? Give it a voice: "I'm like . . . what?"

C: I'm the pain? [T: mhm]

T: Be the pain.

C: Be the pain. Well I start somewhere at the pit of my stomach, and I spread all over. [T: mhm] Lots of deep colors. Browns and blacks. And I'm suffocating. [T: mhm]

T: Say this again.

C: I'm suffocating. [T: yeah] And I'm trying to get out. [T: yeah] And you won't let me. You're just holding it all in. You're just tightening up and keeping me in as tight as possible. You'll scream. You'll yell, you won't let me out in any way. You're just trapping me inside here.

T: Change. Be the trapper. The squeezer. How do you do this? [Differentiate self interrupter]

C: How do I do this? [T: mhm] Well, because I am stubborn [T: yeah] I know nobody cares . . .

T: Tell her this. Nobody cares.

C: Nobody cares. There's nobody out there anyway to hear the screams. And if they did hear, they wouldn't understand. [T: yes] They would . . . they might punish me.

T: So therefore, just hold it in.

C: Yes. There is no place to go. [T: mhm]

T: You won't be heard. There's nothing.

C: No. All I can do is hold you in. That's my only power. [T: right, right]

T: Tell her again. [Intensify arousal of interrupter]

C: I'm just gonna squeeze you as tight as I can. Just keep you inside. [T: Because . . .] Because no one will hear. There's no point. There's no point letting you out. [T: mhm. no one . . .] No one will hear.

T: There's nothing there. No one . . . again.

C: No one will hear.

T: What do you experience?

C: Well, I feel resignation. I know there's nobody there, I know it. [T: mhm] It's very obvious to me. [T: right] Nobody will be there, and if they are they won't understand.

T: So therefore, just . . . what are you doing with your hands?

C: Yes (*laughing*), they're holding on.

T: Mhm, mhm. Describe this holding on. Do it some more. [Intensify arousal of interruptor]

C: I'm squeezing. [T: describe this] Squeezing. Just holding on very tight, so I won't . . . [T: mhm] I guess this is . . . I'm just steeling myself . . . for the inevitable.

T: And the inevitable is . . .

C: Well, the inevitable is just being here.

T: Mhm. Again.

C: There's pain and . . . isolation. [T: yeah. Can you tell this to me? I want to scream but no one will hear me scream.] [Identify interrupted expression]

C: Can I tell you that? [T: mhm]

T: Yeah, that no one will hear me.

C: I don't know. Cause I know, I mean, if I tell you, I know that's not true. I know I do cry, and people *do* hear.

T: But somehow there's this . . . tell her "no one will hear." [Differentiate interruption]

C: Well. I guess, yeah I guess I've always known . . . that ultimately there's nobody there. That moment to moment you're here, [T: mhm] that other people are here, but, but if you were to really probe and really strip back to the essentials, then there's nothing.

T: Tell her this. There's ultimately no one.

C: Ultimately there isn't anything. No one who cares.

T: Uh-huh, cares. [C: mhm] Ultimately nobody really cares for you, or will care, in the way you need to be cared for.

C: Well, it's even beyond that [T: mhm] They're not even there to care. It's not like they are there and they don't care. [T: right] They're not there. [T: right] There's nothing ultimately.

T: Ultimately, there's nobody there to care for you. [C: yeah] Right? And . . . [Differentiate self interruption]

C: And ultimately you're completely alone. (*unintelligible*) . . .

T: Change. What do you need in that aloneness? [Stimulate felt need]

C: What do I need in that aloneness? [T: yeah] Well, on the one hand, it's comfortable [T: yeah] because I feel, uh yes, here I am again. This feels real. I know this isn't playacting. [T: mhm, mhm, mhm] It feels completely real. I feel . . . I feel I'm back to myself [T: mhm] I'm back to what I've always known.

T: So it's a very real, vital, non-phoney part [C: yeah] that . . . and yet it's very painful to be so alone.

C: Oh, it's awful.

T: Somehow to be wanting for there to be someone out there to hear the scream or the need or the pain. [C: mhm] Just having had the experience, and feeling that there's nobody out there who's really looking at me, looking . . . after me. Just seeing me, seeing my pain, seeing my struggle.

C: Yeah, noticing.

T: Nobody noticing, [C: yeah] Yeah. The scream somehow is "I want to be noticed." [Stimulate assertion of the need]

C: Yeah. A scream would just bring punishment. Yeah, a scream would bring something different. The scream would bring some other kind of notice. [T: yeah, yeah] but it wouldn't be . . .

T: The notice I need.

C: Well, it wouldn't—notice wasn't really happening. It'd be another diversion—a scream would bring on another diversion.

T: mhm, mhm. While what was really happening was some sort of vulnerability, or just a need to be cared for. A need—what was the need? [Stimulate felt need]

C: Well, I guess I needed to be taken out of there [T: mhm] To be shown that that wasn't so. [T: yes] That it never happened. And still doesn't.

T: So somehow it's a need to be taken out of . . . [C: yeah] . . . the pain.

C: mhm. I can't do it on my own. All I can do is hold on. [T: mhm]

T: To just hold, and then kind of, just try to make it . . . as small as possible, [C: yeah] so that it doesn't—

C: And then maybe fall asleep.

T: Yeah. That's a very painful . . . as you say, sort of a resigned feeling of "and nobody will take me out. I can't get out."

C: No, yeah. I can't get out. If there is anybody there, they could get me out, but there isn't. It's not like there's people walking around while I'm there—there aren't, there isn't. There's not, [T: mhm] there's nothing out there, there's no noise, there's nothing, [T: right, right] so I just hold myself tight.

T: Somehow, holding tight like this, and not really feeling like there's anybody out there, it's very hard to scream out or to reach out. [C: Yeah, it's . . .] And say I need to be held, I need to be comforted. [Support emerging assertion of felt need]

C: When I am there, there isn't anybody to say that to anyway. First of all now I don't feel it unless there's nobody there. [T: yeah, yeah] Uhm, when there's somebody there I don't usually feel it because I'm playing (*laughs*) or doing, I'm doing my other life. [T: Yeah, yeah] which is [T: I understand] . . . so I don't have to be there [T: mhm] I guess though I don't like . . .I never liked to need.

T: Yeah.

C: I refused to tell anyone I need anything.

T: Can you tell this to me? "I refuse to need support."

C: Okay. I refuse to tell you I need anything. Just nice and tight. I don't need anything I just go about and do my business.

T: I just go around and hold myself tight. How do you do this? Can you come over here and do this, make her tight. How do you do this? [Awareness of self interruption]

C: Hold everything in. Well, I'm . . . I've done it long enough, I can continue. I don't need anything.

T: Come over here and hold everything in. Actually do it. [Promote awareness of agency]

C: (*Client pushes and squashes her imagined self in the chair and breathes out*)

T: Yes, do it some more. Can you make a sound? [Intensify arousal as agent]

C: UUUHH! (*effort, full sound*)

T: Now put some words to it.

C: Don't need anything and even if you do, don't ask. Goddamn it, don't ask! Just get on with your business. Don't ask.

Contact

T: OK, good. Can you change? What happens here, what's it like? [Awareness of passive aspect]

C: I feel so bound up in . . . It's awful. I can't breath here. I don't have needs. Of course I have needs. I needed someone to comfort me then in the emptiness.

T: Tell her, tell her what you need. [Stimulate assertion of need]

C: I do need support. I need comfort and support.

T: Can you bring this into contact with me? Tell me about your needs. [Experiment with interpersonal expression of need]

C: I need support. Yeah, I want your support. I want . . . I need people to respond to me, to sooth my pain, to help make it go away.

T: Uh-huh, say this again. I need comfort. [Support emerging assertion of felt need]

C: Yeah, I need comfort, I need help sometimes when I am afraid or alone. I need people, I don't want to be all locked up in a basement all on my own. I really want help.

T: Yeah, this is important. It's important to need and to be able to ask. Who could you ask in your life for what you need? [Support assertion and empower]

C: A number of people. My boyfriend for example.

T: OK, let's put him here in the chair and ask him. [Experiment with interpersonal expression of need]

C: I need your support. I have needs. I'm going to ask you for support when I need it.

CONCLUSION

Again it is important to emphasize that this is a process of facilitation, not of instruction or modification.

EMPTY-CHAIR WORK AND UNFINISHED BUSINESS

ONE OF THE WAYS in which organisms handle situations and emotional experiences that are too overwhelming, painful, or frustrating is to hold back from feeling, including blocking both the expression of the feelings and the needs from which the feelings emerge. Unmet needs do not, however, fully disappear. Rather, they and the situation become encoded in memory and remain as "unfinished business" (Perls et al., 1951) for the individual, often interfering with the person's ability to respond adaptively to current situations. Unfinished business may thus result when needs are not satisfied. There is no completion to the natural sequence of the arousal and expression of the emotion, leading to the awareness of the need and to action to meet one's need and cope with obstacles encountered. When this sequence is not completed, there is an arousal of excitement and tension, but it is not reduced. Emotion mounts, but when obstacles are too great, the person gives up. When the need/goal is unmet, dissatisfaction remains, often accompanied by complaint. Resentment constitutes the most common and one of the most important manifestations of unfinished business.

WHAT NEEDS TO BE CHANGED? THE UNDERLYING PROCESSING DIFFICULTY

Unfinished business represents the encoding in memory of the unsuccessful resolution of some kind of emotionally based need/goal-oriented interaction with the environment. It is the emotional equivalent of the push for completion, the Zeigarnik effect, found in the interruption of cognitive tasks (Zeigarnik, 1927). The unexpressed feelings, aroused in the situation, remain in schematic emotional memory and can be readily reevoked. The feelings seem to linger because they are often reevoked, and, when evoked, they push for expression and resolution. However, not every incomplete need/feeling/action-resolution sequence is coded into deep schematic memory. Only highly salient or traumatic experiences or repeated instances of similar frustrations are likely to become structured and stored as emotion schemes.

Of particular significance are those unfinished experiences built up over time in relationship to others who have been significant to us in the major developmental tasks of life—tasks such as developing trust, autonomy, competence, identity, intimacy, and generativity. This class of unfinished business develops in the realm of interpersonal relations with parents, siblings, lovers, spouses or friends, or between people who have intense or longstanding relationships that affect a person's sense of well-being. This type of unfinished business often involves difficulty in separating and ending, and it results in a "hanging on" reaction to a terminated relationship with a significant other. In this difficulty, the person continually tries to rework issues that were never fully dealt with in the relationship, including unexpressed emotions and unmet needs. It is as though the person is left with the accumulated unexpressed emotions, the old resentments, frustrations, hurts, guilts as well as unexpressed appreciations and love. Essentially, suppressed feelings that remain at the termination of a relationship result in an unfinished relationship. What is needed is to finish the emotional relationship internally and to let go and separate.

Another class of unfinished experience arises in traumatic, stress-inducing situations, or victimization experiences involving tragic loss, violence, death, disaster, or abuse. Probably the most damaging unfinished business occurs when the trauma involves a significant other. Loss of, or abuse by a significant other produces the most overwhelming and imprinting of experiences. These situations generally involve the arousal of powerful feelings of grief, rage, disgust, powerlessness, or terror. These are often unable to find expression and be dealt with in the situation but, rather, become encoded in memory and then return as intrusive images, thoughts, and feelings, as aspects of posttraumatic stress.

Individuals at different times and for different reasons, restrict complete expression and experience of emotion, often to significant others. Emotions such as anger, hurt, resentment, disappointment, grief, and sometimes caring and love are restricted for reasons that include the need to cope, fear of the effects of expression on others, and avoidance and fear of painful, unwanted emotions.

As long as expression remains incomplete, the action tendency unimplemented, and the need unmet, the individual will not be able to achieve closure of the situation or relationship. An unexpressed feeling, an unmet need, and a forever-hopeful expectation will remain in schematic memory. This results in some aspect of the person's current attentional allocation and processing capacities remaining involved in either the reliving of the experience, or in misperceiving or overreacting to current situations in terms of the unfinished business.

Most commonly, emotional expression is interrupted because of social and internalized prohibitions against expression of intense emotions and because of the fear that expressing strong emotions will hurt self or other. Interruptions become chronic in situations in which people were originally aware of strong desires, but the desire was frustrated, or there was a perceived danger to satisfaction (Perls et al., 1951). The person then deliberately inhibits the desire and awareness of the desire in order not to suffer and to keep out of danger. The whole complex of need, feeling, expression, gesture, and the sensory impression is rendered inactive by a complex set of internal operations. Because the traumatic situation is unfinished in significant ways, considerable energy is expended to prevent its reactivation in related present situations. The organism is active in this attempt to suppress or contain the evocation of the scheme, the interruption at first being deliberate and later automatic.

Interruptions that help maintain unfinished business involve muscular restrictions such as holding back tears, swallowing anger, or immobilizing the tendency to flee. These activities eventually take place automatically, out of awareness. Thus, unfinished business involves the nonrelease of tension, the storage in memory of the event, and the interruptions of expression as a familiar way of coping with the difficulty. This pattern limits the possibility for new responses. For example, people may continue to ruminate about the hurt or loss, and each time they remember, the feelings and the tears well up or the anger rises.

The cognitive/affective processes involved in current experiences of unfinished business can be viewed as follows. Cues in the present situation activate schematic emotional memories of the unfinished situation. The activated scheme governs current awareness and generates the associated emotional and expressive responses, as well as the interruptions to these responses. The person experiences the situation as containing the frustration or danger of the past. As a result, the past is remembered, and the whole sequence of arousal and interruption takes place again and again, leaving the person feeling tense, dissatisfied, resentful, resigned, or helpless.

Thus unfinished business is experienced with the triggering of schematic emotion memories of significant others with whom one has unresolved emotional reactions. Painful feelings are reexperienced whenever the scheme is evoked. Thus, when one thinks of or imagines the other person, unresolved feelings ensue. It is this scheme that needs to be changed, containing the situation with the significant other, including unresolved feelings, needs, and perceptions of self and others. The unfinished business needs to be reexperienced in order to allow the emotion and the action tendency to be expressed. It must run its course and be reprocessed in the safety of the therapeutic situation; this in turn will lead to closure and reconstrual of self and other.

OPPORTUNITIES FOR INTERVENTION: MARKERS OF UNFINISHED BUSINESS

Clearly defined experiences of unfinished business emerge as clients talk in therapy about their past relationships and life experiences. For example, a client may complain bitterly of the way in which she was treated by her father or a client may express long-standing bitterness or resentment toward an ex-spouse for a betrayal or abandonment. The marker of this type of unfinished business with a significant person has the following components: (1) the presence of a lingering, unresolved feeling such as hurt or resentment; (2) this feeling is related to a significant other who has been developmentally significant, such as a parent or spouse; (3) the feelings are currently experienced; (4) the feelings are not fully expressed, and there are signs of interrupted or restricted expression.

The important feature of these experiences is that the person currently feels the unresolved feeling but is stuck, feeling either helpless or resigned or unable to get release or relief by talking about it. In these instances, the client is experiencing unfinished business with the significant other. We have found that resentments and hurt are the most common signs of unresolved feelings. However, resignation and hopelessness are also signs of unfinished business, reflecting the emotional quality of having tried unsuccessfully to resolve the feeling and given up, rather than being the experience of the original unresolved feeling itself. A complaining quality is often present in relation to those on whom the client was dependent for need satisfaction or for approval. This complaint represents a fusion or confluence of unexpressed anger and hurt. In addition, unresolved grief represents another type of unfinished business, one in which it is feelings of loss that are unresolved.

A prototypic marker indicating both anger and resignation follows.

> I have a lot of anger towards my mother. She always criticized me and kind of hovered over me. Sometimes I just wanted to yell at her but I never could.

Even to this day, I can feel this urge to yell—but it was so long ago. What's the use of yelling now? It'll never change.

Finally, other less-direct markers of unfinished business are the signs of longings, sadness, resignation, and hopelessness. Or, they may include signs of the interruption of the feelings evoked in relation to a significant other, but without a full statement of the lingering bad feeling. Examples would be the longing in talking about an ex-spouse, indicated by mentioning how much one wished for a sense of family and that the kids had two parents; or the sadness in talking about a deceased parent; or beginning to "tear up" as one talks in the cool objectivity of an "I don't care" statement about a parent's neglect. These are all signs that it would be productive to engage in a dialogue with the significant other, to express one's evoked feelings and complete the unfinished business.

HOW DOES CHANGE OCCUR?

The basic assumption in this intervention is that having the person express unresolved feelings to the significant other in an empty chair will lead to arousal and completion of previously restricted affect expression towards the other; this helps resolve or reframe remaining relationship issues, generally resulting in an acceptance of the relationship as it is, or was. This process involves resolving past interpersonal relationship issues or bringing traumatic experiences to closure by reliving them, actively expressing the previously unexpressed feelings, acknowledging the unmet needs. It may involve confronting distress-producing dysfunctional beliefs about need satisfaction and attaining closure. The dialogue offers an opportunity to express feelings fully and to allow them to run their course rather than be interrupted; this results in relief from the tension and pain of holding back. Thus, the intervention involves the *arousal* of emotion and the *expression* to completion of what was previously restricted. This process of intense expression leads to *relief and recovery*.

Marcus (1976) described Empty-Chair work with a client whose mother chided him for his "insistent demands upon her." She told him to be a good boy and stop whining. In the therapy setting, the client reencountered his mother in fantasy in an empty chair in front of him and began to feel his once inhibited anger towards her. He remembered her chiding, admonishing words and felt again his impulse to be quiet and be a good boy. Then he experienced a strong press of anger and expressed clearly that he was not going to be a good boy and that he demanded and insisted that she hear him.

Empty-Chair work of this type facilitates the client's awareness of and attention to new information and meanings associated with old emotional experiences. This includes information that previously had been unavailable because of the interruptive process. The release of tension gained in expressing the previously restricted emotion seems to free people to continue clarifying the meaning of the experience, a process that appears to have been impeded by the tension and discomfort of unexpressed feelings in that area.

In addition to the relief and recovery experience, the dialogue offers an opportunity for a schematic reorganization based on the emergence of new reciprocal views of self and other. This occurs by incorporating new information into the scheme of the other and the situation. Sometimes a new understanding of the other emerges, incorporating both good and bad features. At other times, clients change their views of the other as powerful and themselves as weak and possibly discard distress-producing beliefs (e.g., self-blame) related to the experience and the other. The activation of the related schemes of the other, self, and situation thus provides the opportunity both for the arousal and expression of emotion. This allows for the restructuring of the schemes.

For emotional change to take place, the relevant schemes must be accessed. It is not sufficient that the client conceptually discuss difficulties with the significant other in a purely conceptual manner. The scheme in *all* its conceptual, emotional, motivational, and expressive motor aspects must come alive in order to enhance the possibility of change at all these levels. The experience is then reprocessed utilizing present resources and capacities to promote schematic restructuring and closure.

Generally, when the scheme of the significant other is evoked, the person initially feels the emotion and then restricts the experience or expression resulting in a complaining, unsatisfied feeling. It is the purpose of the intervention to allow the person to experience and fully express the feelings to the significant other in an empty chair. This helps to remobilize the suppressed need and the sense of entitlement to the need. Mobilization and acknowledgment of the need then empowers the self to be able to separate appropriately from the other.

What is required for resolution of unfinished business is not that every unsatisfied need be met, but that one's feelings and needs be expressed fully and be acknowledged. Perls et al. (1951) describe what occurs when a person truly confronts the environment:

> In the whole-hearted striving to gain what is desired, in desperation and perhaps in rage, one may get what is needed or give up the need for the impossible...by tantrum and the labour of mourning the need for the impossible is annihilated. (p. 362)

Thus, out of this struggle, the organism makes the creative adjustment to the situation. Through the Empty-Chair dialogue, the client is given the opportunity, in the safety of the therapeutic situation and with the presence of a supportive therapist, to express fully to the imagined other all that has been interrupted and to struggle to create a new solution. Contact is created between the need and its object. This contact provides for the possibility of the creation of a new solution.

Resolution occurs in this process ultimately in two ways. First there is change in the self-related schemes. This may involve affirming the self, which involves separating oneself from the other, holding the other, rather than the self, accountable for wronging the self, and accepting and validating one's own actions. Second there is change in the other-related schemes. This may involve coming to see the other in a new light by either achieving a better understanding of the other (possibly including forgiveness), or by seeing the other as less intimidating, powerful, and dominant.

Empty-Chair work begins with a marker of unfinished business. When the marker emerges, the therapist helps the client engage in a dialogue between the self and the significant other, who is enacted by the client. The focus in this intervention is on having the client express previously interrupted feelings, rather than on having a dialogue with the other or the teaching of skills of interpersonal conflict resolution. The other chair is occupied far less frequently in this intervention than in Two-Chair Dialogue for conflict splits. It is generally occupied only at two major points in the dialogue: initially to help evoke emotion and later to check for resolution. The major mode of engagement in this task is that of active expression. The major goal is to have the client actively express the interrupted feelings and to mobilize and express needs.

In this intervention, the therapist directs the client to imagine the other's presence and to describe salient details of the other's appearance and manner. This imaginal representation is used to stimulate the emotional response (i.e., to activate the relevant schemes). At this stage, the client is also encouraged to enact the other as specifically as possible, particularly those aspects of the other that were the most troublesome. This could be a patronizing look on the face or a complaining tone in the voice. These expressive motor methods enhance the use of imagery in increasing the effectiveness of the image as an evoker of relevant emotional schemas.

The process of resolution in this dialogue has been rigorously modeled to determine the components of resolution that discriminate resolution and nonresolution dialogue (Greenberg 1991; Foerster, 1991). The model of resolution is shown in Figure 12-1. The resolution path can be seen as involving three stages: Arousal, Expression, and Completion.

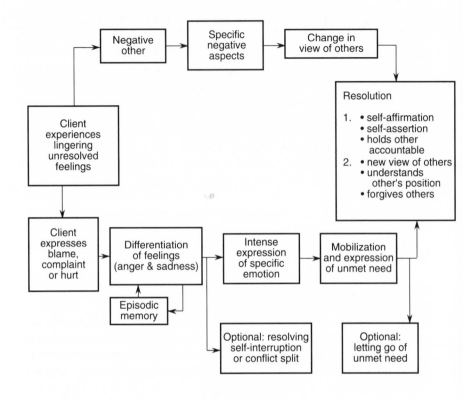

FIGURE 12-1. Resolution of unfinished business.

These are described in detail below. In addition, a short form of a rater's Degree-of-Resolution Scale devised for research purposes is shown in Table 12-1. This indicates six degrees of resolution and can be used as a guide to estimate how far along in the resolution process one has progressed.

The first step in this process involves the client's expressing to the other his or her unresolved feelings. The person is unable to accept the way the relationship was or is. There are expressions of complaint, bitterness, or regret accompanied by discomfort and bad feelings. The person often begins the dialogue by blaming, or complaining to the other, or expressing hurt about the treatment received. The other is reproached for what he or she did not do. The hurt, if expressed, has a constricted quality. At this point, the client generally moves to the other chair and enacts the negative other, capturing the troublesome features of the other's behavior and demeanor. The client draws on his or her internal representation of the other based on previous experience with the other.

TABLE 12-1. Degree-of-Resolution Scale (Short Form): Unfinished Business

1. Client blames, complains, or expresses hurt or longing in relation to a significant other.

2. Client makes contact with the other and expresses unresolved feelings, often resentment or hurt.

3. Complaint is differentiated into underlying feeling, and the relevant emotions, generally sadness and anger, are experienced and expressed with a high degree of emotional arousal.

4. The client's unmet need is experienced as valid and is expressed assertively.

5. The client comes to understand and see the other in a new way, either in a more positive light or as a less powerful person who has problems of his or her own.

6. The client affirms the self and lets go of the unresolved feeling either by forgiving the other or holding the other accountable.

Thus the client may enact a discounting or disconfirming other. As the client's schematic memories of the other are accessed, the representation of the other becomes more specific. The client enacts the other in greater detail, capturing the negative tone and look as well as the harsh, rejecting words of the other.

The client then responds to the enactment of the negative aspects of the other. At first, the feelings are more global, but as the client ventures to express these reactions, they become clearer, more differentiated expressions of emotions. The mixture of anger and sadness in the complaint and hurt become differentiated into expressions of pure anger or pure sadness. Resolution seems to require an intensity of emotional expression that is proportionate to the felt intensity. The expression of intense emotion involves unrestricted expression accompanied by matching expressive behavior such as weeping, mourning, shouting, kicking, or stroking the other chair until there is completion of the expression. This is accompanied by statements such as, "I felt betrayed," "I hate you," or "I felt so lonely," which symbolize and express the feeling. For example, after completing, the expression of the anger at violation or the sadness at loss will often emerge. On the other hand, after expression of sadness, anger may emerge, accompanied by an assertion of one's autonomy and rights and the creation of boundaries. This process is illustrated in the following example.

A client in an Empty-Chair Dialogue with her sickly mother expressed her resentment toward her about having been made to parent her and to grow up too quickly. The client reevoked a memory from when she was 6 years old—her mother had come to meet her on the way home from school, and she had seen mother in "her 90-pound body" being blown away by the wind. Amid the tears, and the pain and anger of that experience, she said, "I resent you for not being able to stand up to the wind." After expressing the resentment, she expressed her feelings of helplessness and differentiated them into the feelings of how she was "doing fine walking home from school until my mother came into sight, and I felt guilty that my mother had come out for me and was being blown about by the wind. But even more important, now I felt responsible for having to take care of my mother." This led to a clear feeling of anger toward her mother. For this client, who had in her own words, always "bent over backwards" to be good to her mother, this anger became important in helping her to define herself more clearly and to separate from her mother.

Of particular interest in the resolution process is that once the client has fully expressed feelings of (for example) anger and resentment, he or she can begin to acknowledge the other's weaknesses, frailties, limitations, and admit this information into the internal representation of the other.

The next step in the dialogue in the self chair involves the mobilization and expression of the unmet need associated with the emotion. Often these are needs that were never expressed in the original relationship because of a feeling of lack of entitlement. Now the client expresses these heartfelt needs to the imagined other. These needs flow from the intensely expressed emotions and are generally related to the satisfaction of basic interpersonal needs for attachment or separation and for self-esteem. The needs are owned as one's own and expressed as belonging to and coming from the self, rather than as deprivations or accusations of the other. They are expressed with a sense of entitlement and a sense of legitimacy. It is often important to help clients get to their ability to assert their boundaries, to say "no" to the intrusion and to reassert their rights. In situations in which the need cannot or will not be met by the other, clients who resolve come to recognize their right to have the need met by others. At the same time, they let go of having to have it met by the significant other.

One of the aspects of resolution not yet fully captured in our empirical research and in the model is that, in working with the aroused emotion and the expression of need, clients often confront a dysfunctional belief about their needs or the situation in which the needs were thwarted. Legitimizing needs involves the overcoming of beliefs that prevent the mobilization and acknowledgment of the need. Thus, in a dialogue in which a client was disciplined by an alcoholic father with a revolver, she confronts the dysfunctional belief that she must have been bad enough to deserve this treatment. She claims "it wasn't me who was bad, it was you who was sick."

Another client who was working on sexual tension in her marriage, reworked a date rape experience in which the man had told her she deserved it. She had carried the belief around for years, but when she relived the experience and felt the legitimacy of her feelings and needs, she said, "I didn't want this nor did I do anything to deserve this. It was you, not me who is to blame." Similarly, people in traumatic situations who form the belief "I should have died" or "I was a coward for living" confront this type of dysfunctional belief empowered by the legitimacy of their own feelings and needs.

The next stage in the dialogue involves a shift in the representation of the significant other in the empty chair. Through the arousal of emotion by expression and the strengthening of the self through the increased sense of legitimacy of one's needs, the client is now able to identify previously less salient and often more positive aspects of the other. The individual can expand his or her former overly constricted view of the other. A different representation of the other is now enacted, generally either a more affiliative or a less dominating other. The "other" scheme changes in one of two ways: either the previously held, negative other changes to a more positive, caring other, or the bullying, dominant other becomes weaker and is seen in terms of inner failings. The other expresses more love and understanding of the client and/or expresses regret that he or she was unable to meet the client's needs. The other may articulate aspects of his or her life situation that left him or her inadequate to meet the client's need. The other may ask for understanding and forgiveness of the client. Abusive others may be seen for their sickness or dysfunction and may accept accountability for their actions.

The final step in the dialogue is the client's experience of resolution in the form of self-affirmation and self-assertion and/or in the form of a forgiveness or greater understanding of the other without necessarily condoning the other's actions. Self-affirmation means clients know that they themselves were not bad and that it was not their fault that the other could not meet their needs. Often there is a sense of accomplishment of having succeeded in spite of the difficulties and of having built satisfying lives for themselves, plus a sense of pride in their own strengths and attributes. Self-affirmations may also involve a clearer sense of separating from the other and holding the other accountable. The client confronts the other and the situation with the other, which frustrated need satisfaction. He or she recognizes that the relationship did not provide what was needed and declares the legitimacy of those needs.

Clients let go of expectations of having their needs met and in effect accept the other for what they could and could not provide. Sometimes resolution states are characterized by the explicit expression of increased understanding of the other. Clients may express acceptance of the other, acceptance born of newly experienced understanding of the other's difficulties in providing what was missed. Clients also express appreciation for what was given and forgiveness or acceptance of what occurred in the past.

The crucial resolution processes in this task appear to be: (1) the intense emotional arousal and completion of emotional expression accompanied by the mobilization of the need; and (2) the shift in the internal representation of the other. The change process seems to be one of shifting one's role relationship position with a significant other such that one feels more powerful and tolerant. In a study of resolution sessions, resolvers reported feeling more powerful and tolerant than nonresolvers (King, 1988). In order for a person to shift self–other role relationship perceptions, he or she needs to feel empowered. This appears to occur by expression of the powerful feelings and needs that had previously been unacknowledged or disowned and by recognition of the legitimacy of these needs.

Therapeutic Intervention to Bring About Change

The intervention involves encouraging the client to engage in a dialogue with an imagined significant other or to reenter the traumatic situation until the interrupted feelings are reexperienced and expressed. The therapist facilitates the arousal and expression of the unexpressed feelings. The process goal is to complete the expression of the emotion to enable the person to mobilize the previously unmet need and to change his or her view of the self and other or situation. In the past, when the emotion scheme was evoked, the feelings were suppressed and never allowed full expression. As a result, there was never an experience of release of tension and relief, nor the opportunity for a schematic restructuring. In this intervention, the unresolved emotions are aroused, expressed, and allowed to run their course.

Therapeutic intervention involves promoting intensified expression and mobilizing and validating of previously unmet needs. The therapist's task is to stimulate the expression of the unexpressed emotion. The therapist needs to help the client move beyond the secondary reactive feelings of blaming, complaining, and feeling hurt to more primary expressions of anger and sadness. The therapist listens for what is most primary at any moment and intervenes to bring this expression into the dialogue. When the feeling has begun to be accessed, the therapist promotes intense expression of the emotion. This may involve the use of expressive motor experiments to help the client fully experience, express, or let go of the feeling. Thus, hitting, yelling, or kicking may be encouraged to express anger, whereas sobbing and grieving may be encouraged, to express sadness. Deliberate expression of the feeling is encouraged, and graded experiments are used to help the client intensify expression of the feeling. In this intervention, the client is asked to deliberately speak and act in an angry or sad manner in order to evoke the feeling. As Berkowitz (1990) has shown, deliberate expression can evoke feelings. The art is in encouraging the person sufficiently until the feeling flows spontaneously and then facilitating this authentic expression. The therapist needs to shift between directing the client to actively express and helping the person try to attend to the experience. The oscillation between expressing and attending helps to bring the emotional experience alive.

In addition to attempting to arouse unexpressed feelings, the therapist is also alert to the way in which expression is prevented. Two major methods of blocking expression of unfinished business involve the two different types of conflict splits (see Chapters 10 and 12). Either self-evaluations or "shoulds" against expression, or self-interruptions, which involve more muscular and automatic holding back of expression, are found. The self-evaluations or "shoulds" against expression of feelings are generally noted by the therapist. But rather than explicitly working on them, the therapist attempts to counter the "shoulds" and overcome performance anxiety by suggesting that it is appropriate and important to express the emotions. This is done gently and is usually effective. However, if the client experiences a major conflict over the expression, or a strong value that expression would violate, then work needs to be done to deal with resolving this conflict. There are two circumstances when self-interruptive split resolution takes precedence over completion of unfinished business. First is when the block to expression involves an automatic interruption of the experience and the expression, such that it is there one moment and gone the next. Second is when the person is cut off from the start, literally unable to experience (as opposed to feeling he or she shouldn't). Under these circumstances, resolution of the interruptive split is viewed as a subtask necessary to enable the arousal of intense emotion necessary for the resolution of unfinished business.

A major subgoal is arousal of expression. It should be emphasized that the process in this experiment is not the promotion of a highly interactive back-and-forth dialogue between the self and significant other but, rather, the expression and completion of the unfinished business with the other. A back-and-forth dialogue tends to promote a role play of interpersonal conflict. Although some taking of the role of the negative other is useful to help stimulate the arousal of feelings, the purpose is not one of arguing back and forth. Once the unexpressed feeling has been contacted, the goal is to promote its expression. This is done primarily by keeping the client in the self chair and working with the arousal of expression and assertion of need.

After the mobilization and assertion of the need, the client is again asked to play the role of the significant other to gauge the response of the other. If the other's position has not shifted, then more expressive work needs to be done. If the other shifts in stance, then the dialogue between the two is facilitated. At this stage, the client is asked to respond to the other. Either spontaneously or in response to therapist inquiries, clients tend to reevaluate their position. This may include whether they understand, forgive, or hold the other accountable and whether they are able or unable to let go of expectations. Clients are then asked to say "goodbye for now" to the other, as a means of ending the work and are asked to come back to themselves and check out how they feel. They are thereby grounded in their current sensory experience. The meaning of what occurred in the dialogue is discussed and processed further where necessary.

THERAPIST OPERATIONS

Therapeutic intervention facilitates the client engaging in a dialogue with the significant other in order to express previously unexpressed and unresolved feelings. The therapist facilitates the client in expressing these feelings to the other until the client experiences some relief and is able to complete their expression. The process goal is to complete or let go of the unresolved feelings. In life these feelings are often kept to oneself and seem to fester and sour, rather than disappear. In this intervention, they are brought into the open and expressed to produce schematic restructuring.

Therapeutic work involves arousing the emotion to an intensity that matches the degree to which it has been felt and to have it expressed toward its correct target. The therapist's task is to promote sufficient arousal to enable emotional relief and recovery and to bring about change in view of self and other and the relationship. This is done so that the client is able to let go of the feelings and unmet needs and carry on with his or her life in a less-burdened fashion.

Therapeutic work can be divided into three core phases, Arousal, Expression, and Completion, plus pre- and postdialogue stages. Each involves a number of specific types of therapist operations, which are shown in Table 12-2 and are discussed below.

TABLE 12-2. Therapist Operations

Predialogue Stage
    1. Establish collaboration.
    2. Structure the experiment.

Arousal Stage
    3. Evoke the sensed presence of the significant other.
    4. Establish contact between self and significant other.
    5. Facilitate the taking of responsibility.
    6. Access client's initial feelings in response to the significant other.
    7. Facilitate enactment of the significant other and intensify the stimulus value of the significant other.
    8. Evoke a specifically recalled event or episodic memory.

Expression
    9. Differentiate feelings toward significant other.
    10. Promote full expression to significant other of differentiated primary/ adaptive emotion by graded experiments of expression.
    11. Help client maintain a balance between expression and contact with inner referent.
    12. Facilitate expression to significant other of unfulfilled needs and expectations in regard to significant other.

Completion Stage
    13. Identify with other and support emerging new representation of other.
    14. Support emerging new understanding of other and of relationship with other.
    15. Empower the client.
    16. Close contact with the other appropriately.

Postdialogue Stage
    17. Create meaning/perspective.

Predialogue Stage

As in the other tasks, the therapist begins with the two prerequisite steps.

Establishing Collaboration

On the appearance of a marker, the therapist suggests the unfinished business as a focus for work and obtains the client's agreement to work on it.

Structuring the Experiment

The therapist suggests a dialogue, pulls up a chair, and invites the client to begin a dialogue in whatever way seems most appropriate.

Arousal Stage

Evoke the Sensed Presence of the Significant Other

Using the client's preferred sensory modality, suggestions are given to evoke the significant other's presence. The therapist might suggest bringing him or her into the room, imagining that individual sitting here, perhaps pointing to the empty chair. If needed, the therapist asks the client to describe the other, particularly his or her face, or to imagine the sound of the other's voice. The therapist checks with the client by asking, "Can you see her?" "Can you hear his voice?" followed by "What do you feel?"

Establish Contact between Self and Significant Other

The therapist instructs the client to react to the imagined presence of the significant other by directing statements to the significant other in the empty chair.

The therapist guides the client in evoking the presence of the significant other (in the empty chair) using sensory images. The client is directed to respond to the other and express to the other whatever he or she is experiencing at the moment. The therapist attends to the client's expression, noting whether the client's expression is spontaneous or deliberate, whether the affect being expressed is primary (such as genuine anger, sadness, or hurt), reactive, or instrumental (such as reactive anger, whining, defeat, or helplessness). Often the client expresses a complaint, representing feelings that have remained undifferentiated, as well as unexpressed. In that case, it is the therapist's task to help the client both differentiate and express these.

Facilitate the Taking of Responsibility

To discourage the client from hurling accusations toward the other, and to help the client to identify with and take responsibility for his or her own experience, the client is guided to speak from his or her own experience and to express feelings in terms of "I" statements.

Access Client's Initial Feelings in Response to Significant Other

As needed, the therapist helps the client focus inward in response to the imagined presence of the significant other. In the process, the therapist looks for the authentic complaint, often undifferentiated hurt or resentment. In order to arouse the client, the therapist may suggest that he or she repeat or intensify some of his or her nonverbal expressions, particularly if these are spontaneous and reflect primary affect.

Facilitate Enactment of the Significant Other and Intensify the Stimulus Value of the Significant Other

This is done by heightening the figural, negative, verbal, and nonverbal expressions of the significant other through repetition, exaggeration, and enactment. In order to increase the client's emotional arousal, the therapist directs the client to enact the significant other in the empty chair. The therapist instructs the client to focus on and represent, in both verbal and nonverbal expression, the key negative aspects of the significant other. It is important for the therapist to recognize that at this point, the "bad" other in the empty chair, is a powerful ally for stimulating and arousing the client's level of affect.

Evoke a Specifically Recalled Event or Episodic Memory

Sometimes the client will remember a specific situation that remains particularly painful and unfinished. If so, the therapist helps the client reenter the situation and evoke it vividly in the present by helping the client describe and enact the particulars of the event in detail, using present tense language. Otherwise, the therapist inquires whether the client recalls a specific relevant situation or event that remains particularly unfinished, helping the client to evoke an episodic memory. In either case the vivid retelling of this episode in the present and the enactment of the self and the significant other in the remembered context will further stimulate and enliven the client's experience.

Expression

In this stage, the therapist facilitates the client's full differentiation and expression of emotion in relation to the significant other.

Differentiate Feelings toward Significant Other

The therapist brings the client's attention to the expression of feelings toward the significant other, attending to:

- The microsignals of emotion themselves, bringing to the client's awareness his or her primary adaptive emotions.
- The expressive signs of the avoidance or interruption of emotional experience and expression.

If the client has remembered and evoked a past, unfinished situation, the therapist will encourage the client to respond to the other as him- or herself within that situation, allowing the client the opportunity to reexperience and differentiate the full range of feelings that the client felt then.

Promote Full Expression to Significant Other of Differentiated Primary/Adaptive Emotion by Graded Experiments of Expression

In fostering full expression of the unfinished emotion the therapist starts small (shake your fist again) and builds in a step-by-step fashion to larger and more comprehensive expressive actions (hit the pillow). As this proceeds, the therapist focuses on the emergence of client expressions that are spontaneous rather than deliberate. The therapist also gives the client ample opportunity for verbal and nonverbal expressions of emotion. In the process, deliberate expression of reactive-instrumental emotion (such as whining, defeat, or helplessness) is bypassed or discouraged. Instead the therapist validates and supports the client's authentic, spontaneous expressions of grief, pain, anger, and sadness.

Help Client Maintain a Balance between Expression and Contact with Inner Referent

As the expressive process moves forward the therapist helps the client alternate between expression and inner experiencing. In doing this, the therapist looks for congruence between client's experience and client's expression. The therapist ensures that expression is authentic by helping the client maintain a balance between contact with the other and contact with his or her inner experience. The therapist attends to the microsignals of emotion expression, to the client's signs of avoiding emotion, and to the client's repertoire of emotion expression. For example, a therapist might note whether the client expresses anger or whether the client is able to allow him or herself to experience sadness. By bringing these to the client's attention, and by directing the client to focus inward, the therapist helps him or her to access the underlying, unacknowledged, primary emotion. The therapist then encourages the client to express the emotion to the other and helps the client to put the anger, the disgust, or the longing in contact with its object. This allows the emotion to be completed.

Facilitate Expression to Significant Other of Unfulfilled Needs and Expectations in Regard to Significant Other

At this point, the therapist specifically instructs the client to tell the imagined other what he or she needed (or still needs) from the other or what he or she had missed. With the therapist's help the client articulates what he or she wanted or needed from the other but did not receive. The therapist ensures that the client receives ample time for full expression to the other of whatever has been accessed. The therapist pays attention to boundary definition, helping clients to assert themselves and to say "no" in situations in which they had been intruded on or violated.

Completion Stage

In this stage, the therapist supports and promotes the letting go of the unfulfilled expectation in relation to the significant other. Letting go often seems to follow naturally from the full expression of anger or lingering resentment, hurt, or disappointment. When it does not, the therapist helps the client explore and evaluate whether the unfulfilled expectation can realistically be met by the other, and, if not, the therapist helps the client explore the effects of hanging on to the expectation. Here the therapist might suggest that clients experiment with expressing to the other something like "I'll never give up wanting you to meet my need" and to see how they feel doing this. This often produces a shift.

Supports Emerging Positive Representation of Other

At this point the therapist directs the client to enact the other in the empty chair once again. This time, the therapist supports the emergence of a different, more positive, or less controlling representation of the other. This often follows quite naturally after expression and letting go have occurred.

The therapist also supports the other's inclination to admit his or her own inadequacy and request forgiveness, if this is present.

Supports Emerging New Understanding of Other and of Relationship with Other

The therapist recognizes when a shift has occurred for the client, perhaps a softening of feeling toward the other or the articulation of a resolve by the client never to forgive the other. Regardless of the nature or direction of the shift, the client is enabled to assert the new-found view. This step may involve supporting the offering of forgiveness to the other, perhaps followed by an expression of appreciation for the other. Alternatively, acceptance may involve the resolution not to forgive. In any event, resolution of the relationship involves the client's letting go of any remaining unfulfilled expectations in regard to the significant other.

Empowers the Client

In the event that the client cannot let go of unfulfilled expectation of other and has an unmet need, the client is asked what he or she might *do* in order to get the remaining need satisfied.

Close Contact with the Other Appropriately

The therapist next assesses the extent to which the client has completed expression of the need and let go of the unfulfilled expectations and whether client might benefit from further empty-chair dialogue work with the significant other.

This step involves helping the client say good-bye to the other in some suitable fashion that fits the client's experience and need. The therapist may ask the client if there is anything else that he or she wants to say or wants from the other. This may be a literal good-bye or the building of a bridge to the future with the statement of the desire to resume the dialogue at another time. Thus, if more work is needed to complete expression of emotion and need, to let go of unfulfilled expectations, and/or to accept or otherwise resolve the client's relationship with the other, a temporary good-bye is appropriate. On the other hand, if the client has completed this work, then a more final good-bye is appropriate.

Postdialogue

Creating Meaning/Perspective

Finally, the therapist helps the client where necessary or appropriate to integrate this new experience of self and the significant other into his or her real-life experience of the other. This helps the client to resolve the relationship, either through closure or through a decision to take some appropriate action in relation to the other. Thus, the therapist discusses the client's dialogue experience or suggests that the client sit with the experience and reflect on it in order to help the meaning to emerge.

Example of a Complete Dialogue

The following dialogue comes from a midtreatment session with a 45-year-old woman who had been feeling depressed over the past week partly as a function of having talked about her relationship with her mother in the previous session. The segment begins about 8 minutes into this session. This transcript could sound controlling and directive depending on how one reads the transcript. It is important to understand that both the manner and tone with which the interventions are made are empathic and concerned. The style is not distant and authoritarian but caring and egalitarian.

Predialogue Stage

C: I feel stupid to say this, it feels like I can't be happy until I feel accepted. And I never felt accepted, especially by my mother. I would just like her to have accepted me, liked me.

T: Uh-huh, never feeling truly accepted, especially by her. I think it might be helpful to bring her in here and kind of have a dialogue with her. [Structure the experiment]

C: Dialogue with my mother?

T: Yeah, are you willing to try that? It can often be quite helpful. There's a lot there, and it might be helpful to express some of that to her. [Establish collaboration]

C: OK. You want me to talk to her?

Arousal Stage

T: Yeah, put her here. Can you imagine her here. [Evoke presence of the other]

C: I don't know. It's like I don't even want to look at her.

T: What's the feeling?

C: It's anger and hurt all balled up together.

T: Uh-huh, so do this some more; make the sound. [Access feelings]

C: I can't.

T: It's just this bad feeling.

C: I mean, I don't want to push her away. Umm.

T: Can you tell her this? [Establish contact]

C: Well, it's funny you know. It's like I have the most incredibly . . . (*mutters to self*) Well, I guess I could tell her this. (*to other*): I have the most incredible jumble of feelings about you. You were an absolutely *impossible* woman. Do you have any *concept* of how impossible you were? You always said you weren't going to be like your father, and, damn it all, you were. You were at least as bad as he was. Stubborn! God damn it, you were stubborn.

T: So tell her. (*client grimaces*) What happens then?

C: Oh, I feel so frustrated that you couldn't use that stubbornness to live instead of to die. You fucking well told me at 50 that you were going to die at 70. I thought your whole world would have changed around if you'd gotten past your birthday, and you managed to die 6 months before it. You were a woman of incredible will!

T: What's your frustration? Your face is very . . . It's like there is an appeal to her: "I needed you to have been more . . ." [Facilitate taking responsibility]

C: Yeah. Why couldn't you *live*? Why did you just have to give up?

T: She left you without what?

C: Without a mother. Without a grandmother. That really hurt.

T: So tell her about it.

C: I'm angry that you could never, never accept that even though you didn't like my husband he was really an OK man.

T: Can you see her? I'm not sure if you're in contact with her. [Evoke presence and make contact]

C: Yeah. I don't know. It's partly that I can't stand to see her the way she was before she died.

T: So what is it that's too difficult to see, that you can't stand?

C: I can't, I couldn't stand to see you looking so thin, so gray.

T: So will you try looking at her now. [Make contact]

C: I don't want to see her like that.

T: Uh-huh. I'm not sure, are you saying it's too painful to look.

C: No. If I look I'll want to reach out, and she won't be there.

T: Uh-huh.

C: It's useless. It's pointless. I've tried for years to get her acceptance. I, I mean I had three kids. It wasn't exactly to please her, but, you know people are supposed to like their grandchildren. Right? Wrong. She didn't like me. Why should she like her grandchildren any better. It was kind of stupid. [A split emerges]

T: Sounds like you're kind of mad at yourself for wanting acceptance. Can you come over here and tell her this. [Sets up the two-chair split subtask involved in preventing contact]

C: Well, how many times do you have to hit your head against a brick wall before you find out that it's harder than you are. You just get hurt.

T: So . . .

C: So give up. Give up wanting it. It's not going to happen. She died and it didn't happen, so forget it.

T: Change. (*pause*) So what happens to you?

C: It's true.

T: But . . .

C: It doesn't even feel like a "but" . . . it's just true.

T: What happens to this wanting, this wanting acceptance?

C: Ummm. I think I'm still more in that chair. It's like you're a big girl now, you know.

T: Change.

C: You know, I'm grown up. I can take care of myself and a lot of other people too. I'm competent, responsible, so what's the point of flogging a dead horse? [Laugh] That's a funny image when it comes to my mother. [T: Umm-hmm]

T: So what are you experiencing? [Attending]

C: There's something just happened for me about my mother and horses, and somehow, it's like. (*Shakes head, gestures to move back to the other chair*) Can I put my mother in there?

T: Sure. [Reestablish contact with mother and Unfinished Business]

C: It's a real piss-off that you paid any attention to Dad when he said that you should give up horseback riding. It really is a piss-off. It was really stupid. I know Grandpa got really badly hurt. But you really loved it. It's the only thing in your life that you ever really loved, was that horseback riding. Doing it with your Dad. I mean every morning for years and years . . . And it was me. Oh shit! [crying]

T: Breathe, breathe.

C: Was it my fault? That she had to give it up? My father told her that she was a mother now and that she shouldn't ride horses anymore. It was too dangerous . . . (*crying*) I feel I could never make up for that.

T: Tell her this.

C: It was my fault. It was my fault you didn't ride.

T: Change.

C: You weren't much of a substitute.

T: Say this again. You're not a substitute for. [Enact significant other]

C: You're not. I told you so. I liked the pekingese better than I liked you. I sent you off to nursery school when you were two so that I wouldn't beat your brains out. If I ever had two kids, I said, I'd probably hit their heads together. No, no you weren't a substitute. You were never the joy that she was.

T: Go with this, tell her. "You're . . ." [Enact significant other]

C: You weren't a joy. I don't know. That's not quite right. You're a bother.

T: Yeah, yeah.

C: You're a bother. I mean little kids. I don't like little kids much.

T: Will you go with the expression on your face? It's like, "Yuck," that's the message. "You're a bother." Try to really be her. How did she convey it? The nonverbal? [Identify with the other]

C: Bleak. Tight, tight. Hard jaw.

T: Hard jaw, right? Tight? Now what's the message from that?

C: I don't like you.

T: Yeah, just say it again.

C: I don't like you. I like animals better. I don't like people much. I don't like messes and you made messes. [silence]

T: What's happening?

C: I guess I'm just experiencing that, this walled in, hard feeling of not, I mean, just, what an awful place to live . . . I didn't know what to do with you. You made me feel inadequate. I mean, what do you do with a baby? I mean I sure didn't want you nursing, I mean.

T: Yeah, do that again, 'cause there's the disgust. Express some of this. Put a sound to it. [Intensify the significant other]

C: Yuck. Umph. No way. I mean motherhood is not what it's cracked up to be. If you are the sole produce of my life, I don't feel very good about it. I mean, as a person you really weren't too bad.

T: What's at the center of all this. What's the central message, right, "you're . . . You get in my way. You're in my way. You're a bother." [Intensify significant other]

C: You're a bother. Grow up, grow up fast. I don't like little kids. I really don't like little kids. I want you to grow as rapidly as possible, so that I do not have to have a little kid any longer than is absolutely necessary.

T: Change.

C: Oh, I did.

T: What's it like to receive that message? "You're a bother. You get in my way" . . . what happens? [Access feelings]

C: It sort of immobilizes me. I feel like, what do I do? I mean I guess you couldn't help it if you didn't like kids, but I was your kid, and it really wasn't too good for me.

T: What was it like for you? [Differentiate feelings]

C: It was awful. I mean, really being your little kid was just bloody awful. I mean you did have some of the weirdest ideas of how to take care of little children. You know, mother, you do not leave little kids in houses alone when they are 6 years old. It is too scary.

T: What was it like for you?

C: I was terrified. You shouldn't have done that.

T: Stay with the child. Because you sort of become the critical parent. It was scary for you to be left alone. [Access feelings]

C: Damn right. I was in the house. The Indians would come by, and they threw rocks against the house, and the dog barked, and there wasn't anybody there. Over and over and over.

T: So she just left you, and you had to fend for yourself. [Empathize to evoke the episodic memory]

C: At night.

T: At night. So you felt both frightened and really abandoned.

C: I mean you and Dad, both, I mean really. How could you both be so stupid?

T: Do you hear your voice? What happens? What do you hear? [Attend]

C: Well, I hear the me that knows about taking care of kids, judging that this was just unutterably stupid.

T: Right. There's the exclaiming "How could you do this?" (*pause*) Tell them what it was like for you. What were you feeling? "I felt unloved, uncared for, unsupported." [Access feelings]

C: Yeah. I did feel all those things. I was just a little girl, and I really was a little girl, and it was OK to be a little girl. (*voice change to that of a child from here on*) I would have liked a little while longer to be a little girl. I was kinda cute. If I had a little girl like me, I would have taken better care of her.

T: Um-hmm. Say this again.

C: If I had a little girl like me, I wouldn't have left her alone at night.

Expression Stage

T: Yeah. What would you have seen that she needed?

C: I would have seen that she needed somebody there, and she needed a big hug when I left, and she needed to know that it was hard when your Mummy and Daddy went out and left you, and I'd know that if she cried in the dark that she was scared, and it didn't matter whether there wasn't anything there.

T: Tell her. I was scared when I cried. [Differentiate feelings]

C: Yes, I was. I wasn't just making up things to be bad. I did see shadows, and they were scary.

T: Tell her what you needed. [Express unfulfilled need]

C: I wanted you to be like my aunt. She left the light on in the hall and the door open . . . It was OK to be a little kid in her house. It wasn't OK with you.

T: Yeah. Tell her what else you needed.

C: I needed lots of cuddles. [T: Yeah] I needed you to like me better than the dog. I needed to be able to tell you what was going on on the bus all the way to school every morning. And I was scared then too. It was a long ride. [T: Yeah]

T: What happened?

C: Well those kids next door were really mean, and it was a long way. It was 12 miles, and I was only 6.

T: So what did you want from her?

C: I don't know. Maybe you were kind of helpless too. I wanted you to understand.

T: Say this, I wanted you to understand.

C: I wanted you to understand, not always to tell me that it wasn't so bad. (*deep sigh*)

T: Breathe again . . . I'd like you to change.

C: Can I stay here for a couple more minutes. [T: Um-hmm] It feels really good to be so little. I don't think I almost ever felt so little in my whole life.

T: Right. So what do you want to tell her? "I needed to feel this little."
[Balance of expression and internal experience]

C: Yeah. I'm a nice little girl. It's OK to be little when you're little. I would have cuddled you back. I would have liked to have sat in your lap. But I'm glad for all the stories you read me. We liked that together. I needed you to know what it was like when I was sick.

T: Tell her that.

C: You took care of me, but I don't think you ever understood how horrible those hallucinations were when I looked at you and you kept getting littler and littler until you only looked this big. (*Sigh*) And I just, so scared.

T: What did you want from her then?

C: I think I got some of what I wanted. I think that was one of the few times that I really did. Yeah, you really were pretty good when I was sick. It's a wonder I'm not a hypochondriac . . . [T: Uh-huh] I really appreciated cold cloths on my head, and I liked when sometimes you gave me little back rubs. I liked that. But you shouldn't have to get sick to get that stuff.

T: "I, I shouldn't."

C: I shouldn't. I wish I didn't have to get sick.

T: Tell her, tell her, "I shouldn't have to get sick to get your comforting and care."

C: Yeah, yeah, that's the only time I remember you really being there. Was when I was really sick. And then I felt like you cared. That maybe it was important to you. (*adult voice resumes*)

T: I want you to take a step now. It wasn't my fault about the horses and riding. Can you do that? "It wasn't my fault you gave up horses." [Empowering the client]

C: Yeah, it wasn't my fault. I'm sorry. I am sorry, but it wasn't my fault.

T: What do you feel when you say this to her?

C: It's true, it wasn't my fault, and sad that she bought that crock of shit.

T: Whose fault was it? Tell her.

C: My father's.

T: Just put him there for a moment and tell him.

C: Oh, I don't want to be mad at my father. Yeah, actually, I thought that was really stupid. I mean for Pete's sake she'd been riding horses since she was 5 years old. That was really dumb of you. Didn't you know how much she cared about it? You don't make people give up things that they really love.

T: Tell him what it did to you.

C: It made her resent me. It made her.

T: "I wish you hadn't done . . ."

C: Yeah, I really wish you hadn't done that. That was a very bad idea. I think you really did drive a wedge in between us.

T: Go back to your mother. Tell her it wasn't your fault. [Empowering]

C: Yeah, that was between you and Dad. It wasn't me. I mean 2-year-olds don't tell you not to ride horses. It wasn't my fault.

T: Tell her again.

C: I would have liked to have ridden with you. I wish you had taught me how to ride too. And you did a little bit out in Texas, and I loved it. That's something we could have shared. 'Cause I liked horses too. It wasn't my fault, I hope.

T: What happens? What does she say?

C: Well, if it wasn't for you, I wouldn't have given it up.

T: It's still powerful for you. So what do you say back to her?

C: I say that Dad would have found some other reason if Grandpa hadn't gotten hurt, and you would have given in anyway, even if I had never been born. I don't think it was my fault.

T: Again.

C: I don't think it was my fault. I really don't think it was my fault. I *know* it wasn't my fault. [Empower client]

T: Again, "it wasn't my fault."

C: It wasn't my fault. If it was anybody's fault, it was your fault for not standing up to Dad and telling him to take a hike, that you were going to go ride horses [T: Right] until you were 65 and some horse bucked you off a bridge, and it would have been a better way to go than the way you went. That's for damn sure.

T: So now the anger comes up again, about how she died. So tell her, "I'm angry at you." [Promote full expression of a primary emotion]

C: I am, I am. I'm angry at you. That has to be one of the dumbest ways to die I've seen in a long time.

T: So tell her how angry you feel.

C: Yeah, I'm mad, real mad. I mean, you drink yourself to death, and you don't eat, and you get thinner and thinner, and your bones break, and so then you have a broken hip and a broken leg, and God knows what else. You were one tough cookie that you could have done to yourself what you did for so long and not died until you were 72. You are impressive in that way. But do you know that you could have lived to be 90?

T: So that killing herself was like the final rejection.

C: Oh God, yeah.

T: Tell her. "That was like the final . . ." I think that's what you're saying.

C: You're right, you're right. You're absolutely right. It just went, (*strikes stomach*) hits me right in the pit of the stomach.

T: Tell her how it hit you. [Promote full expression of primary emotion]

C: I just felt so rejected, so uncared for.

T: OK, will you change? Can you tell her, do this to her, this ultimate rejection?

C: You weren't worth living for. You weren't. There you were with your nice, tidy little household, and I come to visit, and I always feel on the outside. And your husband goes around opening all the windows, cause he doesn't like my smoking, and no, no you weren't, you weren't worth living for.

T: Say, you're not.

C: You're not, you're not worth living for. You're not enough to make it worth living my life any longer. I have had it with my life.

T: In the present, "I've had it with my life. I don't want to live for you." Somehow that's the message. [Identify with other]

C: Um-hmm. I've had it with my life. I don't want to live for you. There isn't anything in my life that's worth living for. I am done with this life. Maybe there is something after this life and maybe there isn't, but, enough of this. It really is enough of this. I'm lonely, I'm bored. At least drinking helps me forget that some of the time. And, I don't want to live anymore.

T: So what do you want from her? [Identify with other]

C: I want you to stop wanting from me what I can't give you.

T: Say this again to her.

C: I want you to stop wanting from me what I can't give you. I can't give you what you needed. I knew I couldn't give you what you needed, and I told you that. In a way, I think I even told you I am sorry. When I told you I wasn't very good with kids, I was trying to tell you that I wasn't very good with you.

Completion Stage

T: Tell her this, what it was like. [Support emerging representation]

C: I don't think I was cut out to be a mother. I think I would have been a good executive. You really weren't, I mean, I like you, except when you're on my back, on my case all the time. But you're always trying to improve me. But beyond that I really quite like you. As a kid you were not too bad.

T: Tell her, "I'm sorry."

C: I'm sorry I couldn't give you what you needed.

T: Again.

C: I am sorry that I couldn't give you what you needed and what I needed too. Whatever kept me from loving you and being with you the way I wanted to be, kept me away from everything in my life. And I got tired of living in back of that wall. [T: Yeah] And I didn't want to live any more. And your kids weren't going to get through it either and I'm too old. I'm too old to ever do, to ever get past this.

T: And what do you want from her?

C: I want you to let me go. (*long pause. Crying*)

T: Breathe. "I did let you massage me. I even asked you for it."

C: It was time for you to hold me. You did it better than I did. Do you understand? I want to die.

T: So what do you say?

C: I guess, can you let me go?

T: Also I guess you said "I let you into my wall." [Supports new understanding]

C: Yeah. I did. You're the closest. You got closer than anybody else. It was a near thing.

T: Tell her again. "I let you closer than I ever let anybody"

C: Yeah, I think I did. I think I let you closer than I ever let anybody. Any person. You were right about the animals. But I wasn't scared of them.

T: Tell her what you want her to understand. "I want you to understand . . ." [Supports new understanding]

C: That I loved you. Maybe it wasn't all the things that you needed it to be, but it was the best I could do. And I did really care. And we had some good times together.

T: What are you experiencing?

C: Ah. I'm quiet.

T: Come back, if you want. What do you say?

C: Yeah, I guess I knew that. It was hard though.

T: What?

C: Oh, some kind of. She was a character. [to other]: You were, you were a character. (*smiling*) You really were something else. Much as I was ready to beat your brains out, I really sort of like ya.

T: Tell her what you liked. [Empowering the client]

C: I don't know. I don't know how you did it. To fire nine nurses when there's hardly anything of you left. You had everybody so intimidated, but you know it was a neat quality too. You were tough. You were a tough lady. And I guess I like that about myself too sometimes. Cause I can be a tough lady. And you were smart. You were really bright. And I like it that you liked that about me. And, before things got so tense between us, I liked the talks that we had. I liked talking to you. And I have a lot of good memories about that. I liked going on holidays with you. That was fun. I think you did the best you could. And I'm glad that you're not alive anymore rather than be in the place you were in, cause that was just awful, and I couldn't do a thing about it. But it was awful. It was a zoo. You lived in the middle of a zoo. I don't know how you gathered all these characters around you. It was a menagerie. But nobody was your equal. I was the only one. I don't know about Dad. I think I was the only one, that was almost equal, that you got anywhere close to.

T: What else do you want to say to her? Can you say good-bye for now? [Closing contact]

C: I don't disapprove of you. I did, but I don't anymore. I think that for whatever reasons, your life was really, really hard for you.

T: So can you say, at some level I can accept that that's how it was?

C: Yeah. I can. I hope you're not mad at me up there wherever you are cause I got you a modern, brass urn instead of a French provincial one. (*laughing*) [To therapist: I guess what I'm doing right now is, that I'm back after she died, yes, and where I am is holding that urn, which I in fact did, by myself, and putting it in that niche next to my father, that I'd never seen.] I'd never seen that place. I thought that mausoleums were all dark and gloomy. The sun was streaming down. The beautiful marble. I put you next to him, and there you are in your modern urn next to his French provincial one, and it seems kind of fitting, and it seemed kind of fitting then. I guess I see them put the marble up, turn down the screws, and I said good-bye to you then, and I regret that we couldn't have had more fun as adult women together. That's a loss for me, and I think that it was probably a loss for you too.

T: Can you say good-bye to her?

C: Yeah. I hope you're some place where things are easier. Or maybe you started over again, and you'll do it better next time, however it happens. I give you a hug. And for me I'm sorry you're gone. My image is of (*clasps arms together*) putting my cheek against hers and giving her a hug and turning away.

T: So come back to yourself and feel your own place.

C: I made good use of this handkerchief.

T: Good. Do you have a sense yet of being back in here?

C: Not quite.

T: It will take some time. How would you like to stop now? Are you...?

C: Reassembled?

T: Right. Just sit for a while and absorb this until you're able to begin the process of going out in the world. [Beginning to promote the creation of a meaning perspective]

CONCLUSION

The intervention is more directive, especially in the expression stage, than the Two-Chair intervention but it still involves facilitation and stimulation rather than training.

EMPATHIC AFFIRMATION AT A MARKER OF INTENSE VULNERABILITY

W E END THE SECTION on specific tasks by going full circle and returning to the importance of empathy. This time however, we emphasize its role in a specific task, that of providing empathic affirmation of the vulnerable self. We see this task as being of fundamental importance and of taking precedence over other tasks.

Some of the most powerful moments in therapy occur when clients allow themselves to experience and express extremely painful self-relevant emotions. Such emotions as deep hurt, despair about the future, intense shame, feelings of anger and bitterness, or a sense of total isolation from others, are felt as intensely personal. Although they may have been evoked by some external events, they are extremely self-relevant, and the negative emotion is felt as being about oneself rather than being simply a function of an external stimulus. Thus people feel extremely vulnerable about having these feelings. Moreover they are feelings that, in our culture, are often considered to be "abnormal" and unacceptable to others or even to oneself. It is therefore crucial that the therapist recognize and empathically affirm the person's experience at these moments of vulnerability.

Although the negative emotions are intense, clients may be reluctant to reveal them in their full intensity. In fact it is often the intensity of these feelings that leads clients to fear them. Clients often fear that if they reveal themselves and fully express these painful emotions, or other seemingly unacceptable aspects of themselves, that the therapist will judge them, feel alienated from them, or even reject them. They fear that they themselves will be viewed by the therapist as unacceptable, abnormal, defective, or even frightening. There is thus often an attempt to close down, or hold off, dreaded feelings or aspects of self and to avoid dealing with them. For some clients there is even the fear that if they fully acknowledge these dreaded negative feelings, these emotions will be bottomless and engulfing, and they will lose control and will, themselves, be overwhelmed by them.

Our assumption is that at times of intense vulnerability such as these an attempt to engage the client in an exploratory process, such as experiential search or a process of active expression, is not likely to be productive and may even be disruptive or threatening to the client.

WHAT NEEDS TO BE CHANGED? THE UNDERLYING PROCESSING DIFFICULTY

In any good Process-Experiential Approach, emotions are of central concern, signalling to the therapist a potentially important place to focus. But different therapy theories take different positions on the nature of these signals and on how best to respond to them. As we have emphasized throughout this volume, in our view, emotion is central in therapy. But the complex connections among emotion, motivation, and cognition suggest that emotion schemes may best be accessed and changed by means of different processes at different times. These different potential change points can be recognized by different markers.

A clear distinction can be made between markers of "vulnerability" and other markers, such as those for conflict splits or problematic reaction points. Markers for times of intense vulnerability present an important opportunity for an empathic, highly affirming interpersonal experience with the therapist. For instance, the following two client statements represent vulnerability markers. The first client expresses a feeling of loss and a type of envy and bitterness related to this that she finds difficult to integrate. "I wanted so badly to have a child myself, and I can't (*sob*). And now my sister-in-law is having one, and its terrible I just *can't feel glad for her. I even have bad feelings about the baby.*" Another client, who had experienced a loss, expressed a feeling of deep, overwhelming emptiness— "Nothing seems to have any meaning any more." In both of these examples the clients express painful feelings that are difficult to assimilate, and in their voice and manner of expression, there is a sense of intense vulnerability.

If one can fully express a feared, dreaded aspect of experience, such as intense despair, and have it fully received by a therapist who is sensing the feeling in it's full intensity and is clearly valuing the client with no reservations, this can be a powerful experience that promotes change. Markers indicating a time of intense client vulnerability are extremely important, taking precedence over other kinds of markers and task processes. If they arise in the process of engaging in other tasks they need to be responded to in an empathically affirming manner. Therefore it is crucial for therapists to be alert in recognizing these markers whenever they emerge.

At vulnerability markers like the ones described above, it is the expectation that others will find these painful feelings totally unacceptable that needs to be changed. For many people intense negative emotions are viewed as being beyond the limits of normality, and their expectation is that if these negative emotions or aspects of self are fully acknowledged and expressed, they would be totally unacceptable and perhaps frightening to others. For instance, the feeling of intense hopelessness may have the expectational quality of being "beyond forgiveness," or intense anger may be viewed as "frightening and dangerous." The experience is often one of feeling that one is fundamentally or irremediably "defective" or "flawed," possessing what Goffman (1959) has referred to as a sense of "stigma." Therefore, accessing such schemes involves not only accessing one's own fear or disgust about these emotions, but also the expectation that these extreme negative emotions will be viewed by others, including the therapist, as shameful, abnormal, or even frightening.

At some other time in a successful therapy these vulnerable feelings of shame, intense anger, or despair will become the explicit exploratory focus of therapy, involving the reexamination of the source and nature of these emotions, leading to the restructuring of some relevant emotion schemes. In the present event, however, the exploration of the emotion and its sources is *not* the primary focus. It is the person's intense vulnerability related to the feelings that needs to be addressed. The crucial first step at a vulnerability marker is for clients to experience the Empathic Affirmation and acceptance of the therapist. This occurs when the client makes full contact with the deeply feared aspects of his or her own experience while simultaneously being fully accepted and valued as a worthwhile person. The intense emotions, previously felt to be beyond the limits of normality, are then fully recognized and accepted as a shared human experience, involving understandable human emotions. This breaks the sense of personal and existential isolation. It can also alleviate a sense of self-rejection or fragmentation and restore clients' confidence in their own potential as worthwhile people.

The client's mode of engagement in these events is one of expressing current feelings of intense vulnerability while making interpersonal contact with the therapist. As the client moves deeper into the dreaded experience, there may be some experiential search, but the focus is on revealing rather than exploring. The product of this event is the crucial interpersonal learning that one's experience is acceptable, leading to greater self-acceptance.

In this whole process, clients are confirmed by making contact and being accepted as they are. They are helped to become unique selves by the therapist's confirming them in their uniqueness. It is the existence of the self as a separate center of experience and agency that is confirmed by the therapist's Empathic Affirmation of the client's unique inner experience. Accepting clients as they are in their vulnerability or despair does not imply their remaining that way or that the therapist has given up hope for their growth. Instead, the continuing Empathic Affirmation of the whole person while the individual is experiencing and revealing these painful aspects of him- or herself helps the individual to differentiate this aspect of self from the total self. The person ceases to feel as overwhelmed by the vulnerability and can see the feared aspect as a part, rather than as the totality, of him- or herself. The person then feels stronger, empowered, and more able to cope. This strengthened sense of self makes possible further changes and growth.

OPPORTUNITIES FOR INTERVENTION: VULNERABILITY MARKERS

For most people in therapy there is some sense of vulnerability, embarrassment, or shame in revealing their most personal and vulnerable aspects. There is a sense of risk in sharing experiences that are uncomfortable and private. Nevertheless, the usual relationship conditions in a process-experiential approach, of empathic attunement and communicated genuine empathy and prizing, establish an atmosphere of acceptance and safety that enables people to explore uncomfortable feelings and experiences that would not normally be shared with others.

At times, however, when the client is approaching a feared aspect of experience involving negative emotions such as shame, rage, or despair, the sense of vulnerability can become very intense. For some clients there is even the fear that, if the emotion is fully experienced, it will be overwhelming. At such times it is the interpersonal experience with the therapist that needs to be the central ingredient. Genuine Empathic Affirmation at such times indicates that the therapist is sensing the feeling in its full intensity, is not judgmental, and is clearly continuing to value the client with no reservations.

The markers for these times of intense vulnerability usually involve four aspects:

1. The person is expressing an intense, self-relevant negative emotion and is clearly feeling vulnerable at that moment. This sense of vulnerability may involve fear of the therapist's criticism and rejection, or even fear of being overwhelmed by the feeling.

2. Even if the emotion is evoked by a particular event or experience, the feeling seems to be a more pervasive one that colors a variety of experiences.

3. There is a sense of deep reluctance to express the feeling, a sense of being at risk. In the voice and manner there is a sense of holding back and, often, a quality of the feeling being expressed for the first time.

4. There is one further related aspect that is hard to describe in words, but it comes through in vocal quality, posture, sighing, and facial expression. These signs indicate the intensity of the vulnerability, even a feeling of being "at the end of the road," and of the self being highly at risk. Some examples of these are:

- "When I've been talking with friends, I don't even try to tell them how bad I feel. They wouldn't understand." (deadness in voice)
- "I feel total despair, but there's no point in talking about it—nothing is going to change."
- "I just feel so full of regret, like there are so many things I've done I deeply regret. And now all I have are the consequences."
- "There's something—I've never told anyone. I've been so afraid to let anyone know."

HOW DOES CHANGE OCCUR? THE MODEL

The model for vulnerability events is shown in Figure 13-1. Change in the client can take place in two different ways. For some clients the understanding and valuing responses at this marker lead rather quickly to the client's experiencing the safety of the therapist's full acceptance of these dreaded negative feelings. Thus, although still involved in the negative feelings or the dreaded or shameful aspects of self, the client begins to move into a real exploration of the emotion and its personal content.

This seems to be an indication that the client's intense vulnerability has been eased and that he or she is now motivated and ready for an exploratory process involving relevant emotion schemes. The person feels understood and supported and is now ready to explore the sources of the feeling (Stages 2B and 3B in Figure 13-1).

On the other hand, after the initial period of Empathic Affirmation by the therapist, the client may continue to be clearly disturbed by the

1. The Marker
The client is experiencing some intense negative self-related feeling and is clearly disturbed by it.

2A The feeling deepens in response to Empathic Affirmation from therapist.

2B Empathic Affirmation is followed by some reduction in anxiety.

3A Increasingly intense expression of negative self-experience.

3B As anxiety is reduced, there is some indication of client's readiness for moving into exploration.

4A Client seems to touch bottom. Experiences the feared emotion or the painful aspect of self in its full intensity. Seems to be expressing the most dreaded or painful aspect of the experience.

5A Begins to feel calmer. No longer fragmented. A more agentic sense of self and one's possibilities. ("I'm acceptable as I am").

FIGURE 13-1. Empathic Affirmation at a vulnerability marker: Client performance model.

intensity or depth of the feelings of fear, shame, or despair, as indicated by voice and manner as well as content, or is holding back in an effort to stifle the feelings. If this is the case, then clearly the anxiety about the negative self-experience is still primary. At such a time the empathic understanding and valuing from the therapist continue to be the most important ingredients. This empathic understanding then leads (as shown in Figure 13-1 in Stages 3A to 5A) to an intense expression of the negative self-experience, then to expression of the most painful aspect, and finally to feeling calmer and more integrated.

As the emotional expression deepens and continues to be empathically received by the therapist, the client begins to feel that what was previously viewed as a totally unacceptable aspect of experience can be seen as an understandable, humanly acceptable feeling. The anxiety that has previously inhibited the full sharing of these experiences is reduced, and they can be expressed in their full intensity. It is as if going to the very bottom, fully feeling the experience, and not being overwhelmed by it, enables the client to start up again and move toward personal growth. Thus, the main focus of the entire session is on the empathic understanding of the client's experience, with consistent valuing of the client, leading eventually to a more positive and agentic sense of self. The client is now able to feel the whole experience in its full intensity, leading to a sense of relief and acceptance and integration of the entire experience into his or her sense of self. The energy that has been used to ward off the negative feelings can now be used for more positive, constructive self-exploration. The session may conclude with some exploration, but usually the focus of the entire session is on the full experience and expression of the emotion followed by a sense of relief and wholeness.

THE FUNCTIONS OF THE THERAPIST AT DIFFERENT STAGES OF THE MODEL

As we have said, it is extremely important for the therapist to be aware of vulnerability markers and to attend to them whenever they emerge. In our view a true vulnerability marker should take precedence over other kinds of exploratory processes, even if it emerges while a client is engaged in some other kind of task. It is crucially important because the whole fabric of the process-experiential approach depends on the empathic attunement of the therapist and on the client's experience of feeling fully received and valued.

At times of client vulnerability the therapist's empathic responses have a special quality. They do not usually have the exploratory, "open-edged" quality that serves to stimulate further exploration. On the other hand, they should not simply be "parroting" the client's statements. The therapist is not trying to dampen the feeling, nor is he or she trying to expand it. He or she is trying to sense the particular flavor of the client's experience, confirm that this *is* the client's experience, and to convey a receptive and accepting attitude to the client. At a vulnerability marker, the therapist's reflection of the client's message is *not* an attempt to push for deeper exploration or clarification. It is, rather, an explicit recognition of having received the client's expressed message with full empathy and consistent prizing.

The therapist needs to be responsive, not only to the initial marker, but also to the nature of the client's responses to the therapist's empathic reflections. If there is a sense of the client's retreating and clamping down on the feelings, then the therapist may be acknowledging and reflecting them in a form or manner that is too intense. At this point the genuine Empathic Affirmation by the therapist should continue but without too much poignant emotional arousal. When the client begins to feel more integrated, and a sense of agency or new-found energy emerges, the therapist recognizes this and follows with a growth-oriented reflection picking up the new sense of possibility.

If the client begins to move into exploration, as in Stage 3B in the model (Figure 13-1), the therapist begins to follow this exploratory track, as in any good empathic exploration. It is especially important to continue to be empathically attuned and clearly prizing, as the client moves into this exploration, since it is clearly a difficult and vulnerable area to explore.

A brief example of Track B in the model is shown below.

C: I guess I just don't have much to say. Nothing comes to mind.

T: Nothing you especially want to talk about?

C: No. Not really. (*flatness in voice*)

T: I'm not sure . . . feeling down . . . ? [Empathic conjecture]

C: Yeah, I guess I've been realizing I don't have any goals any more. I took care of Sam while he lived. It wasn't easy, but I knew it had to be done.

T: It was hard. but I guess you're saying you were needed, and you *did* it.

C: Yeah. I did. But now it's over. There's nothing I want to do.

T: You've got time. But what for? Who cares?

C: Yeah. I'm not needed any more. I have nothing left to live for. [Vulnerability marker]

T: Uh-huh just like what's the use of carrying on—I'm not needed any more by anyone.

C: Yeah. Sometimes I think of something to do, but then I feel . . . why bother?

T: Just for a minute you might think of something you might want to do, but . . . I'm not sure . . . It's just too much work?

C: It's more like would that be worth doing?

T: Uh-huh, just feeling—would it be worth the effort?

C: Yeah, like I'm spent, just nothing left to give. [Hits bottom]

T: Uh-huh, just all out of steam, just . . . no more . . . nothing left to give.

C: Yeah. (*sighs, takes a deep breath*) I have an idea for a story I want to write, and I get kind of interested, but then I'm not sure I . . . ah . . . have the energy.

T: It would take a lot of energy, but it sounds as if you're sort of intrigued by it. [Growth-oriented reflection]

C: Yes, I even get sort of excited.

The therapist in this event is not trying to anticipate the point at which the client will "touch bottom," nor is he or she attempting to hasten it. But it is important to recognize when this point has been reached and to share the client's sense of having expressed the worst and beginning to feel less burdened. If the client's sense of relief is directly expressed, or clearly present in the voice, then one can share in the client's new feelings and his or her emerging sense of agency.

If the client does not move into exploration but continues to go deeper into his or her negative self-experience, then the therapist continues to feel and express an empathic sensing of these feelings with continuing and genuine respect (side A in Figure 13-1). One continues to follow the client's level of intensity, neither attempting to play it down, nor to intensify it, but to remain genuinely empathically attuned to these feelings.

A condensed example of Empathic Affirmation taken from Rogers with Miss Mann is shown below (Rogers, 1983):

C: I was thinking the other night . . . I was feeling very blue about the way I felt. I thought, well, maybe . . . I wish I had my mother here in the way that she was. Because she used to be sort of reassuring when I was ill then, and . . . she would do little things . . . make some special dish, like custard or something. And it was sort of reassuring to have her around. And of course I know she isn't able to be that way any longer . . . I don't know what that all means . . . but for a minute I thought . . . well, I really *miss* her, and I sort of *need* a mother at this point . . . and yet . . . it's sort of impossible.

T: But even though it's factually impossible, the feeling was "Gee I *miss* her. I wish she was here to take care of me and to look after me." (*pause*)

C: And yet at the same time I thought, well . . . A little later I thought that wasn't what I needed . . . maybe it was a more *adult*, sort of . . . companionship, in some way, rather than a mother. But I needed something and somebody.

T: You really didn't feel sure in yourself whether . . . what you wanted was someone to really give you close mothering . . . or whether you wanted some more grown-up kind of relationship.

C: Mhm. And then in another sense, I thought "well . . . maybe it's just something I have to go through alone."

T: Maybe it's just hopeless to wish that I could really be in a relationship with anybody . . . Maybe I *have* to be alone.

[There is a short part omitted here, relating to the client's appointment with her doctor.]

C: And I'm frightened . . . because I kind of feel that they're having to be sure that it isn't cancer. And that really frightens me [T: Mhm] terribly . . . and . . . I think it's when I've let that thought come to me . . . "maybe it is and what if it is" . . . that's when I felt so *dreadfully* alone. [Vulnerability marker]

T: Mhm. Then . . . if it's *really* something like that . . . then you just feel *so* alone. (*pause*)

C: And it's really a frightening kind of loneliness . . . because I don't know who could be with you. (*unintelligible*)

T: Is this what you're saying? Could *anyone* be with you in . . . in . . . fear . . . or in loneliness like that?

C: (*weeps, pause*)

T: It just really cuts *so* deep.

C: (*long pause*) I don't know what it would feel like . . . if there was somebody around that I could feel sort of . . . as though I *did* have someone to lean on, in a sense. I don't know whether it would make me feel better or not, but I was trying to think "well, this is something that you just have to grow within yourself" . . . to just sort of *stand* . . . even just the thought of it. It'll take two weeks before they know. Would it help to have somebody else around . . . Or is this something that you just have to . . . really be *intensely alone* . . . in? That's . . . well I just felt that way this week . . . so dreadfully, *dreadfully* . . . all by myself sort of thing.

T: Just a feeling as though you're so terribly *alone* . . . in the universe, almost . . . and whether [C: mhm], whether it even . . . whether anyone *could* help . . . whether it would help if you did have someone to lean on or not . . . you don't know.

C: (*long pause*) I guess probably *basically* . . . there'd be a part of it you *would* have to do alone . . . I, I mean you just couldn't maybe take anyone else along in some of the feeling . . . and yet . . . it would be sort of a comfort, I guess . . . not to be alone.

T: It surely would be nice if you could take someone with you a good deal of the way into your . . . feelings of aloneness . . . and fear.

C: (*pause*) I guess I just have. (*pause*)

T: Maybe that's what you're feeling right this minute.

C: (*long pause*) I think it *is* a comfort. (*long pause*) And I guess the feeling I have now is . . .well . . . I'm probably looking at the very *blackest* part of it. And maybe there's no real need *for* that, you know. It may just take time to reassure me. And then this'll all be sort of unimportant [T: mhm] . . . although it's something (*laughs*) I shan't forget, I'm sure. [T: mhm. mhm] . . . the experience. [T: mhm] (*pause*) But it's been sort of hard to be optimistic about it. Usually I can see the bright things of it. This has been something that's thrown me, I guess.

T: I guess you feel as though you've really . . . lived with the blackest possibilities even though the facts may turn out to be quite otherwise. C: mhm] But it *has* been *hard*.

Rogers here made no attempt to reassure the client or to play down her fear. He has acknowledged her deep dread in its full intensity. When the client moves into her awful sense of being all alone in this time of intense dread, here again the therapist makes no attempt to reassure her. But the full sensing of the intensity of her fear and loneliness, and the genuine empathic caring in his voice and manner are clearly received by her. She still has the fear, but she can manage it. She is no longer alone.

At times, in this type of event, there will be a sense of the client having fully expressed the dreaded aspect or feared emotion, but no upward move takes place during the session. At such times the therapist may express a genuine sense of respect that the client has had the courage to fully share this difficult experience. The real upward move may not be made until the next session, but here again the therapist will share in the client's new sense of possibilities but not impose them.

The experience of having one's disturbing and seemingly unacceptable feelings empathically heard and feeling valued and confirmed by the therapist can be a very important change experience, involving greater self-acceptance and integration of the previously disowned experience into the self, leading to a changed and stronger sense of self.

PART IV

CONCLUSION

APPLYING THE PROCESS-EXPERIENTIAL APPROACH

I N THIS CHAPTER we describe how the Process-Experiential approach is put into practice. First, we consider a number of general clinical issues important to implementing this approach in actual clinical situations. We attempt to answer questions such as: Are some clients more (or less) suited to this therapy? How does the therapist begin treatment? What blend occurs between relationship and tasks and across tasks? What common problems occur? How are these best dealt with? How should therapists be trained for the Process-Experiential approach? After this, we present two case studies illustrating how therapeutic task interventions and treatment principles are integrated with particular clients.

SELECTION OF CLIENTS AND SUITABILITY ISSUES

Some clients seem to enter therapy with processing styles that allow them to engage almost immediately in the empathic exploration and experiential search processes so important in experiential treatment. These clients may not start out immediately focusing on their moment-by-moment inner experience, but they quickly respond to empathic interventions by turning inward and exploring. This suggests some predisposition or set of available resources on their part. Clinically, such clients may present with various problems, including depression, anxiety, low self-esteem, internal conflicts, and lingering resentments toward important others. This highlights that it is not the diagnostic category or problem class into which they fall that determines their exploratory resources but, rather, some individual style of processing.

In our experience, not all clients enter treatment with this ability to focus in on and search out the edges of their own experience. In fact, much of the challenge and art of the Process-Experiential approach comes in adapting the treatment to meet the needs of a variety of clients with various processing styles. For instance, some clients seem to be persistently focused on external factors such as unsupportive others or financial or medical problems, to which they return repeatedly, in the face of the therapist's best efforts to help them focus inwardly. They have difficulty turning their attention inward and are often unable to describe their feelings except in global terms such as "bad," "upset," or "frustrated."

Other clients enter therapy seeking expert guidance or advice. These clients may experience the Process-Experiential therapist's failure to give advice or interpret the causes of their problems as the withholding of help. Often, even though the therapist has encouraged them to focus inwards, and they have tried, they will find themselves almost automatically turning back to the therapist for expert guidance.

Nevertheless, the Process-Experiential approach can still be used successfully with clients whose styles are generally external or interpersonally dependent. For these clients, the therapist needs gradually to create an internal focus, in part by consistently empathically searching for their inner experience and in part by directing their attention inward, often using experiential teaching. In addition, treatment with these clients may over time emphasize the use of the more process-directive tasks that utilize Attending (Focusing) and Active Expression (Chair work) to stimulate deeper experiencing. These techniques often help a client to access inner experience when he or she has been unable to do so with empathically facilitated exploration alone.

This treatment is best suited to outpatient problems. Unsuited for this approach to therapy, or for major aspects of it, are clients with major thought disorder or schizophrenia, or severe borderline or antisocial personality patterns. Some form of Process-Experiential approach might be useful with clients with these and similar severe acting-out problems. However, major adaptations in the treatment outlined in the manual would have to be made, both through increasing the degree of emphasis on the relationship and by focusing on specific task markers and interventions that suit the particular population. Clients with borderline personality patterns, for example, benefit more from the relational conditions and Empathic Prizing than from specific use of tasks, especially early in treatment.

In addition, we are not inclined to impose this treatment on those few clients who develop strong negative reactions to the internal exploration and self-autonomy foci of the treatment and who find the therapist's nondirective stance of neither advising nor interpreting to be unacceptable. If an initial task collaboration has not been established by the third to fifth sessions, we will recommend that such clients seek out other forms of treatment that will better suit their needs and refer them on to a more suitable form of treatment. However, this situation occurs only rarely in our experience.

TREATMENT PARAMETERS

Treatment Length

As we envision it, a Process-Experiential approach is most appropriate for use in an outpatient clinic or private practice setting with clients experiencing mild-to-moderate levels of clinical distress and symptomatology. As described here, the Process-Experiential approach is appropriate as either a brief therapy, or a long-term treatment, although the balance between task and relationship elements will probably vary with treatment length. As a brief therapy the treatment will usually be more active and emphasize task interventions appropriate to the client. On the other hand, as a long-term (i.e., 50+ sessions) treatment of chronic personality or interpersonal difficulties, a Process-Experiential approach will tend to emphasize relationship aspects more, although task interventions will certainly be used where appropriate.

A useful strategy is to view treatment as composed of three stages. First, client and therapist arrange to meet for approximately three initial sessions to give the client a chance to determine whether the relationship and treatment approach seem likely to prove beneficial. We suggest that part of the third session should be devoted to discussing the client's views of how treatment is progressing. At this point, if the client feels he or she cannot come to trust or feel safe with the therapist, or that the treatment approach is not what is wanted or needed, then he or she can be referred elsewhere. It is important, and quite in keeping with the treatment principles, for the therapist to respect the client's experience and support their client's autonomy in this decision. In addition, allowing clients to make this decision freely enhances their commitment and involvement in the treatment.

Next, client and therapist can make a tentative agreement on the number of sessions appropriate to the client's presenting problem. After this agreed-upon number of sessions is completed, client and therapist can take stock of the client's progress and experience of the treatment to this point. If the client's problems were primarily acute, symptomatic, or situational, the treatment will generally have been successful in helping the client to overcome them, or it will be clear that several more sessions at most are all that is needed to "tie up loose ends." If, on the other hand, the problems were largely chronic, stylistic, or personality-based, then the client will still feel in need of treatment, and a longer or open-ended course of treatment can be agreed upon.

Session Length and Frequency

In a Process-Experiential approach, standard session length and frequency of 50 to 60 min once a week is typical. Sessions shorter than the standard therapeutic hour are not recommended because of the amount of time required by many of the task interventions and because the longer time increases the likelihood of completing therapeutic tasks (cf. Task Completion principle, Chapter 6). In some contexts it is desirable to use a flexible session length ranging between 50 and 90 min (i.e., by scheduling sessions at hour-and-a-half intervals) in order to allow for the completion of therapeutic tasks.

Sessions will generally occur on a weekly basis, particularly in brief treatments, in order to maintain continuity. But the therapist should be flexible and allow for client autonomy within the limits imposed by scheduling. Additional sessions can be scheduled, where possible, if a crisis emerges between regular sessions. In long-term treatments or toward the end of treatment, frequency of sessions may be reduced at the client's request in order to encourage client autonomy and a tapering off of the support offered by treatment.

Beginning Therapy

In beginning treatment, the general stance of the Process-Experiential approach is one of "contact before contract" (Gendlin & Beebe, 1968). In other words, in the first session, the most important tasks are for the therapist to connect with the client's experience, to form an emotional bond with the client, and to begin helping the client explore his or her issues. Thus, the relationship tasks of establishing Empathic Attunement, Therapeutic Bond, and Task Collaboration are the first priority. Information about the client's situation, presenting problems, and symptoms generally emerge out of empathic exploration. If any information is needed in addition to what the client has provided, this is asked for toward the end of the session, after empathic contact between client and therapist and experiential contact with self have been created.

In the first session, the therapist begins to communicate both in manner and style that the client is viewed as expert on his or her experience and that the therapist's task is to understand and to help the client focus in on this inner experience. At the end of the session, after a brief discussion about how treatment will proceed, it is generally advisable to see how the client has reacted to the session and to respond to any questions or concerns he or she might have about therapy.

Early Sessions

As a rule, in the early phase of treatment, the therapist works almost exclusively in the "basic mode" of empathic exploration, avoiding the use of task interventions until the working alliance is well established. Beyond this, during the course of these first two or three sessions, it is important to explore and establish general agreement between client and therapist regarding the treatment goals. Explicit goals are not set, but the focus of treatment or the client's presenting concerns are often discussed, and an agreement is established to work on these. Thus, early in treatment the therapist explores and implicitly or explicitly communicates understanding of the client's goals. At the same time, although the therapist has agreed to work with the client on the presenting problems, he or she is attuned to the evolving nature of these problems.

By the third or fourth session, it is important that clients feel comfortable, at least provisionally, with the general therapeutic task of experiencing and exploring feelings and that they try engaging in the various forms of therapeutic activity such as Active Expression and Experiential Search. As treatment progresses, the therapist provides clarifying information when questions or problems arise, often in the context of proposing new task interventions.

Adapting Therapy to Clients

In the Process-Experiential approach, the goal is to be empathic and support the client's emerging sense of self. Therefore, the therapist avoids directive interventions such as advisement, interpretation, or confrontation and generally employs what might appear to be a fairly restricted range of response modes. These are primarily different forms of reflection, open questions, and process suggestion. Nevertheless, the preferred responses offer a very wide range of options in the form of both basic and task interventions; this makes it possible for therapists to adapt what they do to a wide range of clients.

For example, research on humanistic and experiential therapies suggests that the client's internal resources and style of processing, and the interpersonal style that clients bring to treatment, are the most important predictors of outcome. In some cases, these interact differentially with different forms of Experiential Therapy (Beutler et al., 1991; Greenberg, Elliott, & Lietaer, in press). Research and clinical observation suggest that there are at least three global dimensions of client variation that are likely to affect client response to experiential treatment; these include client internal versus external focus, degree of interpersonal independence, and degree of client distress, with internal clients preferring less direction and more dependent clients preferring structure. Although we emphasize differential interventions for different momentary states, these more global characteristics also need to be taken into account. These styles need to be addressed by varying the degree of process directiveness, proposed modes of client engagement, and the degree of affect stimulation and evocation.

In our view, it is important to note, however, that client individual differences are not viewed as constant, immutable personality traits; instead, the same client may vary from session to session and even within sessions from one time to another. In other words, the therapist does not "pigeonhole" the client on these dimensions and expect him or her to always respond in the same way or need the same kind of intervention. At certain moments, even the most externally oriented client, for example, may turn inward and engage in a poignant experiential search. Perhaps the best way to think of these dimensions is as useful indicators of what is needed initially with different clients; that is, it is generally important to "join" with clients early in treatment in ways that complement their strengths and predispositions, before beginning gently to foster alternative modes of engagement.

TREATMENT COMPOSITION

If required to provide a single characterization of the relative weight of treatment components, we would suggest that a 50/50 split between purely empathic exploration and task-focused work would best convey the flavor of the treatment. Of course this varies with clients and across phases of treatment, with early and late phases in each therapy being more empathically oriented. This holds for sessions as well: tasks are generally introduced in the first 20 mins and definitely before the midpoint of a session to allow enough time for them to be completed. In our characterization of a 50/50 split between purely Empathic Responding and task-focused intervention, our intention is to convey our belief that the relationship and the task resolutions contribute equally to therapeutic change. In addition, this description roughly represents the actual proportion of time spent in the different modes in an average treatment.

As we have already said, the first two or three sessions are generally focused on empathic exploration. However, from the third session tasks begin to be introduced. The ongoing sessions will vary widely, with some being purely empathically oriented and others being predominantly task-oriented. Depending on the client's presentation of markers and the nature of the therapy, the middle phase of treatment would be characterized by more task sessions than purely relational sessions. The proportion of task-to-nontask sessions is highly dependent on the unfolding nature of the treatment, and the emphasis certainly could be in either direction. In addition, within each task session, the first 10 min would generally involve empathic exploration until contact had been made both between client and therapist and internally within the client by attending to his or her own internal experience. Finally, the later and termination phase of treatment would again become less task-oriented, with the last sessions generally more empathic in style.

As to the blends of the different tasks, three basic patterns occur. One is a pattern in which all tasks are used equally with no one task predominating. The other is a pattern in which, after a time, one particular task becomes predominant. This is the task that appears to have most relevance to the client and becomes predominant. A third pattern is one in which different treatment phases focus on different tasks.

In general, our process-diagnostic approach leads us in the first phase of treatment to respond to whatever markers appear, according to our judgment of the clinical appropriateness of engaging in tasks at that time. Having sampled the different types of processes, the client often spontaneously veers toward involvement in some particular marker/task that is most relevant. Thus, clients particularly troubled and puzzled by their inexplicable reactions will produce markers of their problematic reactions. Others, troubled by conflicts or unfinished business, will focus on these. In addition, the therapist, having observed how the client engages in the different tasks, might selectively focus on markers of a particular problem. For example, if Focusing had seemed particularly helpful, this task might be used regularly when the client feels an unclear felt sense, or if clients seem to repeatedly interrupt the expression of their experience, the self-interruptive process may be focused on particularly when this emerges.

DIFFICULTIES AND DILEMMAS

In the presentation of the different tasks, clear examples of successful task interventions were provided as models of how the tasks work. Of course, not all interventions lead to instant, one session resolutions. Nor do all interventions necessarily lead to major change. In many instances, tasks can and do get only part way to resolution, and the client can become stuck at many points along the path to resolution in each task. At these points the therapist relies on the basic mode of empathic responding to overcome difficulties and blocks, attempting to understand client's experience and listening for what is most alive for the client at that moment.

It is important to note that different types of difficulties in the different tasks are treated differently. Difficulty in initial engagement in the task is one of the major problems that may arise. As pointed out in the task chapters, a degree of structuring of the task is needed. But if the client is hesitant or reluctant, the therapist may decide that a bit of gentle encouragement is needed. Thus, when important issues are involved, and the client and the alliance appear to be strong enough, then the therapist may begin by offering empathic support ["I know it may seem silly/awkward at first . . ."]. This may be followed by a bit of teaching about the purpose of the activity ["but it is often useful to try this"]. The therapist then suggests, in an appropriately gentle, accepting but confident tone, that the client give the activity a try ["I have the feeling that this may be important. Perhaps we could try it for a bit and see where it goes"].

Therapist and client may, however, decide that the limits in the state of the therapeutic alliance or in the client's ability to engage in or sustain intense exploration requires a backing off. This is particularly true if the therapist has attempted the task intervention too early in treatment or if the client is feeling too highly distressed or fragile. In these instances, empathic prizing is always the response of choice.

Once clients have agreed to participate in a task, the next issue is one of facilitating experiential engagement in the task. By their nature, all the tasks initially engage clients in deliberate exploration or enactment relevant to the presented marker. Clients with an external focus may find it difficult to focus internally as the tasks require. Here is where the therapist needs to use all of his or her skill in listening, looking, and sensing what the client is experiencing most vividly in the moment. The therapist needs to help the client attend to this inner experience by empathically responding to it or by directing the client's attention to internal experience. The client's vocal quality and expressive style are often the best indicators of what is currently most poignant or alive. On occasion, the use of Active Expression with some external clients may help to stimulate sufficient internal arousal to make experience more salient, whereas with others, the use of Focusing may produce the attentional concentration needed to symbolize experience.

Crises

Crises of various sorts are handled with flexibility and respect for the client's needs, even if this means deviating from the usual Process-Experiential approach of focusing on internal experience. For example, if clients become suicidal, the therapist should explore this experience but should also take appropriate steps such as advising clients about lining up external supports and asking them to make a contract with the therapist to contact the therapist if they feel that they will harm themselves.

Alliance Ruptures

Major disruptions, produced by the client or therapist feeling that treatment is not helpful, or by the client not liking or trusting the therapist, are viewed as ruptures in the Therapeutic Alliance and are handled within the Process-Experiential frame. That is, the therapist encourages the client to describe the problem and then encourages a mutual exploration of the situation, including an honest examination and disclosure by the therapist of his or her own role or responsibility for the problem.

At the same time, the therapist does not try to persuade the client to stay in treatment. Not only would this risk violating the client's autonomy, but it also overlooks the fact that at points like this the client is usually ambivalent about remaining in treatment and might benefit from an exploration of both sides of the issue. This helps the client to come to a decision with which he or she feels comfortable.

TRAINING OF THERAPISTS IN THE PROCESS-EXPERIENTIAL APPROACH

Training is typically broken down into a series of modules. Training in basic empathic responding (including the prizing task) is central. Without this, in our view, training in the other modules will be hampered, as they rely on both the ability to attend empathically and the relational attitudes of prizing and genuineness. Training within each module, Evocative Unfolding, Focusing, Two-Chair Dialogue/Enactment, and Empty-Chair work proceeds on a number of levels. In addition to training in the overall relational *attitudes* and the ideas of facilitating change by process diagnosis and process directiveness, three components of training are emphasized: *didactic* learning of both the underlying theory and typical client steps to successful resolution; *perceptual* training involving practice in recognizing markers, experiential states, and emerging signs of resolutions. Training in *skills* involving exposure to *examples* of skilled performance (i.e., modeling). This may include viewing films and demonstrations, training in the *microskills* of the different interventions, and most importantly *experiential learning* by engaging in both therapist and client roles as part of training (Greenberg, 1979; Greenberg & Sarkissian, 1984). In learning to do the task interventions, it is often as helpful to experience the process as the client as it is to experience it as therapist. Finally, training requires supervised *practice* with actual clients.

Training in each major component of the therapy begins with a didactic component, including reading and discussion of theory and technique and viewing of sample audio- and videotapes. This is followed by practice of techniques in a directly supervized peer-counseling format (i.e., trainee therapists practice on each other). An experiential workshop format is often used, in which trainees practice microskills and stages of the technique in small groups while the trainer moves from group to group modeling intervention skills for the therapist. Alternatively, trainees can practice with each other independently, then review tapes of these practice sessions in small-group supervision sessions with the trainer. As mentioned above, an important aspect of the training is the trainee's experience in the client role, ensuring that the intervention skill is learned from the "inside" as well.

Hands-on experience with actual clients is also essential for deepening, fine-tuning, and integrating skills. Therefore we have found that it is essential that therapists see at least two training cases to begin to be able to practice this style of treatment. In some instances, more cases may be required for the therapist to be adequately trained.

CASE EXAMPLES OF A PROCESS-EXPERIENTIAL APPROACH

In the final section of this chapter, we present two case examples illustrating the treatment principles and task interventions presented in earlier chapters. We show how the different elements of the treatment are integrated in actual practice. Brief summaries of each session are presented as a means of providing a picture of how different interventions are integrated into an overall treatment.

In reading this session-by-session account of the two treatments, it is important to remember that the treatment is guided by process diagnoses of current states. Each session is thus in some way an independent event. The thread that binds the sessions together is the client's experience. If the client forms a focus based on work in a session, then this will act to focus the treatment. The therapist's focus is on entering the client's frame of reference and being attuned to any marker that may emerge in the session. For this reason the cases should be read as a series of events strung together predominantly by the clients' experience and the clients' and therapists' shared understanding of the clients' difficulties. In the first case, we present an example of how the different tasks are used to deal with the many different aspects of the client's problems. In the second case, although different tasks are used, the treatment begins to focus on the use of one specific task, Two-Chair Dialogue, because of its suitability in addressing the client's issue of self-criticalness.

Sharon: Brief Process-Experiential Therapy with a Client Suffering from Clinical Depression

Sharon, a 31-year-old, divorced office worker and part-time student, responded to a newspaper ad for a study on therapy for depression. After screening, she was diagnosed as suffering from a current Major Depressive episode and was accepted into the 16-session treatment. She described her main problems as a negative outlook on life, procrastination and lack of motivation, dissatisfaction with her appearance, social isolation, and various problems in relationships with men. As she was one of the first clients treated in the study, the therapist approached the first session with excitement and uncertainty.

Session 1

In the first session, the therapist concentrated primarily on entering the client's frame of reference (Empathic Attunement), on establishing an empathic, genuine, supportive relationship, and on helping the client begin the process of self-exploration. Sharon revealed that she was nervous about treatment failing and was in fact feeling worse than she had during screening because she had just broken up with a man she had been seeing for some months. Their relationship had centered around drinking together, and she was worried that this meant that she would become an alcoholic like her father. She then began exploration of a series of related conflicts (to which she would return throughout treatment): her sense of hopelessness versus her desire to accomplish things in her life; her feelings of hatred versus loyalty toward her parents; her obligations versus her desire to be free of responsibilities; and the competing wishes of wanting to be with a man versus wanting to be her own person.

She then explored her sense of being a failure and having something basically wrong with her. She revealed that she had had a previous unsuccessful therapy, and that was the reason she feared that this treatment would fail as well. She said that she was afraid that her problems were too much for a brief treatment such as this one. At the conclusion of the session, the therapist disclosed his sense of excitement about working with her; Sharon then said she was feeling somewhat better than she had at the beginning. On her postsession forms, she rated the therapist as very warm and trustworthy and rated feeling understood as the strongest impact of the session. On the open-ended Helpful Aspects of Therapy (HAT) form, she wrote that the most helpful part of the session was "being able to confront feelings about myself that I usually try to push back and ignore."

Session 2

Sharon opened the next session by nervously reporting that she was feeling better and was afraid that she would have nothing to talk about. After responding empathically to this, the therapist proposed that they use Focusing to help her find a therapeutic focus. Proceeding through the Focusing steps, Sharon was able to label an internal sense of aloneness, heaviness, and yearning for a man as the task she wished to address. As she began to explore these feelings, she quickly moved into unresolved feelings of longing and resentment for her ex-husband, Jerry, beginning to weep as she did so. Recognizing this as a marker of unfinished business, the therapist suggested that she imagine and talk to Jerry in the empty chair. As she did this, Sharon began to express anger, then stopped herself. Self-interruptive splits of this type often occur in unfinished business; therefore, the therapist encouraged her to explore this self-interruption. She revealed that her anger was being contained by a part of her that was still convinced that Jerry would come back to her, even though he was remarried.

At the end of the session, Sharon reported that she was left feeling empty and puzzled about why she was not able to let go of Jerry. The therapist suggested that this might be useful to work on further. On the HAT, Sharon referred to the self-interruption:

> At one point when the talking started to bring up feelings of hurt—I wanted to stop. But my therapist, by just asking questions in what seemed like a gentle reaffirming way, managed to get me over the block, and I could talk about my feelings and let them out.

Session 3

Early in the session, the therapist referred back to the puzzlement with which she had ended the previous session, offering her the choice of either continuing with that or working with something else (Growth/Choice principle). She offered an intellectual self-understanding of her difficulty in letting go emotionally of Jerry. The therapist suggested that she evaluate this understanding by using the "checking" step from Focusing. Client and therapist then went through a series of steps with Focusing, eventually symbolizing the difficulty with Jerry in terms of a conflict split: being adventurous versus being safe. At the therapist's suggestion, the client began a Two-Chair Dialogue. However, the adventurous side quickly gave in, and there was an empathic exploration of how her adventurous side needed another person to encourage it. Returning to the Two-Chair Dialogue, the conflict deepened into a struggle between the adventurous part and her internal critic's demand for perfection ("I want everything right—or nothing"). This led to a state of confusion and exhaustion, where the session ended. Nevertheless, Sharon told the therapist that she now saw the problem more clearly, and she wrote on the HAT that it "made me realize that I really do want to change, and the part of me that doesn't [want to change] isn't really stronger."

Session 4

From the therapist's point of view, this session lacked a central focus. Early in the session, the client reported getting upset at seeing Jerry driving with his new wife. The therapist helped Sharon to explore her reaction in detail, which led her to express clearly her feeling of being still married to him and her fantasy that he would come back to her. As she described this, she said she was aware that her hands were shaking. In response to the therapist's focusing probes, she was able to symbolize the shaking as a caged, frustrated feeling tied to the adventure-versus-security conflict. In further discussion of this conflict, Sharon explored the security-oriented part and her desire to escape from her financial and other responsibilities. Her postsession HAT description suggested that the session seemed actually to have had a positive effect on the client: "I realized that my problem with my Ex is *not* the biggest one I'm dealing with."

Session 5

The next session centered around a single task and set of issues, and the therapy entered its main "working" phase. Early in the session, Sharon presented a PRP of being puzzled by her habit of impulsively driving by Jerry's house. As client and therapist unfolded a particular incident, she reached an understanding of a sequence of events in which she first felt tired and lonely, then wanted to be held, next thought of Jerry, and suddenly decided to drive by his house to look for some sign of hope. Sharon's exploration then broadened to a consideration of her sense of not being whole or real without a man. This led to an exploration of previous relationships with men, especially her use of sex to feel close and whole and her sense that "there's something wrong with me that I feel this way." On her HAT, she wrote, "The more I talk to my therapist, the deeper I seem to go into my thoughts. So my actual problems are coming up instead of superficial problems."

Session 6

Client and therapist agreed that this session was the turning point of the treatment. Sharon began by reporting that she had stopped driving by Jerry's house, but she was left with the sense that "something feels unfinished" with him. The therapist had her begin by speaking from the part of her that still wanted Jerry back and then suggested that she imagine Jerry in the empty chair and speak to him. For the rest of the session, Sharon alternated between speaking to Jerry and narrating and exploring her relationship with Jerry, including specific harrowing episodes of physical abuse. She expressed hurt with much weeping, as well as anger, bitterness, and puzzlement at why he left her. During this, the therapist generally encouraged exploration and dialogue with Jerry, but offered empathic affirmation at several points of client vulnerability.

Towards the end of the session, the therapist facilitated Sharon's identification with Jerry in the empty chair by suggesting that she speak not as he had acted toward her, but as the "real Jerry inside," the man she had loved. Then, speaking as this "real Jerry," she revealed that after Sharon had insisted on an end to the abuse, Jerry had gotten bored with the relationship and left because "things weren't exciting enough." Sharon was quite struck by this insight and mused thoughtfully as the session ended. Afterwards, she wrote that it "made me stop to question 'Was it really all my fault, or was some (or most) really his immaturity and self-centeredness?'"

Session 7

Sharon began the next session by saying that she now felt finished with Jerry and saw that the divorce was mostly his fault; as a result, she said, she found that she was less desperate to find another man. The therapist responded empathically to this, and they briefly explored her sense of relief.

She then said that she was uncertain about what to work on next in therapy. Taking this as an unclear felt sense, the therapist suggested the initial "clearing a space" step from Focusing to help her select an issue to work on. As a result, Sharon identified her puzzlement at her general "laziness" as a task to work on. When the therapist suggested that she describe a particular example, she identified not working out at her health club. Client and therapist then evocatively unfolded this PRP, reaching the meaning bridge of her understanding the particular incident. However, Sharon stated that she was still puzzled about other times when she was lazy, so she and the therapist then proceeded to unfold a "lazy Sunday" in which she did nothing. A meaning bridge for this PRP, too, was reached, in that she realized that she simply enjoyed "being lazy" and not having to do anything for anyone. Having sensed this process operating in two different contexts, she proceded to explore her enjoyment of being her own boss and the times when she felt free of responsibilities. Because sessions in this treatment generally ran 90 min, there was also time to do some Two-Chair work when a split between an active "do something" part and a "lazy" part emerged several minutes later. The key moment in the session came when Sharon suddenly recognized the "critic" as her mother:

> At one point, in my mind I could picture my Mom telling me what I *should* do and my feeling that for once, instead of doing it because I'm *supposed* to, that I'm just not going to. Even though I do put things off, it might be because in the back of my mind I'm "rebelling" against my Mom, Dad, or ex-husband.

Session 8

At the start of this session, Sharon announced that Tom, a married male friend, was staying with her and that her female co-workers disapproved of her for this. What she wanted to work on was being bothered by their disapproval. She wrote: "When the girls I work with verbally attack my sexual views, I get very angry with them. Through the Two-Chair therapy, I discovered part of my anger isn't really against them, it's against myself."

Thus, the initial attribution split evolved into a conflict between a rule-following self and a rebellious, sexually promiscuous self. Although this conflict was not resolved during the session, it was clarified.

Session 9

In the next session, Sharon continued to explore her sexual behavior and began to look at her relationship with her father. She began the session by presenting unfinished business with her father; however, when the therapist suggested she imagine him in the empty chair, she refused, later describing this as a hindering event: "When my counselor tried to get me to do the chair [work], having my father in one, I froze and couldn't deal with the thought of talking to my dad.

Instead, she gave a narrative of her relationship with her father, describing his alcoholism and emotional absence, but particularly his derogatory sexual comments about Sharon, her mother, and women in general. As the therapist responded empathically, Sharon then explored her own flirting and sexual behavior, including her awareness of how much she seeks male attention and approval through sex. At the end of the session, Sharon pondered the importance of the connection between her relationship to her father and her general attitudes toward men. Client and therapist agreed to work on the issue further, and the therapist suggested the potential usefulness of chair work for this task.

Session 10

Because Sharon was so nervous about having to explore her feelings about her father, she and the therapist briefly explored whether she was willing to go through with it or not, and she decided that she was. The therapist helped her ease into the exploration by suggesting that she imagine and describe a recent interaction with him. Because she was still unable to express her unresolved feelings directly to her father in the empty chair, Sharon at first told the therapist what she felt and wanted from her father, and the therapist expressed these to the father for her. Then, after she distinguished between "good" and "bad" aspects of her father, Sharon was able to express her hurt and anger directly toward each of these parts of her father. At the end of the session, Sharon was struggling with a conflict between her desire to help her father and her desire to avoid him completely, but she appeared to be less angry with him. In a surprised tone, she remarked, "I sure kept this one hid from myself"; she said she now saw that she was trying to obtain from other men what she had not been able to get from her father.

Session 11

Sharon began by reporting that she felt that her issues with her father had been largely resolved after the previous session; she reported that the therapist's not taking sides between her and her father had been particularly helpful. With the therapist responding empathically, Sharon then explored how difficult it had been for her to be caught in the middle of conflicts between her two sisters over how the father should be treated.

Sharon next reported that she felt that her major issues had been resolved and that she now wanted to work on "fine tuning" relatively small problems that she feared might grow large (e.g., her discomfort at her boyfriend's drinking). She and the therapist then explored her conflict over whether it was right to work on small issues in order to please herself, with the therapist disclosing support for this at the end of the session.

Session 12

Sharon came into the next session all "bubbly" and not sure she wanted to be there; she said that she would rather be at home with Tom, the friend with whom she had now developed an intimate, romantic relationship. The therapist listened empathically and explored for remaining issues, but it was clear that Sharon was simply enjoying the experience of feeling good. The therapist empathically affirmed her good feelings, and she explored how this relationship compared with previous ones, less supportive relationships. The session continued in a less formal vein than previous sessions, with client and therapist discussing academic advising issues. At the end, the therapist disclosed his enjoyment of her happiness. On the HAT, Sharon wrote that she "just talked to T, almost as a 'friend.' I wanted him to know how *happy* I felt."

Session 13

Sharon announced that she wanted to work on her procrastination problem, particularly on her school work. The therapist helped Sharon explore a particular incident of putting off her work. This led to a clearer expression of the underlying conflict split between the critical, coaching "nagger" and the experiencing "naggee." Two-Chair Dialogue led to a sense of dissatisfaction with her current college major and an exploration of her career plans. Although these issues were not resolved at the end of the session, Sharon wrote "In the process of sorting out my reasons for not studying I realized that there is more to the issue than just studying, [It] made me understand how much it means to me to be happy in my life and work."

Session 14

This turned out to be the last session of therapy. Sharon started by saying that she had nothing to work on and felt fine. Client and therapist explored her sense of feeling finished with therapy for now, including her feeling that the procrastination was not going to change and was not really a problem for her. The therapist then guided her through a

Then–Now Exploration, an intervention used to help clients to appreciate change and growth in their life. That is, client and therapist alternately explored what she felt like now versus what she had felt like before therapy and the emotional difference between the two. For example, she no longer felt "squashed" by her responsibilities.

The therapist then offered her various options for handling the rest of treatment, and Sharon decided that she was ready to end two sessions early. The therapist asked her how she felt about ending therapy, and she said that, in contrast to her previous treatment, she felt that the therapist had understood her, that she hadn't had to do things to please him, and that it had been a success because now she felt changed *inside*. The therapist disclosed his pleasure at how well she had done, and therapy ended.

Clinical Status and Helpful Aspects of Treatment

From midtreatment (after session 8) through 18-month follow-up, Sharon's scores on all major change measures (e.g., BDI, SCL-90) showed her to be no longer depressed or otherwise clinically distressed, to have generally resolved her presenting problems, to have developed very positive self-esteem, and to be functioning adequately in her intimate, work, and family relationships. At her 6-month follow-up, Sharon reported that she now had a generally happier outlook on life, had gained patience, and now cared what happened to her; she attributed all these changes to therapy.

When asked to describe the most helpful aspects of therapy at her 6-month and 18-month follow-ups, Sharon pointed to

- The sessions in which I *had* to deal with feelings about my father and couldn't bury them as I had before.
- The session in which my mother came into my mind.
- The nonjudgmental attitude by my therapist.
- Reflections of my words and feelings, which helped me think through my statements.
- A feeling of closeness with my therapist, feeling that he really cared.

Commentary

The case of Sharon illustrates several common difficulties and strengths of the Process-Experiential approach. One principle of the approach is to facilitate task completion. However, in this treatment, when a new marker emerged, the therapist and client on occasion shifted tasks sometimes leaving earlier ones unresolved. This then left a large part of the task resolution up to the client. Achieving the right balance between task completion and following the emerging markers is a difficult issue for Process-Experiential therapists. This case however, does illustrate the creative combination and interweaving of different task interventions, with Focusing often setting the stage for Evocative Unfolding or Two-Chair Dialogue. The process nature of the treatment shines through with each session focusing on what emerges for the client rather than the therapist imposing a focus on the treatment.

Margaret: Brief Process-Experiential Therapy with a Client with Procrastination, Anxiety, and Depression

Margaret, a married 36-year-old mother of a preschool daughter, a writer of history, sought therapy for her problems of procrastination and depression. She described her main problem as one of being powerless and out of control of her life and being unable to finish a book she had been writing on and off for 3 years. Her problems, on a target complaints measure, were to rid herself of her self-criticalness, to overcome her paralysis and be able to act, and to be able to remember, and integrate, her childhood into her adult life.

Session 1

The first session was not tape-recorded but involved an introductory meeting in which the client explored entry into therapy, and a reduced-fee therapy that could be used for research was negotiated. This session involved the creation of a therapeutic bond by means of the therapist's empathic responding to the client's presenting concerns involving her inability to write and her feelings of being extremely self-critical and thereby unable to act. She had written one book that had been recently published to good reviews, but she now felt both unable to write and that the time of reckoning had come. She would either have to write or abandon the book. Having first made empathic contact with her sense of distress and her difficulties, a contract was made to engage in a brief treatment of at least 12 weeks.

Session 2

The second session began with Margaret reporting that she felt positive for once. She proceeded to say she had noticed during the week that it was not just writing on which she was blocked, and it was a major struggle for her to just get herself to her desk. After empathically exploring her dread about having to do anything (such as to respond to the mail, or answer her phone messages), she expressed puzzlement about her inability to respond to a letter from a close friend of hers. The therapist recognized this as a problematic reaction, reflected her sense of puzzlement and then used systematic Evocative Responding to unfold the problematic reaction. Once the scene of sitting at her desk to reply to the letter had come alive, she became aware of her need to protect herself from disappointing others.

After broadening this into an exploration of fear of failing, Margaret connected her fear of disappointing others to her family, saying that her sister and father were very self-critical and had placed high expectations on her. This was a partial new view of herself. She then proceeded to expand upon her childhood, explaining that a year after having lost her mother, her father had remarried. She felt unloved by her stepmother, and as a way of coping with this began to censure herself. She stopped asking for anything and withdrew rather than feel the pain of being unloved and neglected. The therapist responded by being empathically affirming of her in her deep sense of vulnerability and abandonment, and the session ended. Although she had presented both a self-evaluative split and unfinished business within the problematic reaction, the therapist elected not to deflect from the exploration of the PRP by engaging in other task interventions. Instead, he elected to focus on resolving the PRP. Further, the therapist focused on establishing a safe, empathic and prizing environment.

At the end of the session, the client and therapist completed the Working Alliance Inventory, the Helping Alliance Questionnaire, and the Barrett Lennard Empathy Scale. All were high, showing that a good empathic bond had been established as well as collaboration on the goals and tasks of treatment.

Session 3

Margaret began by saying what she had taken away from the previous session was a strong image that what blocked her now, her self-censure and withdrawal, had initially been a very positive strategy for survival. Now, however, it was acting against her rather than for her. She described how, as a preadolescent, she had almost literally decided to stop talking. She had engaged in a campaign of willful resistance as a way of protesting against her father's withdrawal from her. The therapist, after reflecting how painful this must have been, suggested a dialogue with her father. She rapidly engaged in a dialogue with the father in an empty chair and became the 12-year-old who expressed both her need for him and her defiance. She then expressed her sense of abandonment and worthlessness at his turning away from her. Enacting her father in the empty chair, she identified with his sense that he had let people down, that he was a jinx to people close to him and, therefore, couldn't give to her and didn't want her to need him. At this point, she wept deeply and expressed her unmet need, saying that her needs were not unacceptable and disgusting, as he had made her feel they were. She just needed him to love her. This represented a definite movement toward resolution of her unfinished business with her father, in that she felt more entitled to her needs and saw him in a new light.

Session 4

This session focused on her inability to write. Margaret said she didn't mind talking about her past, as she had last week, but that it was difficult to let the therapist into her present life difficulties. The client disclosed how foolish she felt about her problem, and the therapist responded genuinely that he did not see her as foolish and encouraged her to explore this experience of feeling foolish. She then referred back to her unacceptable needy part, which she had talked about in the last session. She said she felt stuck in these feelings. She proceeded to talk about what a difficult time she was having now that her husband was away. She also discussed how she felt after she dropped off her daughter at school each day and with the pressure she felt of having to make a life for herself. She said that after dropping her daughter off, she didn't want to go home, that home felt like a prison of her own making. She didn't know why, but she didn't like being alone in the house. This was explored as a problematic reaction in which the scene of entering the empty house was vividly reevoked. She described her response as one of being paralyzed. She equated this experience of paralysis with one of having withdrawn and hidden under a bed after her mother had died and with having virtually stopped talking as a preadolescent because she had felt so abandoned and had needed to protect her real being. She realized how her current paralysis was a type of withdrawal, protecting her creative self from rejection and criticism. Although she stated that she felt that her problem of withdrawal seemed to be occurring more often, she resolved that she would be able to face this threat and do something about it. This provided her with a new view of her functioning in her paralysis.

Session 5

Margaret started by saying she'd managed to spend the week avoiding her internal life by being busy. The first half of the session involved empathic exploration of the meaning of living a busy, more superficial life versus a deeper, creative life. She then presented a split between a voice that said she should "buckle down" and a part that liked to putter around, visit, talk, read stories, and weave. She engaged in a Two-Chair Dialogue in which she became a harsh critic who told her that she was a disappointment. In this dialogue, she said she despised herself for having destroyed herself in the eyes of others by not living up to her promise. She responded from the self chair saying she wanted to run away, never again to have to face any of those people. She felt despairing and lonely. She commented that in this chair she felt almost heroically, tragically alone and abandoned. Having entered her despair, she emerged from it saying she needed the judgmental voices to say that she had not failed, and to recognize how courageous she was to take on the challenges she had. She ended in conflict between one part saying "you will never measure up" and another saying "I'm paralyzed by being judged" and "I want you to stop being so disapproving and to love me or at least be neutral." This represented a first step in her standing up to her critic.

Session 6

This session involved a combination of Empathic Responding to the client's struggle with feeling inadequate and more work on the split between her critic and herself. This dialogue focused on the demands and expectations to perform and her feeling of impending doom and helplessness. The critic was extremely harsh and perfectionistic saying "I expect you to be perfect," whereas the self desparingly stated, "I need to run away. I need a black hole to hide in." The session, which was very painful for the client, ended with a discussion of how the critical aspect was undermining her sense of herself, and of how this made her feel very weak and confused. By the end of session 6, it was becoming clear that this split was a central issue for the client. The therapist suggested awareness homework for Margaret to become aware during the week of how the critic engaged in undermining herself.

Session 7

This session involved Empathic Affirmation of Margaret's vulnerability. It is imporltant to note that even though homework had been given at the end of the last session the therapist starts this session where the client is and follows whatever emerges as most important for the client. The client began by recounting how on returning from a trip to a funeral of a family member she felt so guilty about not instantly recognizing her own daughter, when she first saw her at the airport because she had judged her as "too gawky." She was shocked and ashamed that she had not recognized her own daughter because her daughter was less perfect than she had remembered. The therapist responded in an empathically affirming manner. This led to her revealing her deep sense of vulnerability at not being perfect herself and her fear of not being able to accept herself or anybody else. Having voiced this thought and having it received by the therapist, Margaret began to feel more hopeful, and ended the session feeling she was beginning to take herself more seriously, able to be herself, do her work, and be separate and differentiated from her husband.

Session 8

Margaret started off the session saying that it felt good to be learning to accept that it was fine to be "regular" and not "super." This represented an important shift for her. She then worked on an attribution split related to proving herself to the world. In this she played the imagined others of her professional world, past and future interviewers, producers of her scripts, staring at her and judging her.

She soon recognized the attributed judgments as her own internal judge and that it was her negative expectations that disempower her and leave her feeling empty. She fought back to a position of demanding that her critic not expect the impossible and support her. She ended by saying she was trying to develop a skin around her to protect herself but that it was very thin and not yet strong enough to defend herself. This was because this part too, wanted to be perfect.

Session 9

Margaret began by saying that the previous session was really good because

"What we did last week we've done many times before like a broken record. It was good to realize that it's still happening, and the most significant thing that I got out of it was this whole thing that every part of me wants to be flawless, needs to be flawless or perfect. I'm starting to see what a ridiculous trap that is. I guess that's one thing I've been carrying around this week with me, saying to myself "Well, what if I didn't have to be perfect?""

She talked about applying for a potential writing job and said she felt excited. When the therapist asked her to speak from the excitement, she said it would be easier to speak from the fear. The therapist asked her to focus on the fear. She emerged from the exploration of her fear with a sense of feeling afraid to expose herself. Another Two-Chair Dialogue ensued in which, from the critical side, she both frightened herself and then was scornful of how frightened she was. From the experiencing side, she then enacted being a wall that protected herself from the scorn. She realized how she had been mistaken in her belief that she was strong in the silence that she adopted to cope with her father's abandonment and her stepmother's neglect. She then ended by dialoguing with her father in the empty chair, and came to realize how she withheld her feelings from him partly to protect herself, but also to protect him. She realized that throughout her life she had tried to protect him and that she no longer needed to do this.

Session 10

In this session the client said that she had bad habits, that she was still a procrastinator and was generally critical of herself for being unable to concentrate and for being low in energy. Although she had begun writing and had produced a good draft, she said she thought of herself as a failure. The therapist Empathically Explored her experience and, in response to her statement that she sabotages her work by monitoring herself so closely, suggested a Two-Chair Dialogue between the monitor and the self. Margaret started the dialogue with "You should" write versus "I can't." With the therapist's guidance, this developed into a differentiated enactment of a perfectionistic monitor criticizing and evaluating everything she wrote or attempted to write. Thus she felt paralyzed. The therapist gave her homework to perfectionistically criticize herself deliberately and to be aware of how she monitors and evaluates her work in the following week.

Session 11

The client returned saying she had been able to overcome her critical judge and to write. This session focused again on a dialogue, with her judge accusing her of not having any backbone. She withdrew in response to the judge and said that she had climbed back into her box and closed the lid. As this progressed, she said she felt claustrophobic in her box and felt like she was in a prison. She felt a great deal of fearful avoidance of facing the litany of failures with which her judge imprisoned her. She then said she refused to defend herself, and again referred to how she felt strong not defending herself, saying that if she defended herself she felt like she would lose her strength, that it was better to withdraw and to go to sleep.

Session 12

In this session she talked about her work and said she was feeling more confident, and that it was as if there was a door in her mind that she was going to be able to open in order to join the two sides of her. This image was worked with as a split. The parts on the two sides of the door made contact, tentatively at first, with the self saying she was scared to come out and be bigger and was afraid of her own chaos and that she needed the other side to provide structure and control. This became a dialogue between her creative self who wanted to get out of the box and of her controllers fear of being overwhelmed by her creative side. The creative part also voiced a fear of being destroyed or disrupted by the controlling side. The controlling critic, after saying she was afraid of the confusion that occurs in her life when she allows the creative side in, said "I need to figure out a way of needing you that is life-giving but doesn't put me in the position of destroying my life as wife and mother that I've built up." She then commented, "There is such a strong desire in me for one or the other side to disappear." The creative self replied, "This side of me doesn't feel threatening. It's because you block me out so much that, when you finally let me in, my exhilaration is so strong that I get carried away, and then you get frightened of me and this hurts both of us."

Session 13

The client began this session by saying that she thought that the last session was really important and had produced quite a breakthrough. The therapist responded with empathic understanding and genuinely shared in the excitement of the client's discoveries. The client reported that the breakthrough had occurred in the session when she had allowed herself to get into her black side, and that it was a side that she remembered having enjoyed. She began to see that it was this side that had developed what was most original in her book and was her "source," and that when she tried to work from the monitoring side, she was merely imitating her meaning rather than expressing it. This led her to "feel fine" about her black side and not to be so scared of it. She then reflected on her struggles of the last eight years and how she was now ready to face her future. She was now able to write and to integrate her superficial social side with her "black," creative side. She could now allow the latter side in, in moderate doses, so as to not create an either/or situation, which had previously resulted in her either not being able to work at all or in her plunging into a totally hermitlike life for more than a year in order to write, which resulted in her feeling so isolated, as though the world didn't exist, that she "couldn't stand it." The therapist ended by commenting on what a journey this had been for both of them, how he hadn't fully realized the effect of the last session, and how pleased he was that she had come to this resolution.

Session 14

This session involved the last Two-Chair Dialogue in which the client said she would like to focus on the two sides that had made contact in the previous session. In this dialogue the critic said "I've been throttling you because I'm scared of you." She invited her "black side" in and offered to allow it to grow up. Her "black" side said that before she had been frightened, but now she was no longer 7 or 12 or 22, but was more mature and had developed a philosophy of how to live. She then talked with the therapist about recognizing how her social, superficial side had skills that her "black" side needed and that the two sides needed to cooperate.

Session 15

The therapy terminated with the client reviewing her progress and stating that she knows she "will step into despair again" but that now she has the knowledge to recognize her despair and to know that it was actually quite life-giving. She said that before she had always felt one side was right and the other wrong, although she used to change her mind as to which side was correct; but now she realized both were important. She felt she now had tools to deal with her issues and was looking at her problem from a different perspective.

Termination and Follow-up

The client changed markedly on the target complaints, on a measure of interpersonal problems, and on a self-esteem measure. In a 5-month follow-up interview by a research investigator, she had maintained her gains. She conceptualized herself as having changed by overcoming her critic and by opening a door between two sides of herself. She commented on how well she thought the therapist understood her and how she trusted him to help her face her terror. She also said how, although she has found chair dialogues difficult, they were most helpful and that the therapist's gentle guidance in these had also been helpful.

Commentary

This case demonstrates how different interventions were used in the treatment and how the client began to focus on a self-evaluative, perfectionistic process, which was resolved with the help of Two-Chair Dialogues. The process nature of the treatment is exemplified in how the therapist at the beginning of each session follows the client's emerging experience rather than imposing a template or focus on the treatment. A focus does develop but this emerges more from the client and her collaboration with the therapist's process facilitation of the split. The client finds this helpful as a way of understanding her experience and adopts it as a way of focusing the treatment.

CHAPTER 15

THE PROCESS-EXPERIENTIAL APPROACH: AN OVERVIEW, RESEARCH, THEORY, AND THE FUTURE

OUR PURPOSE in this final chapter is to provide an overview of the Process-Experiential approach from three perspectives: an empirical view, as provided by systematic research; a theoretical view, exploring the possibility of a common general model for the experiential change process; and a prospective view of emerging future developments.

AN EMPIRICAL PERSPECTIVE

It is beyond the scope of this chapter to review the full range of research relevant to the Process-Experiential approach (see Greenberg et al., in press; Rice & Greenberg, 1984). Thus, we will restrict ourselves to summarizing research on outcome, process, and helpful factors in explicitly Process-Experiential treatments with clinical populations.

Outcome and Process-Outcome Research

The outcome of the Process-Experiential approach has been the subject of six separate studies with clinical populations (Clarke & Greenberg, 1986; Elliott et al., 1990; Greenberg & Webster, 1982; Lowenstein, 1985; Wiseman, 1986; Paivio & Greenberg, 1992). In general, these studies examined both overall treatment and session outcome as well as process predictors of outcome.

In the earliest of these studies, Greenberg and Webster (1982) used a 6-week brief experiential therapy incorporating Gestalt Two-Chair work to treat 31 clients experiencing significant decisional conflicts. Even clients who did not resolve their conflicts improved clinically, but resolvers were found to be significantly less undecided and less anxious after treatment than were nonresolvers. Resolvers also showed significantly greater improvement on target complaints and more behavioral change. After the particular session in which the critic softened, resolvers reported significantly greater conflict resolution, less discomfort, greater mood change, and greater goal attainment than nonresolvers.

Next, Clarke and Greenberg (1986) compared a brief Process-Experiential treatment, again featuring Two-Chair Dialogue, to behavioral problem-solving (D'Zurilla & Goldfried, 1971) in the treatment of decisional conflicts, a type of conflict split. In this study, clients experiencing emotionally significant career decision conflicts were randomly assigned to three conditions: behavioral problem-solving, Two-Chair work, or wait-list control. The Two-Chair method was found to be more effective than behavioral problem-solving or no treatment for reducing indecision.

Lowenstein (1985) investigated a brief Process-Experiential therapy featuring Evocative Unfolding in the treatment of 12 clients with anxiety and interpersonal problems. Therapists used Evocative Unfolding to respond to a PRP marker in either the third or fourth session. The Evocative Unfolding session was rated by the clients as significantly higher than the other two middle sessions on Depth-Value (Stiles, 1980). On final outcome, clients generally showed substantial clinical improvement, but clients who had successfully resolved PRPs typically improved more.

In a further study, Wiseman (1986; see also Wiseman & Rice, 1989) carried out intensive analyses of sessions of five female clients seen for 10 to 15 sessions of a similar Process-Experiential treatment featuring Evocative Unfolding. First, clients showed general improvement over treatment. Second, the Evocative task-focused sessions were rated as significantly deeper and more valuable (Stiles, 1980) than the comparable nontask sessions in the treatment. Clients also rated the Evocative sessions as producing significantly greater shifts in Perspective, New Self-Understanding, and Progress. In a series of sequential analyses conducted on the unfolding sessions, therapist interventions specific to the particular step of the PRP task were found to have the expected differential impacts on client experiencing.

In a recent 12-to-14 session Process-Experiential treatment (Paivio & Greenberg, 1992) using Empty-Chair Dialogue for working on unfinished business with a significant other, clients in the treatment group were found to improve significantly more than a psychoeducational control group on symptoms, target complaints, interpersonal problems, and self-acceptance. In addition, the treatment group reported becoming significantly more affiliative toward the significant other on a measure of interpersonal affiliation.

Finally, Elliott et al. (1990) and Jackson and Elliott (1990) examined an integrative Process-Experiential approach for the treatment of depression. This treatment incorporated Focusing, the various forms of Chair work, and Unfolding within a basic client-centered experiential relationship. Substantial clinical change was observed during treatment, as well as significant clinical change between posttreatment and 6-month follow-up; amount of change was comparable to that reported in a parallel study of cognitive and dynamic treatments (Shapiro & Firth, 1987). The most common posttreatment changes described by clients were improved general mood and optimism, increased independence or assertion, enhanced interpersonal openness or intimacy, improved self-esteem, and greater ability to cope with life situations.

Descriptive Process Research

Adherence measures have been constructed for most of the task interventions. These measures, developed by Greenberg & Rice (1991) and Goldman (1991), have been shown to discriminate these interventions from each other and from Empathic Reflection. Specifically, Goldman (1991) demonstrated that the task interventions predominantly utilize different specific therapist interventions, even though there is a slight overlap. Evocative Unfolding utilized only 0 to 3% of interventions similar to Two-Chair Dialogue and 3 to 6% similar to Empty-Chair Dialogue. There was more overlap between Two-Chair and Empty-Chair task interventions, as would be expected, but they overlapped in only 7 to 17% of their interventions.

In addition, Goldman (1991) also demonstrated that raters could discriminate between Process-Experiential and brief dynamic or cognitive-behavioral approaches, both on specific therapist interventions and on more global experiential relationship skills, such as the therapist's tracking of moment-by-moment experience and empathic attunement to affect.

In terms of client processes, the therapists in Horton and Elliott's (1991) self-report study indicated that clients presented at least one specific task marker in almost every session (96%), most commonly conflict splits and unclear felt sense markers. In addition, therapists reported that client emotional expression was present in almost two-thirds of all sessions in treatment.

Helpful and Hindering Aspects of Therapy

Elliott, Clark, and Kemeny (1991) carried out a content analysis study of clients' postsession descriptions of most helpful events in Process-Experiential therapy. They identified categories of helpful factors having to do with client–therapist actions and therapeutic impacts. By far the most common type of impact was Client Self-Awareness (increased saliency of experience); in addition, clients often also experienced Self-Insight, Problem Clarification, and Positive Self-Impacts. The most common helpful actions described were Client Self-Description and Therapist Basic Techniques (i.e., experiential response modes such as Empathic Reflection). Using quantitative rating scale data from the same study, however, Elliott et al. (1990) found that when clients and therapists evaluated the impacts of significantly helpful therapy events, both gave the highest ratings to relationship impacts, especially feeling understood.

Mancinelli (1992) collected descriptions of helpful and hindering factors from depressed clients halfway through 16-session Process-Experiential treatment. Using a form of qualitative analysis, she identified an "Optimal Helpful Experience" scheme that appears to underlie clients' helpful and hindering experiences in the Process-Experiential approach. Clients appear to evaluate their treatment experiences in relation to this cognitive/affective scheme, which has three sequentially organized, defining features described below. Hindering client experiences, though much less common, were defined by the absence of one or more of the three features.

In the optimal helpful experience in Process-Experiential therapy, the client first experiences the therapeutic context as a *working environment* that is both safe (e.g., confidential, supportive, empathic) and facilitative of client communication (e.g., through the therapist allowing the client to talk or responsively guiding the process). Second, this working environment facilitates a set of *client processes*. Most important is the client getting in touch with and working through feelings (e.g., through role-playing, expression, and release), both inside and outside of therapy. Third, the client experiences a sense of *progress* emerging out of his or her efforts in the working environment. This includes problem clarification (getting clear on what problems need to be worked on), reorganization of experience (scheme change: e.g., insight, changes in views of others), and problem solution and relief (cf. Lietaer, 1992). Some of the results of this study and the previous one are reflected in the general model of the task resolution process, which is presented in the next section of this chapter.

INTEGRATIVE THEORETICAL VIEW: GENERAL MODEL OF THE CHANGE PROCESS

Although the task interventions described in this book emerged out of the study of different important change events, we believe that they have some significant common elements. We believe that these common factors suggest a model of the general change process in the Process-Experiential approach. Although our description of this general model is partly intended to provide a summary of many of the important themes of this book, we also hope that an appreciation of the underlying unity in the diverse tasks described in Chapters 8 to 13 will help deepen the reader's understanding of both the general Process-Experiential approach and the specific task interventions. Such a model, however, is not intended to replace the specific descriptions of client steps and therapist operations needed for resolution of the specific tasks.

Our seven-phase model of the change process in Process-Experiential tasks is presented in Figure 15-1.

Relational Bonding Phase

The model assumes a client enters treatment experiencing a set of general psychological difficulties. The therapist begins therapy by establishing a genuine empathic, prizing emotional bond with the client. In addition, a general sense of collaboration is built between client and therapist on the basis of a shared committment to the client's goals and on the client's perception of the relevance of the treatment to these goals. Although the establishment of the bond is more central during the first few sessions of treatment, it occurs throughout the treatment especially at

1. Relationship Phase (Bond and Collaboration)
2. Empathic Exploration Phase (Involvement)
3. Task Initiation Phase (Marker Identification, Task Collaboration)
4. Evocation/Arousal Phase (Vivid Entry, Priming of scheme)
5. Experiential Exploration Phase (Differential Attending, Symbolizing, Dialectical Construction)
6. Scheme Change or Resolution Phase (Awareness, Understanding, or positive reevaluation)
7. Postresolution or Carrying-Forward Phase (Create a meaning perspective, planning/committment)

FIGURE 15-1. General model of the change process in Process-Experiential task interventions.

the beginning of each session, as client and therapist once again make contact with each other.

Empathic Exploration Phase

Having made contact with the client, the therapist concentrates on entering the client's internal frame of reference and communicating his or her understanding to the client. The therapist selectively attends to that part of the message that is most poignantly expressed and that seems most alive and central to the client's meaning. It is from this inner-focused exploration of the client's experience that the best markers arise. Thus, a true sense of puzzlement about a reaction of one's own, a felt sense of internal struggle between opposing sides, a bad feeling toward a significant other, a sense of deep vulnerability, or an unclear felt sense of something emerges most clearly from the client's empathically facilitated exploration of his or her experience.

Task Initiation Phase

Once relational contact has been established satisfactorily and empathic exploration is under way, the therapist listens for and responds to task markers as they emerge. Whereas the content and form of the markers for the different tasks vary widely, they share some common features: first, they deal with an instance of the client's more general experiential difficulty. Second, the marker signals an inner state of readiness to work on the therapeutic task of resolving the experiential difficulty. In a sense, then, the client can be viewed as posing a literal or implied experiential question, which successful resolution will in some way answer. Markers are thus also direct or indirect client requests for help from the therapist. The help requested is not necessarily in the form of immediate "answers." But from the client's point of view, it may simply be a request for the therapist's attention and facilitation of the client's efforts to explore his or her own question.

Therefore, the therapist's first job in the Task Initiation Phase is to listen for and attend to the client's task markers. There is then a collaborative process in which the therapist confirms his or her understanding of the marker/difficulty and the client's interest in working on it; the next step involves proposing the task intervention; and the third preparing the client for entry into the task.

Evocation/Arousal Phase

Following Task Initiation, all task interventions move through an entry phase, during which two complementary processes occur. On the one hand, client and therapist work together to help the client to *evoke* the difficulty more strongly or clearly. This is done in a variety of ways in different tasks. In Unfolding, the client vividly reexperiences being in the situation in which the difficulty emerged; in Two-Chair Dialogue the client is asked to criticize another aspect of self; in Focusing the client is asked to attend to the whole Felt Sense; and in Empathic Prizing, the client is allowed and facilitated in his or her descent into vulnerability. This evocation acts to prime the emotion scheme and to make it amenable to reprocessing.

As part of this stage, the therapist also helps the client not to engage in processes that may disrupt the client's arousal and interfere with reentry into the difficulty. Typically, these *interfering* processes deflect clients from engaging in the type of processing needed to resolve the difficulty. In therapy, several factors operate to enhance arousal and focus the client on a productive processing track. First, the previously established therapeutic bond helps the client to feel safe and supported, and this provides more attentional resources to engage in the task. Second, the task intervention itself typically provides operations for overcoming interfering self-criticism, embarrassment, or automatic self-interruptive processes. Thus, in Focusing, the client may be asked to "set aside" self-criticism for the moment. In Unfolding, the "reaction to the reaction," after being briefly acknowledged, is not focused on and the client's attention is gently redirected to the task by the therapist directing attention back to the primary reaction. Similarly, reactive defiance and compliance by the self to the critic in Two-Chair work, and blaming and complaining in Empty-Chair work, are not focused on and developed; instead, the client's attention is directed to more primary feelings. In addition, in Two-Chair Dialogue and Enactment, the critic or the negative other is carefully separated from the experiencing part, and both are given equal footing. This paradoxically "contains" the critic while at the same time utilizes it to stimulate experiencing and intensify arousal.

Experiential Exploration Phase

The key phase of the change process in the Process-Experiential approach is a dialectically constructive based exploration process (see Chapter 3) to help clients differentiate and deepen their experiencing to the point where new experiences emerge and core emotion schemes change. In all Process-Experiential tasks, the therapist's strategy involves facilitating experiential processing by helping the client to attend to and focus on different specific aspects of internal experience at different times. This differential allocation of attention to specific aspects of experience fosters increasingly deeper self-exploration, which results in the dialectical construction of the client's essential experience and leads ultimately to the reorganization of core organizing schemes.

Thus, when experiential task interventions are successful, what generally occurs is a process of differential attending to internal experience generated by emotion schemes and symbolizing these meanings to oneself. This is followed by synthesizing new meanings. Each therapeutic task involves different attentional allocation processes, and the processes differ at different times within tasks. We identified four modes of engagement, Attending, Experiential Search, Active Expression, and Interpersonal Contact. All involve the client symbolizing in consciousness their immediate actual subjective reactions and experiences and constructing a new view of themselves and the world from this experience. The content of the final dialectical synthesis of concept and experience, as discussed in Chapter 3, cannot be predicted beforehand. This indicates the truly constructive and emergent nature of this exploration. Thus, common to all of these performances is the process of attending to specific subjective experience and automatic reactions generated by emotion schemes, and consciously representing these to oneself and reflexively examining these representations.

Scheme Change or Resolution Phase

When new experience emerges out of the experiential exploration process described above, the client's schemes of self and other begin to change. These are the impacts of exploration. Depending on the nature of the emerging new experience, research (Elliott et al., 1991) has shown that these impacts may take the following forms: new awareness, such as a new view of self-in-the-world or new view of others; greater understanding; greater self-acceptance.

Thus, in the first process something about oneself may become more salient, obvious, or available to *awareness*. The significance of something about self-in-the-world has now been recognized; that is, it is now experienced as important. An aspect of the self is now "owned" to a greater degree. It is as if the client now says, "That's who I am!" or "That's what is going on!" A second form of change may emerge from the new awareness in the form of a *new understanding* of some process in the self-in-the-world or with another person. Clients may understand how it is they have been construing and reacting, or how they perceive someone else (e.g., a parent) as doing something to them (e.g., neglecting them). It is as if clients can finally say, "*Now* I see how (or why) that happens."

Schemes also change by means of *positive reevaluation*. Thus, the client may experience a change in how he or she evaluates self or another person. Clients may become more self-supporting or self-accepting. They may feel more entitled or empowered to feel and act in certain ways. They may discover that they were "not so bad after all." It is as if the client says, "That's good/OK/my right!" Alternately, as is often seen in successful Empty-Chair work, clients may come to see an important other person in a less negative or more positive light and be able to forgive that individual or at least hate him or her less.

Scheme changes often are experienced by the client as answers to experiential questions or difficulties. However, although these are sometimes answers to the questions originally asked, the original questions have often been revised or replaced along the way. In other words, the result of the change process is frequently unpredictable in nature.

Postresolution or Carrying-Forward Phase

The final stage in experiential task interventions is some form of review of the implications of what has happened. Thus, the client explores the different implications of the change, attempts to create a meaning perspective on it, mulls it over after the session, and begins, often tentatively, to generalize or carry forward the change more broadly into his or her extratherapy life.

Clients in the session may also engage in "carrying forward" in-session task resolution. In more specific terms, they enter, in the session, into a new planning/commitment mode of engagement as they begin to translate awareness or new understanding into additional goals, or life projects to pursue (Problem Clarification), or redirect and commit themselves to change (Problem Solution). In addition, symptom or bodily relief may also be experienced. Thus, reduced anxiety and depression and associated physical and somatic experiences as well as a sense of lightness may be clearly experienced in the aftermath of task resolution.

Postresolution processes may take a variety of forms (Elliott et al., 1990). Thus, a key type of change that is carried forward by the clients is engaging in more generally effective experiential processing. This includes trusting their own experience, making use of a wider range of emotional information, and developing a "disembedded" perspective (Classen, 1991) on their own manner of construing, that is, developing a way of viewing their own way of viewing.

Finally, outside of therapy, clients who have successfully resolved tasks in therapy will generally continue the carrying forward process, putting into practice general changes in relation to their emotional experiencing. They often implement specific changes in their behavior and relationships and experience more general symptom relief.

FUTURE DIRECTIONS

Additional Experiential Task Interventions

There is a strong need for the specification and investigation of additional experiential difficulties and their markers, task interventions, and paths to resolution. As an illustration, we describe briefly Clarke's Creation of Meaning Intervention.

Consistent with the interests of existential therapists, meaning-creation events occur when a patient seeks to understand the meaning of an emotional experience or crisis (Clarke, 1989, 1991). This task involves the linguistic symbolization of emotional experience when high emotional arousal is present. Following a task-analytic procedure for studying events, Clarke (1989) defined the marker for this event as containing three indicators: the presence of strong emotional arousal (positive or negative emotion); an indication of a confronted or challenged cherished beliefs; and an indication of confusion, surprise, or lack of understanding. These often involve loss, disappointment, or other life crises.

The therapist task intervention that facilitates construction of meaning at these points involves a set of meaning-symbolization interventions. These include the use of metaphor, condensation of feelings into words and symbols, synthesizing the relationship between thoughts and feelings, symbolizing the discrepancy between the cherished belief and the experience, and symbolizing the emotional reaction to this discrepancy. Clarke (1991) has developed a model of client task resolution steps and associated therapist interventions similar to those described in this book for other experiential task interventions. The task also appears to fit into the general model described earlier in this chapter. Further tasks of interest are those of Repairing Alliance Ruptures (Safran, Crocker, McMain, & Murray, 1990) and the Empathic Understanding of Misunderstanding (Rhodes, Greenberg, Geller, & Elliott, 1992).

Utility of the Process-Experiential Approach

It is our belief that the Process-Experiential approach shows promise as a model for how to integrate theory, practice, and research in psychotherapy. The task interventions and resolution processes described in this book are based on research and have produced theory development both about human functioning in general, and about specific change processes and how therapists can help their clients to resolve specific experiential difficulties. Furthermore, although not extensive, the available research suggests the likelihood that the Process-Experiential approach is effective in the treatment of clinical depression, interpersonal difficulties, decisional conflicts, and unresolved relationships. In addition, research on other, related experiential therapies suggests that these treatments may be effective in treating a broad range of clinical disorders (Greenberg et al., in press).

Whereas Experiential Therapy is not currently endorsed as a primary orientation by large numbers of therapists, there is some evidence that it has been incorporated by integratively oriented therapists and is a common secondary orientation endorsed by many therapists who label themselves as eclectic or integrative (Watkins, Lopez, Campbell, & Himmell, 1986). The theory, treatment principles, and task interventions described in this book are probably of most direct relevance and interest to these therapists.

However, we suspect that this approach may also be of growing relevance to dynamic therapists, who are becoming increasingly interested in the role of therapist empathic attunement; to cognitive-behavior therapists, many of whom are coming to value emotional processes; and to feminist therapists, who share with the Process-Experiential approach a relational view of self, an advocacy of client empowerment, and an egalitarian client–therapist relationship.

CONCLUSION

When we began to think about this book, some 7 years ago, it was with a sense that we wanted to describe the integrated Experiential Therapy that had evolved out of many years of research and clinical experience. We had found this approach useful with our clients and wanted to record what we had learned about therapy because it seemed to us to be a unique formulation of practice.

Since then, we have spent the last years testing and refining the treatment; developing and clarifying additional therapeutic tasks; analyzing and articulating the underlying theory of function and dysfunction; studying and formulating basic principles and fundamental subtasks; and beginning to describe the common factors behind the different tasks.

We are also aware that there are many additional Process-Experiential tasks, and variations within tasks, that need to be specified, that there are adaptations to particular clients that need to be developed, and that there are many hypotheses in need of further study. Although much more research is needed, there is already an increasingly promising body of process and outcome research that validates the process of change and supports the efficacy of a Process-Experiential approach.

A most striking observation is that in the last decade psychology in general, and psychotherapy in particular, appears to be moving broadly toward a new appreciation of the central role of emotion in human functioning and in the change process, and an appreciation of the utility of experiential methods in helping clients to change. Social/personality, and cognitive psychologists such as Lazarus (1991b), Oatley (1992), and Teasdale (in press) have declared emotion to be a key component in human coping and change. Cognitive therapists have begun to use Chair work to help clients deal with their unfinished emotional business, and Two-Chair work to deal with conflicts; and a new "radical behaviorist" treatment has been developed to help clients accept their feelings (Hayes, 1987). In short, it appears that a major shift in psychology may be under way in which emotion is being redefined not as a source of difficulty but as a complex cognitive/affective–motivational coping process.

It seems crucial to us that the new emphasis on emotion in the change process not become a "new technology of emotional manipulation" (e.g., as now exists in advertising). It seems to us that a key strategy for avoiding this danger is for psychologists and psychotherapists to reconnect themselves to the human facilitation tradition of Kierkegaard, Buber, Rogers, Perls, Maslow, and others, developing a synthesis of the humane and the scientific and of the wholistic and the specific. It is to this end that we have worked.

REFERENCES

Anderson, J. R. (1990). *Cognitive psychology and its implications* (3rd ed.). New York: W. H. Freeman.

Arnold, M. B. (1960). *Emotion and personality* (Vols. 1–2). New York: Columbia University Press.

Arnold, M. B. (1970). *Feelings and emotions.* New York: Academic Press.

Barrett-Lennard, G. T. (1962). Dimensions of therapist response as causal factors in therapeutic change. *Psychological Monographs, 76* (43), Whole No. 562.

Barrett-Lennard, G. T. (1981). The empathy cycle: Refinement of a nuclear concept. *Journal of Counseling Psychology, 28,* 91–100.

Barrett-Lennard, G. T. (1986). The Relationship Inventory now: Issues and advance in theory, method, and use. In L. S. Greenberg & W. M. Pinsof (Eds.), *The psychotherapeutic process* (pp. 439–476). New York: Guilford Press.

Barrett-Lennard, G. T. (1988). Listening. *Person-Centered Review, 3,* 410–425.

Bartlett, F. C. (1932). *Remembering.* Cambridge: Cambridge University Press.

Basch, M. (1976). The concept of affect: A re-examination. *Journal of the American Psychoanalytic Association, 24,* 759–777.

Basch, M. (1983). Empathic understanding: A review of the concept and some theoretical considerations. *Journal of the American Psychoanalytic Association, 31,* 101–126.

Basch, M. (1988). *Understanding psychotherapy: The science behind the art.* New York: Basic Books.

Beck, A. T. (1976). *Cognitive therapy and the emotional disorders.* New York: International Universities Press.

Benjamin, L. S. (1979). Use of structural analysis of social behavior (SASB) and Markov chains to study dyadic interactions. *Journal of Abnormal Behavior, 88,* 303–319.

Berkowitz, L. (1990). On the formation and regulation of anger and aggression: A cognitive–neoassociationistic analysis. *American Psychologist, 45,* 494–503.

Beutler, L. E., Engle, D., Mohr, D., Daldrup, R. J., Bergan, J., Meredith, K., & Merry, W. (1991). Predictors of differential response to cognitive, experiential, and self-directed psychotherapeutic procedures. *Journal of Consulting and Clinical Psychology, 59,* 333–340.

Blaney, P. H. (1986). Affect and memory. A review. *Psychological Bulletin, 99,* 229–246.

Bock, M., & Klinger, E. (1986). Interaction of emotion and cognition in word recall. *Psychological Research, 48,* 99–106.

Bohart, A. (in press). Experiencing: A common factor. *Journal of Psychotherapy Integration.*

Bohart, A., Humphrey, A., Magallanes, M., Guzman, R., Smiljanich, K., & Aguallo, S. (in press). Emphasizing the future in empathy responses. *Journal of Humanistic Psychology.*

Bordin, E. S. (1979). The generalizability of the psychoanalytic concept of the working alliance. *Psychotherapy: Theory, Research and Practice, 16,* 252–260.

Bowlby, J. (1982). *Attachment and Loss: Volume 1. Attachment* (2nd ed.). New York: Basic Books. (Original work published 1969).

Brenner, C. (1976). *Psycholanalytic technique and psychic conflict.* New York: International Universities Press.

Brewer, W. F., & Nakamura, G. V. (1984). The nature and functions of schemas. In R. S. Wyer & T. K. Srull (Eds.), *Handbook of social cognition,* Vol. 1 (pp. 119–160). Hillsdale, NJ: Lawrence Erlbaum.

Broadbent, D. E. (1977). The hidden pre-attentive process. *American Psychologist, 32,* 109–118.

Buber, M. (1958). *I and thou.* New York: Charles Scribner's Sons.

Buck, R. (1985). Prime theory: An integrated view of motivation and emotion. *Psychological Review, 92,* 389–413.

Butler, J. M. (1952). The interaction of client and therapist. *Journal of Abnormal and Social Psychology, 47,* 366–378.

Campos, J. J., Campos, R. G., & Barrett, K. C. (1989). Emergent themes in the study of emotional development and emotion regulation. *Developmental Psychology, 25,* 394–402.

Case, R. Hayward, S., Lewis, M., & Hurst, P. (1988). Toward a neo-Piagetian theory of affective and cognitive development. *Developmental Review, 8,* 1–51.

Cicchetti, D., & Sroufe, L. A. (1978). An organizational view of affect: Illustration from the study of Down's syndrome infants. In M. Lewis & L. A. Rosenblum (Eds.), *The development of affect* (pp. 309–360). New York: Plenum Press.

Clark, C. A. (1990). *A comprehensive process analysis of focusing events in experiential therapy.* Unpublished doctoral dissertation, Department of Psychology, University of Toledo.

Clarke, K. M. (1989). Creation of meaning: An emotional processing task in psychotherapy. *Psychotherapy: Theory, Research, and Practice, 26,* 139–148.

Clarke, K. M. (1991). A performance model of the creation of meaning event. *Psychotherapy, 28,* 395–401.

Clarke, K. M., & Greenberg, L. S. (1986). Differential effects of the gestalt two-chair intervention and problem solving in resolving decisional conflict. *Journal of Counseling Psychology, 33,* 11–15.

Classen, C. (1991). *Self-disembedding: A constructivist view of insight in psychotherapy.* Unpublished doctoral dissertation, York University, Toronto.

D'Zurilla, T. J., & Goldfried, M. R. (1971). Problem solving and behavior modification. *Journal of Abnormal Psychology, 78,* 107–126.

Eagle, M. N. (1984). *Recent developments in psychoanalysis: A critical evaluation.* New York: McGraw-Hill

Ekman, P. (1984). Expression and the nature of emotion. In K. Scherer & P. Ekman (Eds.), *Approaches to emotion* (pp. 329–343). Hillsdale, NJ: Lawrence Erlbaum.

Ekman, P., & Friesen, W. V. (1975). *Unmasking the face.* Englewood Cliffs, NJ: Prentice Hall.

Elliott, R. (1985). Helpful and nonhelpful events in brief counseling interviews: An empirical taxonomy. *Journal of Counseling Psychology, 32,* 307–322.

Elliott, R., Clark, C., & Kemeny, V. (July, 1991). *Analyzing client's postsession accounts of significant therapy events.* Paper presented at Society for Psychotherapy Research, Lyon, France.

Elliott, R., Clark, C., Wexler, M., Kemeny, V., Brinkerhoff, J., & Mack, C. (1990). The impact of experiential therapy of depression: Initial results. In G. Lietaer, J. Rombauts, & R. Van Balen (Eds.), *Client-centered and experiential psychotherapy in the nineties* (pp. 549–577). Leuven, Belgium: Leuven University Press.

Elliott, R., Hill, C. E., Stiles, W. B., Friedlander, M. L., Mahrer, A., & Margison, F. (1987). Primary therapist response modes: A comparison of six rating systems. *Journal of Consulting and Clinical Psychology, 55,* 218–223.

Elliott, R., James, E., Reimschuessel, C., Cislo, D., & Sack, N. (1985). Significant events and the analysis of immediate therapeutic impacts. *Psychotherapy, 22,* 620–630.

Ellis, A. (1962). *Reason and emotion in psychotherapy.* New York: Lyle Stuart.

Epstein, S. (1990). Cognitive–experiential self-theory. In L. A. Pervin (Ed.), *Handbook of personality: Theory and research* (pp. 165–192). New York: Guilford Press.

Fischer, K. W., Shaver, P. R., & Carnochan, P. (1990). How emotions develop and how they organize behavior. *Cognition and Emotion, 4,* 81–127.

Flavell, J. H. (1985). *Cognitive development.* Englewood Cliffs, NJ: Prentice-Hall.

Foa, E. B., & Kozak, M. J. (1986). Emotional processing of fear: Exposure to corrective information. *Psychological Bulletin, 99,* 20–31.

Foa, E. B., & Kozak, M. J. (1991). Emotional processing: Theory, research, and clinical implications for anxiety disorders. In J. D. Safran & L. S. Greenberg (Eds.), *Emotion, psychotherapy, and change* (pp. 21–49). New York: Guilford Press.

Fodor, J. A. (1983). *The modularity of mind.* Cambridge, MA: MIT/Bradford Books.

Foerster, F. S. (1991). *Refinement and verification of a model of the resolution of unfinished business.* Unpublished master's thesis, Department of Psychology, York University, Toronto.

Frijda, N. H. (1986). *The emotions.* Cambridge: Cambridge University Press.

Frijda, N. H. (1987). Emotions, cognitive structure and action tendency. *Cognition and Emotion, 1,* 115–144.

Gazzaniga, M. S. (1985). *The social brain: Discovering the networks of the mind.* New York: Basic Books.

Gendlin, E. T. (1962). *Experiencing and the creation of meaning: A philosophical and psychological approach to the subjective.* New York: Free Press of Glencoe.

Gendlin, E. T. (1967). Therapeutic procedures in dealing with schizophrenics. In C. R. Rogers, E. T. Gendlin, D. J. Kiesler, & C. B. Truax (Eds.), *The therapeutic relationship and its impact: A study of psychotherapy with schizophrenics* (pp. 369–400). Madison: The University of Wisconsin Press.

Gendlin, E. T. (1968). The experiential response. In E. Hammer (Ed.), *Use of interpretation in therapy* (pp. 208–227). New York: Grune & Stratton.

Gendlin, E. T. (1974). Client-centered and experiential psychotherapy. In D. A. Wexler & L. N. Rice (Eds.). *Innovations in client-centered therapy* (pp. 211–246). New York: Wiley.

Gendlin, E. T. (1981). *Focusing* (2nd ed.). New York: Bantam Books.

Gendlin, E. T. (1984). The client's client: The edge of awareness. In F. R. Levant & J. M. Shlien (Eds.), *Client-centered therapy and the person-centered approach: New directions in theory, research and practice* (pp. 76–107). New York: Praeger.

Gendlin, E. T. (1990). The small steps of the therapy process: How they come and how to help them come. In G. Lietaer, J. Rombauts, & R. Van Balen (Eds.), *Client-centered and experiential psychotherapy in the nineties* (pp. 205–224). Leuven, Belgium: Leuven University Press.

Gendlin, E. T. (1991). On emotion in therapy. In J. D. Safran & L. S. Greenberg (Eds.), *Emotion, psychotherapy, and change* (pp. 255–289). New York: Guilford.

Gendlin, E. T., & Beebe, J. (1968). Experiential groups. In G. M. Gazda (Ed.), *Innovations to group psychotherapy* (pp. 190–206). Springfield, IL: Charles C. Thomas.

Gilligan, C. (1982). *In a different voice: Psychological theory and women's development.* Cambridge, MA: Harvard University Press.

Gilligan, S. G., & Bower, G. H. (1984). Cognitive consequences of emotional arousal. In C. Izard, J. Kagan, & R. Zajonc (Eds.), *Emotions, cognitions, and behavior* (pp. 547–588). Cambridge: Cambridge University Press.

Goffman, E. (1959). *The presentation of self in everyday life.* New York: Doubleday.

Goldfried, M. R., Greenberg, L., and Marmar, C. (1990). Individual psychotherapy: Process and outcome. *Annual Review of Psychology, 41,* 659–688.

Goldman, R. (1991). *The validation of the experiential therapy adherence measure.* Unpublished master's thesis, Department of Psychology, York University, Toronto.

Goldstein, K. (1939). *The organism.* New York: American Book.

Goodman, G., & Esterly, G. (1990). *The talk book: The intimate science of communicating in close relationships.* New York: Ballantine.

Goodman, G., & Dooley, D. (1976). A framework for help-intended communication. *Psychotherapy: Theory, Research and Practice, 13,* 106–117.

Greenberg, J. R., & Mitchell, S. A. (1983). *Object relations in psychoanalytic theory.* Cambridge, MA: Harvard University Press.

Greenberg, L. S. (1975). A task analytic approach to the study of psychotherapeutic events. Doctoral Dissertation, York University, Toronto. *Dissertation Abstracts International,* 1977, *37,* 4647B.

Greenberg, L. S. (1979). Resolving splits: The two-chair technique. *Psychotherapy: Theory, Research and Practice, 16,* 310–318.

Greenberg, L. S. (1983). Toward a task analysis of conflict resolution in Gestalt therapy. *Psychotherapy: Theory, Research and Practice, 20,* 190–201.

Greenberg, L. S. (1984). A task-analysis of intrapersonal conflict resolution. In L. N. Rice & L. S. Greenberg (Eds.), *Patterns of change: Intensive analysis of psychotherapy process* (pp. 67–123). New York: Guilford Press.

Greenberg, L. S. (1986). Change process research. *Journal of Consulting and Clinical Psychology, 54,* 4–9.

Greenberg, L. S. (1990). *Integrative psychotherapy. Part V. A demonstration with Dr. Leslie Greenberg.* Corona Del Mar, CA: Psychological and Educational Films, an Everett L. Shostrom Company.

Greenberg, L. S. (1991). Research on the process of change. *Psychotherapy Research, 1,* 14–24.

Greenberg, L. S., Elliott, R., & Foerster, F. S. (1991). Experiential processes in the psychotherapeutic treatment of depression. In D. McCann & N. Endler (Eds.), *Depression: Developments in theory, research and practice* (pp. 157–185). Toronto: Thompson.

Greenberg, L. S. Elliott, R., & Lietaer, G. (in press). Research on humanistic and experiential psychotherapies. In A. E. Bergin & S. L. Garfield (Eds.), *Handbook of psychotherapy and behavior change* (4th ed.). New York: Wiley.

Greenberg, L. S., & Goldman, R. (1988). Training in experiential psychotherapy. *Journal of Consulting and Clinical Psychology, 56,* 696–702.

Greenberg, L. S., & Johnson, S. M. (1988). *Emotionally focused therapy for couples.* New York: Guilford Press.

Greenberg, L. S., & Rice, L. N. (1991). *Change processes in experiential psychotherapy.* NIMH Grant 1R01MH45040, Washington, DC.

Greenberg, L. S., & Safran, J. D. (1981). Encoding and cognitive therapy: Changing what clients attend to. *Psychotherapy: Theory, Research and Practice, 18,* 163–169.

Greenberg, L. S., & Safran, J. D. (1984a). Integrating affect and cognition: A perspective on the process of therapeutic change. *Cognitive Therapy and Research, 8,* 559–578.

Greenberg, L. S., & Safran, J. D. (1984b). Hot cognition: Emotion coming in from the cold. A reply to Rachman and Mahoney. *Cognitive Therapy and Research, 8,* 591–598.

Greenberg, L. S., & Safran, J. D. (1987). *Emotion in psychotherapy; Affect, cognition, and the process of change.* New York: Guilford Press.

Greenberg, L. S., & Safran, J. D. (1989). Emotion in psychotherapy. *American Psychologist, 44,* 19–29.

Greenberg, L. S., & Sarkissian, M. (1984). Evaluation of counselor training Gestalt methods. *Counselor Education and Supervision, 23,* 328–340.

Greenberg, L. S., & Webster, M. (1982). Resolving decisional conflict by means of two-chair dialogue and empathic reflection at a split in counseling. *Journal of Counseling Psychology, 29,* 468–477.

Guidano, V. F. (1991). Affective change events in a cognitive therapy system approach. In J. D. Safran & L. S. Greenberg (Eds.), *Emotion, psychotherapy, and change* (pp. 50–79). New York: Guilford Press.

Harman, J. I. (1990). Unconditional confidence as a facilitative precondition. In G. Lietaer, J. Rombauts, & R. Van Balen (Eds.), *Client-centered and experiential psychotherapy in the nineties* (pp. 251–268). Leuven, Belgium: Leuven University Press.

Hayes, S. C. (1987). A contextual approach to therapeutic change. In N. S. Jacobson (Ed.), *Psychotherapists in clinical practice: Cognitive and behavioral perspectives* (pp. 327–387). New York: Guilford Press.

Hermans, H. J. M., Kempen, H. J. G., & van Loon, R. J. P. (1992). The dialogical self: Beyond individualism and rationalism. *American Psychologist, 47*, 23–33.

Hinterkopf, E. (1984). An interview with Elfie Hinterkopf on "Asking." *The Focusing Connection, 1*(3), 1–3.

Horney, K. (1966). *Our inner conflicts: A constructive theory of neurosis.* New York: W. W. Norton.

Horton, C., & Elliott, R. (1991). *The experiential session form: Initial data.* Paper presented at meeting of North American Society for Psychotherapy Research, Panama City, FL.

Horvath, A., & Greenberg, L. S. (1986). The development of the Working Alliance Inventory. In L. S. Greenberg & W. M. Pinsof (Eds.), *The psychotherapeutic process: A research handbook* (pp. 529–556). New York: Guilford Press.

Horvath, A., & Greenberg, L. S. (1989). Development and validation of the Working Alliance Inventory. *Journal of Counseling Psychology, 36*, 223–233.

Iberg, J. R. (1990). Ms. C's focusing and cognitive functions. In G. Lietaer, J. Rombauts, & R. Van Balen (Eds.), *Client- centered and experiential psychotherapy in the nineties* (pp. 173–203). Leuven, Belgium: Leuven University Press.

Izard, C. E. (1977). *Human emotions.* New York: Plenum Press.

Izard, C. E. (1984). Emotion–cognition relationships and human development. In C. E. Izard, J. Kagan, & R. B. Zajonc (Eds.), *Emotions, cognition, and behavior* (pp. 17–37). New York: Cambridge University Press.

Jackson, L., & Elliott, R. (June, 1990). *Is experiential therapy effective in treating depression?: Initial outcome data.* Paper presented at Society for Psychotherapy Research, Wintergreen, VA.

James, W. (1950). *The principles of psychology.* New York: Dorer. (Original work published 1890).

Johnson, M. (1987). *The body in the mind: The bodily basis of meaning, imagination, and reason.* Chicago: University of Chicago Press.

Johnson-Laird, P. (1988). *The computer and the mind.* Cambridge, MA: Harvard University Press.

Jourard, S. M. (1971). *The transparent self.* Princeton, NJ: Van Nostrand Rheinhold.

Kahn, E. (1985). Heinz Kohut and Carl Rogers: A timely comparison. *American Psychologist, 40*, 893–904.

Kahneman, D., Slovic, P., & Tversky, A. (1982). *Judgement under uncertainty: Heuristics and biases.* Cambridge: Cambridge University Press.

Kernberg, O. F. (1976). *Object relations theory and clinical psychoanalysis.* New York: Jason Aronson.

Kernberg, O. F. (1982). Self, ego, affects and drives. *Journal of the American Psychoanalytic Association, 30,* 893–917.

Kihlstrom, J. F. (1990). The psychological unconscious. In L. A. Pervin (Ed.), *Handbook of personality: Theory and research* (pp. 445–464). New York: Guilford Press.

King, S. (1988). *The differential effects of empty chair dialogue and empathic reflection for unfinished business.* Unpublished master's thesis, University of British Columbia, Vancouver.

Kohut, H. (1977). *Restoration of the self.* New York: International Universities Press.

Kohut, H. (1984). *How does analysis cure?* Chicago: University of Chicago Press.

Kuiper, N. A., & Rogers, T. B. (1979). Encoding of personal information: Self–other differences. *Journal of Personality and Social Psychology, 37,* 499–514.

Lakoff, G. (1987). *Women, fire and dangerous things: What categories reveal about the mind.* Chicago: University of Chicago Press.

Lakoff, G., & Johnson, M. (1980). *Metaphors we live by.* Chicago: University of Chicago Press.

Lang, P. J. (1983). Cognition in emotion: Concept and action. In C. Izard, J. Kagan, & R. Zajonc (Eds.), *Emotion, cognition, and behavior* (pp. 192–226). New York: Cambridge University Press.

Lang, P. J. (1984). The cognitive psychophysiology of emotion: Fear and anxiety. In A. H. Tuma & J. D. Maser (Eds.), *Anxiety and the anxiety disorders.* Hillsdale, NJ: Lawrence Erlbaum.

Laing, R. D. (1969). *The divided self: An existential study in sanity and madness.* London: Penguin.

Lazarus, R. S. (1984). On the primacy of cognition. *American Psychologist, 39,* 124–129.

Lazarus, R. S. (1991a). Cognition and motivation in emotion. *American Psychologist, 46,* 352–367.

Lazarus, R. S. (1991b). Progress on a cognitive–motivational–relational theory of emotion. *American Psychologist, 46,* 819–834.

Le Doux, J. E. (1989). Cognitive–emotional interactions in the brain. *Cognition and Emotion, 3,* 267–289.

Leijssen, M. (1990). On focusing and the necessary conditions of therapeutic personality change. In G. Lietaer, J. Rombauts, & R. Van Balen (Eds.) *Client-centered and experiential psychotherapy in the nineties* (pp. 225–250). Leuven, Belgium: Leuven University Press.

Leventhal, H. (1979). A perceptual–motor processing model of emotion. In P. Pliner, K. Blankstein, & I. M. Spigel (Eds.), *Perception of emotion in self and others* (Vol. 5, pp. 1–46). New York: Plenum Press.

Leventhal, H. (1984). A perceptual motor theory of emotion. In L. Berkowitz

(Ed.), *Advances in experimental social psychology* (pp. 117–182). New York: Academic Press.

Lewinsohn, P. M., Hoberman, H. M., Teri, L., & Hautzinger, M. (1985). An integrative theory of depression. In S. Reiss & R. R. Bootzin (Eds.), *Theoretical issues in behavior therapy* (pp. 331–359). New York: Academic Press.

Lewis, M. (1990). Self-knowledge and social development in early life. In L. A. Pervin (Ed.), *Handbook of personality: Theory and research.* New York: Guilford Press.

Lewis, M. & Michalson, L. (1983). *Children's emotions and moods. Developmental theory and measurement.* New York: Plenum Press.

Lietaer, G. (1984). Unconditional positive regard: A controversial basic attitude in client-centered therapy. In R. L. Levant & J. M. Shlien (Eds.), *Client-centered therapy and the person-centered approach* (pp. 41–58). New York: Praeger.

Lietaer, G. (1991, July). *The authenticity of the therapist: Congruence and transparency.* Paper presented at Second International Conference on Client-Centered and Experiential Psychotherapy, Stirling, Scotland.

Lietaer, G. (1992). Helping and hindering processes in Client-Centered/ Experiential psychotherapy: A content analysis of client and therapist post-session perceptions. In S. G. Toukmanian & D. L. Rennie (Eds.), *Psychotherapy process research: Theory-guided and phenomenological research strategies* (pp. 134–162). Beverly Hills, CA: Sage.

Lowenstein, J. (1985). *A test of a performance model of problematic reaction points and an examination of differential client performance in therapy.* Unpublished master's thesis, Department of Psychology, York University, Toronto.

Mahoney, M. (1991). *Human change processes: The scientific foundations of psychotherapy.* New York: Basic Books.

Mahrer, A. R. (1989). *How to do experiential psychotherapy: A manual for practitioners.* Ottawa: University of Ottawa Press.

Mancinelli, B. (1992). *A grounded theory analysis of helpful factors in experiential therapy of depression.* Unpublished masters thesis, Department of Psychology, University of Toledo.

Marcus, E. (1976). Saying goodbye. In C. Hatcher & P. Himelstein (Eds.), *Handbook of Gestalt therapy.* New York: Jason Aronson.

Martin, D. C. (1983). *Counseling and therapy skills.* Prospect Heights, IL: Waveland Press.

Maslow, A. H. (1954). *Motivation and personality.* New York: Harper.

Maslow, A. H. (1971). *The farther reaches of human nature.* New York: Viking Press.

Mathieu-Coughlan, P., & Klein, M. H. (1984). Experiential psychotherapy: Key events in client–therapist interaction. In L. N. Rice & L. S. Greenberg (Eds.), *Patterns of change: Intensive analysis of psychotherapy process.* New York: Guilford Press.

McGuire, K. N. (1991). Affect in focusing and experiential psychotherapy. In J.

D. Safran & L. S. Greenberg (Eds.), *Emotion, psychotherapy, and change* (pp. 227–251). New York: Guilford Press.

Mitchell, S. A. (1988). *Relational concepts in psychoanalysis: An integration.* Cambridge, MA: Harvard University Press.

Neisser, U. (1976). *Cognition and reality.* San Francisco: Freeman.

Oatley, K. (1992). *Best laid schemes: The psychology of emotions.* New York: Cambridge University Press.

Oatley, K., & Jenkins, J. M. (1992). Human emotions: Function and dysfunction. *Annual Review of Psychology, 43,* 55–85.

Paivio, S., & Greenberg, L. S. (1992). *Resolving unfinished business: A study of effects.* Paper presented at Society for Psychotherapy Research, Berkeley, California.

Panksepp, J. (1989). The psychobiology of emotions: The animal side of human feelings. *Experimental Brain Research, 18,* 31–55.

Pascual-Leone, J. (1969). Cognitive development and cognitive style: A general psychological integration. Unpublished doctoral dissertation, University of Geneva.

Pascual-Leone, J. (1970). A mathematical model for the transition rule in Piaget's developmental stages. *Acta Psychologica, 32,* 301–345.

Pascual-Leone, J. (1976a). Metasubjective problems of constructive cognition: Forms of knowing and their psychological mechanisms. *Canadian Psychological Review, 17,* 110–125.

Pascual-Leone, J. (1976b). On learning and development, Piagetian style. II. A critical historical analysis of Geneva's research programme. *Canadian Psychological Review, 17,* 289–297.

Pascual-Leone, J. (1976c). A view of cognition from a formalist's perspective. In K. F. Riegel and J. A. Meacham (Eds.), *The developing individual in a changing world* (Vol. 1, pp. 89–100). The Hague: Mouton.

Pascual-Leone, J. (1980). Constructive problems for constructive theories: The current relevance of Piaget's work and a critique of information-processing simulation psychology. In R. Kluwe & H. Spada (Eds.), *Developmental models of thinking.* New York: Academic Press.

Pascual-Leone, J. (1983). Growing into human maturity: Toward a metasubjective theory of adulthood stages. *Life Span Development and Behavior, 4,* 117–156.

Pascual-Leone, J. (1984). Attentional, dialectic and mental effort: Toward an organismic theory of life stages. In M. L. Commons, F. A. Richards, & C. Armon (Eds.), *Beyond formal operations: Late adolescent and adult cognitive development.* New York: Praeger.

Pascual-Leone, J. (1987). Organismic processes for neo-Piagetian theories, a dialectical and causal account of cognitive development. *International Journal of Psychology, 33,* 410–421.

Pascual-Leone, J. (1988). Affirmations and negations, disturbances and contradictions in understanding Piaget: Is his later theory causal? *Contemporary Psychology, 33,* 420–421.

Pascual-Leone, J. (1990a). Reflections on life-span intelligence, consciousness and ego development. In C. N. Alexander & E. Langer (Eds.), *Higher stages of human development* (pp. 258–285). New York: Oxford University Press.

Pascual-Leone, J. (1990b). An essay on wisdom: Toward organismic processes that make it possible. In R. J. Sternberg (Ed.), *Wisdom: Its nature, origins and development* (pp. 244–278). New York: Cambridge University Press.

Pascual-Leone, J. (1991). Emotions, development, and psychotherapy: A dialectical-constructivist perspective. In J. D. Safran & L. S. Greenberg (Eds.), *Emotion, psychotherapy, and change* (pp. 302–335). New York: Guilford.

Pascual-Leone, J., & Goodman, D. (1979). Intelligence and experience: A neo-Piagetian approach. *Instructional Science, 8,* 301–367.

Pascual-Leone, J., Goodman, D., Ammon, P., & Subin, I. (1978). Piagetian theory and neo-Piagetian analysis as psychological guides in education. In J. McCarthy & J. A. Easley (Eds.), *Knowledge and development* (Vol. 2, pp. 243–289). New York: Plenum Press.

Pascual-Leone, J., & Johnson, J. (1991). Psychological unit and its role in task-analysis: A reinterpretation of object permanence. In M. Chandler & M. Chapman (Eds.), *Criteria for competence: Controversies in the assessment of children's abilities.* Hillsdale, NJ: Lawrence Erlbaum.

Patterson, C. H. (1990). On being client-centered. *Person-Centered Review, 5,* 425–432.

Perls, F. S. (1947). *Ego, hunger, and aggression.* London: George Allen & Unwin.

Perls, F. S. (1969). *Gestalt therapy verbatim.* Lafayette, CA: Real People.

Perls, F. S. (1973). *The Gestalt approach and eye witness to therapy.* Palo Alto, CA: Science and Behavior Books.

Perls, F., Hefferline, R., & Goodman, P. (1951). *Gestalt therapy.* New York: Dell.

Piaget, J. (1970). *Structuralism.* New York: Basic Books.

Piaget, J. (1981). *Intelligence and affectivity: Their relationship during child development.* T. A. Brown & C. E. Kaegi (Eds. & Trans.). Palo Alto, CA: Annual Reviews.

Piaget, J. (1985). *The equilibration of cognitive structures: The central problem of intellectual development.* Chicago: University of Chicago Press.

Piaget, J., & Morf, A. (1958). Les isomorpismes partiels entre les structures logiques et les structures perceptives. In J. S. Bruner, F. Bresson, A. Morf, & J. Piaget (Eds.), *Logique et perception* (pp. 83–108). Paris: Presses Universitaires de France.

Piper, W. E., Debanne, E. G., Bienvenu, J., Carufel, F., & Garant, J. (1986). Relationship between the object focus of therapist interpretations and outcome in short-term individual psychotherapy. *British Journal of Medical Psychology, 59,* 1–11.

Polanyi, M. (1966). *The tacit dimension.* Garden City, NY: Doubleday.

Polster, E., & Polster, M. (1973). *Gestalt therapy integrated.* New York: Brunner/Mazel.

Posner, M. I., & Snyder, C. R. R. (1975). Facilitation and inhibition in the processing of signals. In P. M. A. Rabbitt & S. Dornic (Eds.), *Attention and performance* (Vol. 5, pp. 55–85). New York: Academic Press.

Raaijmakers, J. G. W., & Shiffrin, R. M. (1992). Models for recall and recognition. In M. R. Rosenzweig & L. W. Porter (Eds.), *Annual Review of Psychology* (Vol. 43, pp. 205–234). Palo Alto, CA: Annual Reviews.

Rennie, D. (1990). Toward a representation of the client's experience of the psychotherapy hour. In G. Lietar, J. Rombauts, & R. Van Balen (Eds.), *Client-centered and experiential theapy in the nineties* (pp. 155–172). Leuven, Belgium: Leuven University Press.

Rhodes, R., Greenberg, L., Geller, J., & Elliott, R. (1992). *Investigation of misunderstanding events*. Paper presented at the Society for Psychotherapy Research, Berkeley, California.

Rice, L. N. (1974). The evocative function of the therapist. In L. N. Rice & D. A. Wexler (Eds.), *Innovations in client-centered therapy* (pp. 289–311). New York: Wiley.

Rice, L. N. (1983). The relationship in client-centered therapy. In M. J. Lambert (Ed.), *Psychotherapy and patient relationships* (pp.36–60). Homewood, IL: Dow-Jones Irwin.

Rice, L. N., & Greenberg, L. (Eds.). (1984). *Patterns of change: Intensive analysis of psychotherapy process*. New York: Guilford Press.

Rice, L. N., & Greenberg, L. S. (1992). Humanistic approaches to psychotherapy. In D. Freedheim (Ed.), *History of psychotherapy: A century of change* (pp. 197–224). Washington, DC: American Psychological Association.

Rice, L. N., & Kerr, G. P. (1986). Measures of client and therapist vocal quality. In L. S. Greenberg & W. M. Pinsof (Eds.), *The psychotherapeutic process: A research handbook* (pp. 73–105). New York: Guilford Press.

Rice, L. N. & Saperia, E. (1984). A task analysis of the resolution of problematic reactions. In L. Rice & L. S. Greenberg (Eds.), *Patterns of change: Intensive analysis of psychotherapy process* (pp. 29–66). New York: Guilford Press.

Rogers, C. R. (1951). *Client-centered therapy*. Boston: Houghton-Mifflin.

Rogers, C. R. (1957). The necessary and sufficient conditions of therapeutic personality change. *Journal of Consulting Psychology, 21*, 95–103.

Rogers, C. R. (1958). A process conception of psychotherapy. *American Psychologist, 13*, 142–148.

Rogers, C. R. (1959). A theory of therapy, personality, and interpersonal relationships as developed in the client-centered framework. In S. Koch (Ed.), *Psychology: The study of a science* (Vol. III, pp. 184–256). New York: McGraw Hill.

Rogers, C. R. (1961). *On becoming a person*. Boston: Houghton-Mifflin.

Rogers, C. R. (1975). Empathic: An unappreciated way of being. *Counseling Psychologist, 5*(2), 2–10.

Rogers, C. R. (1983). *Miss Munn* (AAP Tape Library Catalogue, Tape No. 5). Salt Lake City: American Academy of Psychotherapists.

Rummelhart, D. E., & McClelland, J. L. (Eds.). (1986). *Parallel distributed processing: Explorations in the microstructure of cognition*, Vol. 1. Cambridge, MA: MIT Press/Bradford Books.

Safran, J. D., Crocker, P., McMain, S., & Murray, P. (1990). Therapeutic alliance rupture as a therapy event for empirical investigation. *Psychotherapy, 27*, 154–165.

Safran, J. D., & Greenberg, L. S. (1988). The treatment of anxiety and depression from an affective perspective. In P. C. Kendal & P. Watson (Eds.), *Negative affective condition*. New York: Academic Press.

Safran, J. D., & Greenberg, L. S. (Eds.). (1991). *Emotion, psychotherapy, and change*. New York: Guilford Press.

Sandler, J., & Sandler, A. (1978). On the development of object relationships and affects. *International Journal of Psychoanalysis, 59*, 285–296.

Scherer, K. R. (1984). On the nature and function of emotion: A component process approach. In K. R. Scherer & P. Ekman (Eds.), *Approaches to emotion* (pp. 293–317). Hillsdale, NJ: Lawrence Erlbaum.

Schneider, W. & Shiffrin, R. M. (1977). Controlled and automatic human information processing. I: Detection, search, and attention. *Psychological Review, 84*, 1–66.

Shapiro, D. A., & Firth, J. (1987). Prescriptive vs. exploratory psychotherapy: Outcomes of the Sheffield psychotherapy project. *British Journal of Psychiatry, 151*, 790–799.

Shiffrin, R. M., & Schneider, W. (1977). Controlled and automatic human information processing. II: Perceptual learning, automatic attending, and a general theory. *Psychological Review, 84*, 127–190.

Stern, D. N. (1985). *The interpersonal world of the infant: A view from psychoanalysis and developmental psychology*. New York: Basic Books.

Stiles, W. B. (1980). Measurement of the impact of psychotherapy sessions. *Journal of Consulting and Clinical Psychology, 48*, 176–185.

Stiles, W. B. (1986). Development of a taxonomy of verbal response modes. In L. S. Greenberg & W. M. Pinsof (Eds.), *The psychotherapeutic process: A research handbook* (pp. 161–199). New York: Guilford Press.

Teasdale, J. (in press). *Affect and cognition in change*. Hillsdale, NJ: Lawrence Erlbaum.

Tobin, S. A. (1990). Self psychology as a bridge between existential-humanistic psychology and psychoanalysis. *Journal of Humanistic Psychology, 30*, 14–63.

Tobin, S. A. (1991). A comparison of psychoanalytic self psychology and Carl Rogers's person-centered therapy. *Journal of Humanistic Psychology, 31*, 9–33.

Tomkins, S. (1962). *Affect, imagery and consciousness*. New York: Springer.

Tomkins, S. (1970). Affect as the primary motivational system. In M. B. Arnold (Ed.), *Feelings and emotions* (pp. 101–110). New York: Academic Press.

Toukmanian, S. (1986). A measure of client perceptual processing. In L. S. Greenberg & W. M. Pinsof (Eds.), *The psychotherapeutic process: A research handbook* (pp. 107–130). New York: Guilford Press.

Trilling, L. (1972). *Sincerity and authenticity*. Cambridge, MA: Harvard University Press.

Tronick, E. (1989). Emotions and emotional communications in infants. *American Psychologist, 44*(2), 112–119.

Vanaerschot, G. (1990). The process of empathy: Holding and letting go. In G. Lietaer, J. Rombauts, & R. Van Balen (Eds.), *Client-centered and experiential psychotherapy in the nineties* (pp. 269–294). Leuven, Belgium: Leuven University Press.

Varela, F. J., Rosch, E., & Thompson, E. (1991). *The embodied mind: Cognitive science and human experience.* Cambridge, Mass.: MIT Press.

Watkins, C. E., Lopez, F. G., Campbell, V. L., & Himmell, C. D. (1986). Contemporary counseling psychology: Results of a national survey. *Journal of Counseling Psychology, 33,* 301–309.

Werner, H. (1948). *The comparative psychology of mental development.* New York: International Universities Press.

Werner, H. (1957). *Comparative psychology of mental development.* Chicago: Follett.

Wexler, D. A., & Rice, L. N. (1974). *Innovations in client-centered therapy.* New York: Wiley.

White, R. W. (1959). Motivation reconsidered: The concept of competence. *Psychological Review, 66,* 279–332.

White, R. W. (1966). *Lives in progress.* New York: Holt, Rinehart and Winston.

Whitehead, A. N. (1929). *Process and reality: An essay in cosmology.* Cambridge: The Cambridge University Press.

Williams, J. (June, 1992). *Recovery from depression: Effective problem solving needs effective autobiographical recollection.* Paper presented at the World Congress on Cognitive Therapy, Toronto.

Williams, J., Watts, F., McLeod, C., & Matthews, A. (1988). *Cognitive psychology and the emotional disorders.* New York: Wiley.

Wiseman, H. (1986). *Single-case studies of the resolution of problematic reactions in short-term client-centred therapy: A task-focused approach.* Unpublished doctoral dissertation, York University, Toronto.

Wiseman, H., & Rice, L. N. (1989). Sequential analyses of therapist–client interaction during change events: A task-focused approach. *Journal of Consulting and Clinical Psychology, 57,* 281–286.

Yalom, I. D. (1980). *Existential psychotherapy.* New York: Basic Books.

Zajonc, R. B. (1980). Feeling and thinking: Preferences need no inferences. *American Psychologist, 35,* 151–175.

Zeigarnik, B. (1927). Ueber das Behalten von erledigten und unerledigten Handlungen. *Psychologische Forschung, 9,* 1–85.

INDEX

T

Task collaboration, 109–111
Technical integration, Process-Experiential approach in, 320–321
Temporal focus, 3, 17
 in client-centered therapy, 38
 in problem impacts, 30
Therapeutic change
 creating problem-solutions, 30
 emotion schemes in, 4–5, 63–64, 91–95, 143
 in empty chair procedure, 245–252
 engaging client in, 115
 in experiential approach, 68, 70
 general model of, 315–319
 growth motivation in, 64–65
 impacts experienced in, 29–31
 information processing model for, 7–8, 9–10
 interpersonal effects, 30–31
 in modular self, 62
 outcome research, 311–313
 perceptual, 29–30, 173–174
 recurrent nature of, 8
 role of emotion in, 321–322
 schematic processing in, 46–47
 for self-interruptive splits, 226–227
 in systematic evocative unfolding, 145–150
 tacit emotion schemes and, 143
 theoretical basis for, 3–7
 therapeutic relationship as basis for, 93–94, 102
 therapist's role in, 19–20
 in Two-Chair Dialogue, 191–196
 in vulnerability events, 275–277
Therapeutic goals, 12. See also Treatment principles
 client growth in, 114–115
 development of, 109–110
 in Empty-Chair work, 245–246, 252–264
 in experiential focusing, stages of, 169, 171, 172, 173
 facilitating experiential processing in, 85
 in general model, 317–318
 introduction of, 289
 self-acceptance in, 191–192, 195
 in systematic evocative unfolding, 142–143, 150–151

 as task collaboration, 109–111
 in therapy for self-interruptive splitting, 219, 223
 in Two-Chair Dialogue, 191–192, 197
Therapeutic process. See also Empty-Chair work; Experiential focusing; Problematic reactions; Self-interruptive splitting; Two-Chair Dialogue
 automatic processes in, 44
 carrying forward phase in, 319
 in client-centered therapy, 36–39
 concept of pathology in, 12
 conceptual processing in, 82–83
 content analysis of, 314
 crises in, 293
 in dialectical constructivist model, 56–57
 directing, 15–16, 18, 19, 22–25
 early sessions in, 15, 287, 289
 emotion schemes in, 6, 67
 empathic exploration phase, 316
 evocation/arousal phase, 316–317
 evoking experience in, 85
 in experiential approach, 41–42
 experiential exploration phase, 317–318
 experiential processing in, 82, 83
 facilitating attention in, 6–7, 94, 95
 first session in, 288–289
 general model of, 315–319
 in Gestalt therapy, 41
 intense emotion in, 271–272
 meaning-creation in, 4, 12, 14, 23
 memory processes and, 45–46
 modes of engagement in, 13, 25–28
 moment-by-moment approach, 7–10, 14
 potential difficulties in, 291–294
 as process diagnosis, 13–14, 17–19
 process-focused approach to, 14–17
 relational bonding phase in, 315–316
 resolution phase in, 318–319
 role of markers in, 141
 scheme change in, 95, 318–319
 session frequency, 288
 session length, 288
 stage of, 287–288
 symbolization in, 26–27
 task initiation phase, 316
 temporal location of, 3, 17, 38